Behavior Modificwith Developmental Disabilities: Treatments and Supports

volume I

Edited By:

Johnny L. Matson, Ph.D. , Rinita B. Laud, M. A.
and Michael L. Matson
Louisiana State University

Behavior Modification for Persons with Developmental Disabilities: Treatments and Supports
Volume I

Edited By:
Johnny L. Matson, Ph.D.
Rinita B. Laud, M. A.
Michael L. Matson

Copyright © 2004 NADD Press

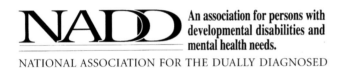

An association for persons with
developmental disabilities and
mental health needs.

NATIONAL ASSOCIATION FOR THE DUALLY DIAGNOSED

132 Fair Street
Kingston, New York 12401

LCCN: 2004114118
ISBN: 1-57256-042-8

1st Printing 2004

Printed in the United States of America

TABLE OF CONTENTS

These Volumes are dedicated to
John W. Jacobson,
May he rest in peace.

FOREWORD

In the last few decades, the field of dual diagnosis as applied to those with intellectual disabilities has boasted a monumental surge in assessment devices and treatment approaches. These relatively recent advances include those in the development of behavior modification principles and procedures that have had a dramatic impact on services for individuals with intellectual disabilities. This book represents the first of two volumes that is designed to update readers on some of these many developments.

This volume is relatively brief compared to what would have been compiled if the same topic areas were applied to the intellectually non-impaired population. However, we have attempted to cover a wide range of topics beginning with the history and current status of Applied Behavior Analysis, current issues and practices in this field, as well as models of service provision. We have also given ample attention to important topics that often co-occur in those with intellectual impairment. These topics include psychotic disorders, stereotyped acts, and self-injurious behavior. Although this book was primarily centered on empirically supported treatments, we have also included chapters on staff training, data collection procedures and observation systems, functional assessment, and rating instruments. These chapters will provide the reader with a good foundation of assessment techniques and procedures common to the field.

We have prepared this edition with the intent of giving clinicians and applied researchers in the fields of psychopathology and intellectual disabilities a clear view of the existing empirical data. We have assembled a group of highly regarded professionals to author chapters in areas where their expertise is well known and respected. It is our hope and purpose that this book will adequately reflect the growing body of behavioral research for persons with intellectual impairment. It is also our hope that this book will serve as a reflection of what we do not know, and can consequently stimulate sufficient interest to assist handicapped individuals in leading happier and more productive lives.

Johnny L. Matson
Rinita B. Laud
Michael L. Matson

History and Current Status of Applied Behavior Analysis in Developmental Disabilities

John W. Jacobson, Ph.D., B.C.B.A.
Sage Colleges Center for Applied Behavior Analysis
Troy, NY

Steve Holburn, Ph.D.
NYS Institute for Basic Research in Developmental Disabilities
Staten Island, NY

Behavior modification, more properly known as operant psychology or applied behavior analysis, occupies a long, distinguished, and central role in the provision of clinical services to people with developmental disabilities. Although clinical application of principles of behavior analysis did not become common until the 1960s, the approach has persisted as a dominant orientation or component of intervention to improve the functioning of people with developmental and psychiatric disabilities, through the shaping and maintenance of simple and complex skills and through the treatment of aberrant behavior. Today the array of applied behavior analysis interventions has grown to include organizational management and development, behavioral safety, community change, and reform of schools, as well as applications in correctional and youth services, and public welfare services, and a variety of disability-specific treatment services (e.g., for traumatic brain injury). Applied behavior analysis has been defined in a number of ways, as a collection of interventions, a specialty, or a discipline, but the most oft-cited definition, to which we refer readers, was presented by Baer, Wolf, and Risley (1968). The nature and breadth of applied behavior analysis is exemplified by the chapters in this book.

The role of behavior modification in developmental services has not, however, been without contention. Behavior analysis, as a model of human performance, is not compatible with common parlance and explanations by the person on the street, and, in clinical application, it has not dealt primarily with subjective aspects of human experience (but see Friman, Hayes, & Wilson, 1998; Kantor, 1950; Moore, 1984). The principles underpinning behavior analysis and, particularly, the emphasis on the transactional nature between observable behavior and the historical and immediate environmental events that explain much of human action and feeling have been intermittently characterized as controversial, dehumanizing, incomplete, or merely passé (e.g., Carr et al., 2002; Chomsky, 1959; Mahoney, 1989). Such criticisms are aimed toward clinical applications in developmental services (e.g., Lovett, 1996) and in the context of services to other service populations, educational applications, and theory. Some concerns about behavior analytic interventions have focused on the use of restrictive (punishment) procedures (e.g., see Repp & Singh, 1990), while others have criticized altering consequences contingently to alter behavior (Cameron & Kimball, 1995) or merely establishing a contingency involving contingent attention (c.f., Bambara & Knoster, 1995; Pennsylvania Code, 1993). Common to most detractors of applied behavior analysis is the uneasiness with applying principles of science to influence our behavior, a suspicion that has been examined in the writings of B.F. Skinner. It must also be acknowledged that there were past instances when restrictive procedures were misapplied, or inappropriately applied (Thompson, Gardner, & Baumeister, 1988), sometimes under circumstances that may be less likely to occur today, or without the degree of scrutiny that is more common in recent years than earlier.

In this brief chapter we touch on the wide range of developments over the past 40 years emphasizing behavior analysis in the field of developmental disabilities, principally in the United States. Limited space precludes an exhaustive analysis of the history of the field, so we have highlighted aspects that seem particularly important or influential, such as the recent increased demand for behavior analytic services. We address the nature and scope of controversies as they have emerged, both with respect to the use of restrictive procedures as a component of treatment, and the development of positive behavior support as an offshoot or variant of behavior analysis.

Behavior Analysis and Developmental Disabilities Before 1960

The antecedents of ABA prior to 1960 are based on experimental laboratory research rather than field application. This was generally true of the field of psychology as a whole; with clinical psychology emerging as a specialty somewhat more distinct from academic settings following World War II. Progenitors of what was to become behavior analysis based on operant principles (e.g, Ferster & Skinner, 1957; Skinner, 1938, 1948, 1953, 1957, 1959) included Itard, Sekhenov and Bekhterev, Yerkes and John B. Watson, and Edward L. Thorndike (whose "law of effect" would presage the principles of reinforcement and punishment). Later contributors were S.S. Stevens, Hull, Tolman, Dollard and Miller, Wolpe, Eysenck, Keller, and Schoenfeld (e.g., Keller & Schoenfeld, 1950). All of these scientists made conceptual or procedural contributions to an evolving behavioral psychology (Boeree, 1998/2000; Lane, 1989). Behaviorism had became a dominant orientation in psychology, at least in research, by the 1940s, co-existing with a clinical orientation that tended to emphasize psychoanalytic models of treatment, or variations thereof (i.e., behaviorism's domination of clinical practice was not so evident).

The inception of behavior analysis in developmental disabilities, at least in terms of applying its principles to intervention involving a person with such disability, is typically traced to Fuller (1949), who used a contingent primary reinforcer (sugar water) to shape a human operant response: An 18 year-old with mental retardation who was characterized as unresponsive was taught to raise his hand. However, earlier studies involving different treatment issues or conditions than mental retardation and involving primarily classical or respondent conditioning, rather than operant conditioning, were also evident (Jones, 1924; Marquis, 1941; Watson & Rayner, 1920). The story of Little Albert, a young boy classically conditioned to fear a white rabbit by Watson and Rayner, has become apocryphal, and has been distorted by Watson, textbook authors, and critics of behaviorism, as well as by behavior therapists (Cornwell, Hobbs, & Prytula, 1980; Harris, 1979; Paul & Blumenthal, 1989). Behavior analysis was not without its critics as early as 1935 (Jastrow, 1935).

By the 1950s, interventions entailing behavioral principles for people with developmental disabilities, or which addressed behavioral disorders seen among people with DD, were increasingly finding their way into professional journals (e.g., Ayllon & Michael, 1959, on behavioral engineering; Azrin & Lindsley, 1956, on reinforcement of cooperation; Bowman, 1957, on contingencies in institutions; Lindsley, Skinner, & Soloman, 1953, 1955, on intervention for psychotic behavior; and Williams, 1959, on extinguishing tantrums). Interestingly, during the 1950s special education became mandated in public schools in America, but there are few or no published reports of educational applications of behavior analysis. The first reported application of operant principles in a special education classroom was demonstrated by

Zimmerman and Zimmerman (1962) who eliminated tantrums and increased academic responding of two 11-year old emotionally-disturbed boys. Soon after, an entire classroom was arranged to facilitate operant strategies through programmed instruction (Birnbrauer, Bijou, Wolf, & Kidder, 1965).

Behavior Analysis and Developmental Disabilities from 1960 to 1980

The 1960s.

During the 1960s the focus of applied behavior analysis within developmental disabilities began to take shape (Risley, 1997), including work with children with autism addressing such issues as functional speech, generalization of treatment gains across situations, alleviation of behavior problems, and longitudinal demonstration, by Montrose Wolf, colleagues, and students, of token economy systems in diverse settings, including schools (e.g., Risley & Wolf, 1967).

During this decade, the defining features of applied behavior analysis, as distinguished from experimental analysis, were established (Baer, Wolf, & Risley, 1968) and evident tangibly in seminal publications involving clinical practice (e.g., Ullman & Krasner, 1965, 1969). Research and practice was extended to many populations that had previously been considered untreatable or resistant to treatment, including people with autism, delinquent behavior, hyperactivity, mental retardation, or psychotic disorders (e.g., Ayllon & Haughton, 1962; Wolf, Birbrauer, Williams, & Lawler, 1965; Wolf, Risley, & Mees, 1964). The influence of systematic and comprehensive alteration of settings through secondary generalized reinforcers was studied and applied clinically through the establishment of token economies (Ayllon & Azrin, 1965; Girardeau & Spradlin, 1964). Much of the applied work during this time period focused on children, including interventions in classroom (Allen, Hart, Buell, Harris, & Wolf, 1964; Birnbrauer et al., 1965; Homme, DeBaca, Divine, Steinhorst, & Rickert, 1963; Zimmerman & Zimmerman, 1962) and in the home (Hawkins, Peterson, Schweid, & Bijou, 1966; Tharp & Wetzel, 1969).

During the 1960s comprehensive and foundational behavior analytic formulations of child development (Bijou & Baer, 1961) and retarded development (Bijou, 1968, concepts later expanded in Bijou & Dunitz-Johnson, 1981) were established, and have since endured. There was particular interest in the alleviation and prevention of developmental (e.g., socio-cultural) retardation, which was evident in emerging national priorities under the Kennedy administration, and in research by non-behavioral clinicians and educators. One such project (the Juniper Gardens Children's Project) remains in operation:

> *"Baer, Wolf, Risley, Hall, Hart, and their colleagues began applying the principles of behavior analysis to the problems of an inner-city community as early as 1964 in the homes, schools, and clinics of Kansas City, Kansas .... This work has continued today, having contributed over the years to the literature of applied behavior analysis, to general concerns in psychology, and to improvements in the lives of community residents"* (Greenwood et al., 1992, p. 1464).

Toward the latter half of the decade, punishment appeared in the literature as a procedure to treat severe problem behavior. It was addressed as a component of intervention (e.g., Risley, 1968; see Sailor, Guess, Rutherford, & Baer, 1968 on contingent presentation of difficult tasks) and with respect to the technical and ethical considerations in the use of such components (Azrin & Holtz, 1966). Although punishment was a component of some interventions for children with autism, these interventions predominantly entailed dense schedules of differential reinforcement and shaping (e.g., Lovaas, Freitag, Gold, & Kassorla, 1965; Lovaas, Freitag, Kinder, Rubenstein, Schaeffer, & Simmons, 1966; Lovaas, Schaeffer, & Simmons, 1965; Lovass & Simmons, 1969). Consistent with the rise in interest of applying operant procedures, at the end of the 1960s, Wolpe (1969) published the first major source of guidance for clinicians on the practice of behavior therapy, a book that was to stimulate new directions in clinical practices, for clinicians in many specialties, including those in private practice. Interestingly, although classical conditioning methods were demonstrated much earlier than operant techniques, the rise in respondent applications lagged behind that of operant demonstrations.

The 1970s.

The 1970s were a critical period in the further development of behavior analysis as a specialty and discipline serving people with developmental disabilities (Hopkins, 1970). Most professionals who are senior and leading behavior analysts today were educated or had their first professional experiences and began conducting research during the 1970s. Most were educated in psychology programs, some clinical, and were trained in both behavior analysis and behavior therapy, as well as traditional psychological functions such as assessment and testing. Somewhat surprisingly, behavior therapy interventions such as desensitization involving people with mental retardation remained uncommon (e.g., Guralnick, 1973), but ABA interventions, particularly for severe destructive behavior, proliferated.

Behavior analysis was often seen, perhaps accurately so, as a service largely confined to institutional settings (Baroff, 1974), and behavior analysts confronted considerable organizational and cultural barriers in attempting to implement treatment services (Reppucci, 1977; Reppucci & Saunders, 1974). This perception was accurate, but there were some indications that ABA interventions were beginning to be implemented in community vocational programs for people with mental retardation (e.g., Gold, 1980; Trybus & Lacks, 1972). Although deinstitutionalization of public mental retardation facilities began in most states during this decade, it began unevenly and neither researchers nor clinicians had as much opportunity to study or serve people living in community group homes as they would later, during the 1980s.

A variety of educational studies continued during the 1970s (e.g., Broden, Bruce, Mitchell, Carter, & Hall, 1970; Broden, Copeland, Beasley, & Hall, 1977; Hall et al., 1971), and included a new focus on pragmatic community use and independence skills training, especially for adolescents with mild mental retardation (Cronin & Cuvo, 1979; Cuvo, Veitch, Trace, & Knoke, 1978; Miller, Cuvo, & Borakove, 1977). Keller (1974) reviewed ten years of progress for the System of Personalized Instruction, which had been implemented in some collegiate, as well as regular school settings. Research and practice also continued in service to children with autism (see Lovaas, Koegel, Simmons, & Long, 1973 on concerns regarding maintenance and generalization that persist today), new comprehensive community services for delinquent children were developed (Phillips, Phillips, Fixsen, & Wolf, 1971), and research and practice with youth and adults broadened to include interventions to increase the responsiveness of people with severe or profound disabilities within social interactions (e.g., Striefel, Wetherby, & Karlan, 1978), and effective rapid training of self-care skills (Azrin & Foxx, 1971).

During this period behavior reduction strategies were implemented that included praise and social isolation (Matson, 1978), overcorrection (Foxx & Azrin, 1973; Ollendick & Matson, 1976), prompting, differential reinforcement, and contingent mouthwash (Matson & Ollendick, 1976), timeout (Barton, Guess, Gacia, & Baer, 1970; Burchard & Barrera, 1972; Foxx & Shapiro, 1978), response cost (Kazdin, 1972), response cost and timeout (Gresham, 1979), response cost and aversive stimulation (Kazdin, 1973), aversive stimulation (Ball, Sibbach, Jones, Steele, & Frazier, 1975), contingent instruction and timeout (Porterfield, Herbert-Jackson, & Risley,

1976), sensory extinction (Rincover, Newsom, & Carr, 1979), and group contingencies (Greene & Pratt, 1972). Generally, these investigations tended to emphasize the effects of consequences on problem behavior, rather than the causes or functions of the behavior as is prominent today, although this was a matter of emphasis, and stimulus control was an important feature of many interventions (see below, and Foxx, 2003). A body of information was developing that indicated which treatments were most effective for which problems, an approach which is still valuable to clinicians today and which is apparent in treatment manuals for treating problem behavior of individuals with developmental disabilities (e.g., Konarski, Favell, & Favell, 1997).

During the 1970s the primary focus of highly restrictive treatment involved aversive stimulation (often entailing use of faradic stimulation), which had clearly increased in use in comparison to the 1960s, was on modification of self-injury or self-mutilation, hysterical or chronic coughing, persistent vomiting and rumination. In a number of instances aversive stimulation was used to treat stereotypic behavior, pica, respiratory problems, self-induced seizures, or aggression. Several studies used aversive stimulation, including shock, to treat behaviors that would not be so-treated today, or so-treated in only exceptional instances; and most of these cases involved non-compliant behavior, or hallucinatory behavior (but see Kircher, Pear, & Martin, 1971). Criticisms of ABA emphasized the absence of evidence for broad and enduring effects of interventions (MacMillan & Forness, 1973), and the need to cast the net of intervention focus to include major modifications to the settings and personnel associated with onset of behavior problems (Holland, 1978). Some of these issues had begun to be addressed during the 1970s (Marholin, O'Toole, Touchette, Berger, & Doyle, 1979; Rogers-Warren & Warren, 1977; Schroeder, Rojahn, & Mulick, 1978; Willems, 1974), but a more ecological focus would presage increased emphasis on contextual factors associated with variability in behavior problems, in the form of establishing operations and stimulus control factors, and the emergence of functional analysis as a convention of ABA practice (e.g., Carr, 1977; Rachlin & Green, 1972).

An influential development in applied behavior analysis during this period was social validity assessment (Schwartz & Baer, 1991; Wolf, 1978), which became an additional dimension of ABA practice and its appraisal. The concept of social importance had been originally presented in the definition of applied behavior analysis by Baer et al. (1968), but it was expanded to include a determination of the importance of the goals, treatment acceptability, and consumer satisfaction. This procedural innovation permitted ways to measure the relevance of behavioral interventions, but social validity itself has not been considered a primary measure of treatment effectiveness.

The 1980s to the Present: Diversification and Controversy

Diversification

From the 1980s into the 1990s, ABA research continued to both pursue established areas of interest and activity, and also extended its focus in response to new opportunities and changing priorities associated with growing community services for adults and children, as well as changing educational services following enactment of the Education for All Handicapped Children Act (EAHC) and later the Individuals with Disabilities Education Act (IDEA). Both these acts and regulations from the federal Medicaid program required, for children, delivery of educationally-related services, and for adults, interdisciplinary services, in both cases including attention to behavioral service needs.

New areas of activity for behavior analysts involved delving into phenomena bordering on areas of interest for behavior therapists, and cognitive-behavior therapists, including subjective states (e.g., Favell, Realon, & Sutton, 1996), and clinical applications of rule governance and verbal relations (e.g., private events, Dixon & Hayes, 1998; Dixon et al., 1998; Hayes & Hayes, 1992; Moore, 2000), all of which contributed to the development operant oriented psychotherapy or clinical radical behaviorism. In the DD sector an explicit emphasis (which was formerly implicit) on preference as a component of assessment and intervention (Bowman, Piazza, Fisher, Hagopian, & Kogan, 1997; Green, Reid, White, Halford, Brittain, & Gardner, 1988; Reid, Everson, & Green, 1999). As services decentralized further, organizational development and staff training activities persisted as key factors underpinning faithful and effective implementation of services (Page, Iwata, & Reid, 1982; Parsons & Reid, 1995; Reid & Parsons, 2000).

Services to prevent mental retardation and other childhood disabilities and to improve the pace of child development for those at risk remained a concern throughout this period (e.g., Hart & Risley, 1981, 1999; Christopherson, Barnard, Barnard, Gleeson, & Sykes, 1981; Mulick & Butter, 2002). Early on in this era there were indications of a growing impetus toward stimulus control procedures as an important component of preventative or ameliorative intervention for severe destructive behavior, when combined with differential reinforcement (e.g., Maurice & Trudel,

1982; Nolley, Buttefield, Fleming, & Muller, 1982; Schroeder, et al., 1982)., More diverse methods were disseminated that assessed the utility of stimulus alteration prior to intervention (Iwata, Dorsey, Slifer, Bauman, & Richman, 1982; Kahng, et al., 1998; Touchette, MacDonald, & Langer, 1985). Numerous developments in classroom management and instructional procedures arose over this period (e.g., basic processes such as stimulus equivalence— Green, 2001; Sidman, Willson-Morris, & Kirk, 1986, and applied procedures such as ecobehavioral analysis— Greenwood, Carta, & Atwater, 1991, classwide peer tutoring—Kamps, Barbetta, Leonard, & Delquadri, 1994, and direct instruction— Nelson, Johnson, & Marchand-Martella, 1996).

During this period there has been a resurgence in professional interest in applied behavior analysis, as well as interest by clinicians in training, and demand for ABA services related to findings of unexpected, or perhaps unsuspected, effectiveness of intensive early behavioral intervention (EIBI) for autism spectrum disorders (National Research Council, 2001; New York State, 1999; Satcher, 1999), coupled with a dramatic increase in the numbers of young children reported with autism (Fombonne, 2001). Follow-up studies had indicated extensive benefits from EIBI (Lovaas, 1987; McEachin, Smith, & Lovaas, 1993; Smith, Groen, & Wynn, 2000). Similar or complementary findings were reported earlier (e.g., Fenske, Zalenski, Krantz, & McClannahan, 1985; Anderson, Avery, DiPietro, Edwards, & Christian, 1987), and reflected longstanding research directions in ABA and autism focusing on specific instructional and therapeutic interventions (Matson, 1994; Matson, Benavidez, Compton, Paclawskyj, & Baglio, 1996). Some studies have been less encouraging with respect of outcomes from their applications of ABA for autism (e.g., Bibby, Eikeseth, Martin, Mudford, & Reeves, 2001). Further longitudinal evaluation findings have been slow in emerging, in part due to the nature of such studies. Generalizability of outcomes for EIBI has been critiqued on methodological grounds (Gresham & MacMillan, 1997; Herbert, Sharp, & Gaudino, 2002), and based on survey findings (Boyd & Corley, 2001), as well as ethical grounds (but see Lovaas, 2000). Some who criticize EIBI on ethical grounds, suggest as alternatives, treatment or educational approaches for which there is little or no behavior science evidence of benefit (e.g., Autism National Commitee, 1999). Presently demand for EIBI services remains high among the families of children with autism (Jacobson, 2000) and demand for services outstrips both supply of qualified therapists and the capacity of professional training programs to rapidly address the demand (Jacobson & Mulick,

2000) creating situations where hiring of unqualified, unskilled, and untrained trainers or teachers may be inevitable, and quality of services diminished.

Bifurcation of the Discipline of Behavior Analysis

In addition to an increase or at least a renewal of interest in autism treatment, during
this era there has been an increasing interest in organizational and situational change
as a means to facilitate individual change, which has become exemplified by person-
centered planning (PCP—e.g., Holburn, 1997, 2001; Holburn & Vietze, 1999) and
positive behavior supports (PBS), the latter best summarized by E. Carr et al. (2002),
Horner & E. Carr (1997), and Horner et al. (1990, an early and primary source), and
briefly and recently described by Anderson and Freeman (2000). E Carr et al. (2002),
as Wacker and Berg (2002) note, characterize PBS as a blend of applied behavior
analysis, normalization principles, and person centered principles. However, whether
a unitary body of knowledge is emerging from this social movement, or perhaps
service delivery model (Wacker & Berg, 2002), is not so clear. J. Carr and Sidener
(2002) have noted that authors identified as advocates of PBS are split almost evenly
in their definitions of PBS with respect to whether it encompasses ABA or is different
from ABA in its inherent nature (e.g., E. Carr, et al., 2002).

What is clear is that PBS has adopted, from the advocacy movement, specific values
that are socially progressive, as well as numerous practices founded on more ideo-
logical formulations of special education ends and means.

> "Positive behavior support (PBS) emerged out of a dissatisfaction
> regarding traditional methods for addressing serious behavior prob-
> lems which were often too narrowly defined, focused exclusively on
> consequences, inappropriate within integrated settings, unaccept-
> ably intrusive, and/or ineffective in helping people to realize
> meaningful changes in behavior and lifestyles" (RRTC on Positive
> Behavioral Support, undated; see also Association for Positive Be-
> havior Support, 2003).

Even cursory reviews of articles identified in PBS bibliographies at websites like
www.pbis.org , indicate juxtaposition with both interventions familiar to and inherent in ABA such as preference assessment (i.e., "incorporating student interests"),
functional behavior assessments, antecedent control interventions, functional communication, and foci that are less familiar involving elements of full inclusion,
nonaversive intervention (a movement that can be considered the progenitor to

PBS), person centered planning, lifestyle modification, parent-professional partnerships, child temperament, and communication alternatives (applied examples can be seen in the *Journal of Positive Behavior Interventions*). To some extent this blending reflects some of the educational sector influences, but it may also represent an embracing of progressive social practices by some behavior analysts, even those practices which may have indifferent, mixed, or poorly understood benefits for people with disabilities (e.g., full, as opposed to individually indicated, inclusion, Kauffman & Hallahan, 1995). If PBS is not a discipline, but instead a service model (Wacker & Berg, 2002), advocating for PBS is akin to advocating for something as molar as the interdisciplinary approach, wraparound services, or psychiatric rehabilitation services, rather than therapeutic interventions like ABA or cognitive behavior therapy.

Very few behavior analysts have been overtly critical of PBS as a movement (but see Mulick & Butter, in press), some have posed concerns about dissemination of PBS that include (1) the adequacy of the research base on PBS for non-restrictive procedures (see Jacobson, 1993; Scotti, Evans, Meyer, & Walker, 1991); (2) the extent to which student outcomes accrue from national PBS training for educators (e.g., Dunlap, Hieneman, Knoster, Fox, Anderson, & Albin, 2000); (3) whether the behaviors treated successfully with PBS are as severe in form as those for which restrictive procedures are eventually used (Foxx, in press-a; E. Carr, et al., 1999a), and (4) whether clinically limited community services can sustain comprehensive and variegated interventions that typify PBS in the ideal situation (E. Carr, et al. 1999b).

Most critically, recent activities at federal and organizational level may have implications both for the bifurcation of ABA and PBS, and for future development of PBS. At the first international conference on positive behavior support, in Orlando, Florida in March 2003, a new organization, the Association for Positive Behavior Support (APBS), was launched, which presumably will compete with ABA for some members. This event may be similar to the formation of TASH (The Association for the Severely Handicapped), which was formed by families, advocates, and educators who were disaffected from AAMR (the American Association on Mental Retardation). Whether there is the necessary critical mass of scientists and practitioners to support two national associations in behavior analysis is uncertain, although APBS may recruit members largely from its trainees, mostly educators, in the national training program. The second event, of significance for both behavior analysts and PBS practitioners, is promulgation of newly proposed amendments to the Individuals with Disabilities Education Act. Although at this writing it is too early to project the final form of this legislation as it will be enacted, there are new provisions that diminish local educational agency responsibility for educationally-related services following suspension or dismissal, removing obligations to consider whether problems in school are related to a child's disability, excision of the term "functional behavioral assessment" and softening of former requirements for "positive behavior support plans" in the bill. These terms, as required activities in legislation had previously provided impetus for training initiatives, consultation, and related PBS initiatives nationally.

Controversy: The Big Picture

During the 1970s most if not all states in the U.S. had enacted regulations or laws regarding applied behavior analysis procedures in the field of developmental disabilities, especially procedures considered to be restrictive. In most instances, these requirements included peer and other reviews of proposed interventions. Some procedures were limited or outright banned, and all known methods for treating aberrant behavior were ranked as to their restrictiveness based on perceived harshness or severity, and ethical concerns pertaining to the potential for misapplication or overuse of a procedure (e.g., contingent aversive stimulation was almost uniformly considered to be the most restrictive procedure). When particular procedures were banned in states, they were those that were typically classified as the most restrictive. The least restrictive intervention framework has been reflected over the years through standards for behavior management services issued periodically by the Accreditation Council (1989), an accrediting body composed of professional organizations, and more recently, federal regulations affecting Medicaid reimbursement for community services have included prohibitive requirements for some procedures. Among the states it appears that more recent regulations and laws have increased the range of banned or limited procedures, but because states periodically revise their behavior management regulations, the handful of studies about these regulations (e.g., Landau, 1993) cannot be readily generalized to characterize present regulatory practices.

By the 1980s, an "aversive controversy" over the use of restrictive procedures erupted and appeared to polarize behaviorally-oriented professionals in the developmental disabilities field. Those who were disinclined to wholesale banning of aversive or highly restrictive procedures formed the International Association for the Right to Effective Treatment (Gerhardt, Holmes, Alessandri, & Goodman, 1991), while proponents of the banning advocated more broadly for what was then termed nonaversive intervention and secured the interest of federal agencies such as the Department of

Education and its Office of Special Education and Rehabilitation Services (OSERS) and the Administration on Developmental Disabilities. This advocacy resulted in two events that contributed to subsequent developments related to the present bifurcation in ABA. The first such event was the availability of grant funds through a cooperative agreement by the Department of Education's National Institute on Disability and Rehabilitation Research (NIDRR) for a consortium of universities to study and develop "Community-Referenced Technologies for Nonaversive Behavior Management." The consortium of universities that successfully competed for this award included the University of California at Santa Barbara, University of South Florida, University of Kansas, University of Minnesota, University of Oregon, and the University at Stonybrook (New York). The initial award for this grant was from 1987 to 1992; subsequent NIDRR grants continuing this work, which has grown to include dissemination of positive behavior intervention, have been made for various periods spanning 1992 to the present, and present activities include additional collaboration with the University of Kentucky and the University of Missouri (see the internet site http://www.pbis.org/english/ links.htm). As such, this series of grants probably represents the largest continuing financial support for <u>applied</u> behavior analysis development and dissemination of related techniques that has been financed by the federal government. Under these grants extensive training programs have been fielded, but peer reviewed publications, as opposed to books and training materials, have been relatively scarce in light of the consortium's dissemination, <u>and behavior analytic roots</u>. For example, we searched the PsycINFO data base online for the period 1990 to 2002, and found that the search terms <u>behavior analysis</u> and <u>applied behavior analysis</u> yielded 1,858 peer-reviewed publications, but using the search terms <u>positive behavior support, positive behavioral support, positive behavior intervention</u>, and <u>positive behavioral intervention</u> we found only 77 (also see J. Carr & Sidener, 2002).

The other event contributing to the present bifurcation was also a federal initiative. The National Institutes of Health convened a consensus development conference on the Treatment of Destructive Behaviors in Persons with Developmental Disabilities held in 1989. The primary conveners of the conference were National Institute of Child Health and Human Development (NICHD) and the Office of Medical Applications of Research (OMAR) and the cosponsors included the National Institute of Neurological Disorders and Stroke, the National Institute of Mental Health of the Alcohol, Drug Abuse, and Mental Health Administration (ADAMHA), and the Division of Maternal and Child Health of the Health Resources and Services

Administration. The statement resulting from the conference, may be found at the internet site http://consensus. nih.gov/cons/ 075/075_statement.htm. The report concluded, among many other specifics, that there were instances when the use of very restrictive procedures may be warranted in the treatment of aggression, self-injury, or property destruction by people with developmental disabilities. It is likely that the nature of the consensus statement as well as key studies involving aversive stimulation during this period (e.g., Landau, 1993; Linscheid, Hartel, & Cooley, 1993; Linscheid, Iwata, Ricketts, Williams, & Griffin, 1990; Linscheid, Pejeau, Cohen, & Footo-Lenz, 1994; Ricketts, Goza, & Matese, 1992), have helped to sustain advocacy for nonaversive intervention and positive behavior support (see Foxx, in press-b).

To what extent did the use of punishment procedures expand in the treatment of people with developmental disabilities in the 1970s and 1980s, and perhaps into the present? To address this question we retrieved and evaluated data from several sources, under the assumption that that the published literature would reflect the degree of professional acceptance of punishment. The first source was the PsycINFO data base maintained online by the American Psychological Association. Table 1 shows the results of a search for each decade since 1950 using the terms "mental retardation and reinforcement" versus "mental retardation and punishment". This search provides a relative count rather than an absolute count of articles using reinforcement or punishment procedures for people with mental retardation, but is illustrative of trends within this constraint. As Table 1 shows, there were no relevant articles found for 1950 to 1959 but in each of the subsequent decades between 8.0% and 12.7% of ABA articles found involved punishment, and the percentage has risen slightly from 11.7% to 12.7% from the 1980s to 1990s and beyond.

Table 1: Journal Articles on "Mental Retardation" and "Reinforcement" or "Punishment"

Type of Article	1950-59	1960-69	1970-79	1980-89	1990-2003	Total
Reinforcement	0	80	298	241	268	887
Punishment	0	7	38	32	39	116
Total	0	87	336	273	307	1,003

Source: PsycINFO online at www.apa.org, April 21, 2003, using keywords only

A second source of information is represented by the data base of articles from the Journal of Applied Behavior Analysis (JABA) maintained at the website http://

www.envmed. rochester.edu/wwwrap/ behavior/jaba/jabaindx.htm. A search from 1968 through 2001 at that site using the terms reinforc*, punish*, and positive beh*, allowing all possible extensions for these words resulted in the cumulative graph shown in Figure 1. This graph indicates few studies involving punishment or positive behavior intervention published in JABA relative to those entailing reinforcement throughout this period, and that while the rate at which new studies involving punishment or positive behavior intervention are published seem relatively stable, during the past 20 years there has been an increase in the rate at which studies relying on reinforcement procedures have been published in JABA.

Figure 1: Cumulative Articles in the Journal of Applied Behavior Analysis: 1968-2001: Procedures

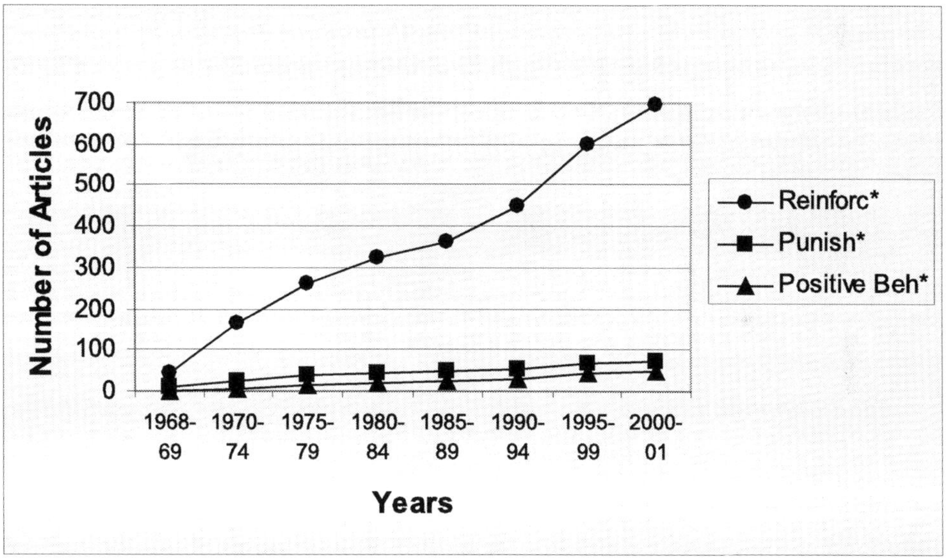

*Note: Use of a search term with an * retrieves all forms of the term searched*

A third source of information consists of online bibliographies, from which we have chosen one at Brandeis University on aversive treatment (see http:// www.brandeis.edu/lemberg/ SGHL/ Subpages/Collections/catalogue.html) and another on faradic shock and other positive punishment treatment in mental retardation services from http://www.effectivetreatment.org/ bibliography.htm. The Brandeis bibliography includes six studies of punishment effects from the 1960s, all of which were data-driven; 12 data-driven studies from the 1970s and 11 commentaries or reviews, the latter including studies of treatment acceptability, 15 data driven studies and 31 commentaries from the 1980s; and eight data-driven studies and 38 commentaries from the 1990s. The articles cited in this comprehensive bibliography appear to suggest that (a) overall, few aversive treatment studies have been published over the period 1960 to the present, (b) there may be a decline in the rate at which articles on aversive treatment are being published since 1980, and (c) it has become far more common to write about aversive treatment than to conduct research on aversive treatment. The latter bibliography, which addresses a narrower range of procedures, lists 15 studies using positive punishment during the 1960s, 43 in the 1970s, four in the 1980s, and 12 from the 1990s to the 2000s. This bibliography appears to indicate that positive punishment publications overall have decreased since the 1970s but increased in the period 1980 to the present.

A number of excellent reviews have been conducted over the years in this area, including Gardner (1969), Harris and Ersner-Hershfield (1978), E. Carr and Lovaas (1983), Matson and Taras (1989), Matson and Farrar-Schneider (1993), and Lerman and Vorndran (2002). Several have noted that while a considerable number of punishment studies were conducted in the 1970s, the rate of punishment publications has since declined, and that behavior analytic punishment-based studies have never represented a major or common focus of intervention reports for treatment of people with mental retardation (e.g., Lerman & Vorndran, 2002).

Other Publication Trends

We also tapped the JABA data base to identify other trends. We found that skill-building interventions have outpaced interventions for aggression or self-injurious behavior from 1968 forward, although the rates at which new studies on these three topics were published have become more similar since 1985 and have perhaps plateaued. We also found that the rates at which new publications in autism versus mental retardation occur have been stable since about 1970, but that the rate has been greater for mental retardation studies from 1968 to the present. We also found that the rate at which studies have focused on observational methods has been lower than the rates for either assessment or intervention studies since 1968, but that since 1990 the rate of publication of assessment studies has increased and cumulatively JABA has now published slightly more studies on assessment than on intervention. Considering only studies of children, we found that the rate at which all studies involving children have been published has consistently exceeded that for either preschool or classroom studies, and that the rates at which preschool or classroom studies have been published has been stable since about 1975. To the extent that JABA publication trends can be treated as an indicator of research trends, and to a lesser extent as a focus of applied work, it appears that ideology (e.g., changes in publications on punishment) and advantageous positioning (e.g., recognition of the effectiveness of EIBI) have not significantly affected the relative level of research interest in a range of areas in which there has been longstanding involvement of behavior analysts in the field of developmental disabilities.

Conclusion

The application of operant principles and the experimental method to the analysis of human behavior problems emerged as a viable approach by the 1960s. By the end of that decade, a smattering of convincing demonstrations became the basis for a new discipline with a mission to solve important social problems in a systematic and individualized manner. Today, the Association for Applied Behavior Analysis has about 3000 members, with a growth rate of about 4 percent per year, and there are over 6000 non-dues-paying behavior analysts represented by affiliated ABA state chapters and national chapters of other countries (Malott, 1999). In addition, the association now oversees an accreditation process for university training programs and a certification organization, the Behavior Analyst Certification Board (Johnston & Shook, 2001) has been established to grant certification to qualified individuals.

Applied behavior analysis has expanded in breadth from institutional demonstrations to mainstream systems in areas such as developmental disabilities, health, education, general clinical practice, and industry; from single variable interventions to complex functional assessment with systemic intervention; and from an appreciation of reliable experimental control of nearly any human operant response to consideration and measurement of consumer satisfaction and acceptability of treatment. Throughout ABA's history, it has retained its hallmark of the experimental method, the foundation for the believability of its effectiveness. This hallmark has been responsible for its success, yet it has curtailed ABA's entry into some areas of significant human problems, and a wide range of problems in particular, in the field of developmental disabilities. Such problems tend to be poorly defined, and they often call for complex interventions with outcomes that have not yet been operationalized. Thus, investigators are challenged to maintain integrity of treatment and reliable measurement of results. Nonetheless, some behaviorally oriented practitioners have taken on some of these problems and will no doubt be discovering new methods for their analysis.

During the aversive controversy in the 1980's, the positive behavior support movement for challenging behavior emerged with principles and practices that extended the purview ABA problems but only by relaxing the experimental rigor endemic to ABA. Today, these applied investigators are facing the difficulties of attaining acceptable levels of believability (by traditional standards) while attacking some of the most significant problems that applied behavior analysts face. At the same time, traditional applications of ABA have advanced at a slower pace, with the exception of some other service sectors, such as early intervention, and instructional design aspects of special education.

References

Accreditation Council on Services for People with Developmental Disabilities [ACDD]. (1989). *Standards for services for people with developmental disabilities.* Landover, MD: Author.

Allen, K. E., Hart, B. M., Buell, J. S., Harris, F. R., & Wolf, M. M. (1964). Effects of social reinforcement on isolate behavior of a nursery school child. *Child Development, 35,* 511-518.

Anderson, C. M., & Freeman, K. A. (2000). Positive behavior support: Expanding the application of applied behavior analysis. The Behavior Analyst, 23, 85-94.

Anderson, S. R., Avery, D. L., DiPietro, E. K., Edwards, G. L., & Christian, W. P. (1987). Intensive home-based early intervention with autistic children. Education and Treatment of Children, 10, 352-366.

Association for Positive Behavior Support. (2003). What is positive behavioral support? Accessed online at http://rrtcpbs.fmhi.usf.edu/apbs/main.html (www.apbsinternational.org).

Ayllon,T., & Azrin, N. H. (1965). *The token economy.* New York: Appleton-Century-Kroft.

Ayllyon, T., & Haughton, E. (1962). Control of the behavior of schizophrenics by food. *Journal of the Experimental Analysis of Behavior, 5,* 343-52.

Ayllon,T., & Azrin, N. H. (1965). *The token economy.* New York: Appleton-Century-Kroft.

Ayllyon, T., & Haughton, E. (1962). Control of the behavior of schizophrenics by food. *Journal of the Experimental Analysis of Behavior, 5,* 343-52.

Autism National Committee [AUTCOM]. (1999). *Alternatives to behaviorism.* Accessed online at http://www.autcom.org/behaviorism.html on 3/22/03.

Azrin, N. H., & Foxx, R. M. (1971). A rapid method of toilet training the institutionalized retarded. *Journal of Applied Behavior Analysis, 4,* 89-99.

Azrin, N. H., & Holtz, W. C. (1966). Punishment. In W. K. Honig (Ed.), *Operant behavior: Areas of research at application* (pp. 380-447). New York: Appleton.

Azrin, N. H., & Lindsley, O. R. (1956). The reinforcement of cooperation between children. *Journal of Abnormal and Social Psychology, 52,* 100-102.

Baer, D. M., Wolf, M. M., & Risley, T. R. (1968). Some current dimensions of applied behavior analysis. *Journal of Applied Behavior Analysis, 1,* 91-97.

Ball, T., Sibbach, L., Jones, R., Steele, B., & Frazier, L. (1975). An accelerometer-activated device to control assaultive and self-destructive behaviors in retardates. *Behavior Therapy and Experimental Psychiatry, 6,* 223-228.

Bambara, L. M. & Knoster, T. P. (1995). *Guidelines: Effective behavioral support.* Harrisburg, PA: Pennsylvania Department of Education, Bureau of Special Education.

Baroff, G. S. (1974). *Mental retardation: Nature, cause and management.* Washington, DC: Hemisphere Publishing.

Barton, E. S., Guess, D., Gacia, E., & Baer, D. M. (1970). Improvement of retardates' mealtime behaviors by timeout procedures using multiple baseline techniques. *Journal of Applied Behavior Analysis, 3,* 77-84.

Bibby, P., Eikeseth, S., Martin, N., Mudford, O. C., & Reeves, D. (2001). Progress and outcomes for children with autism receiving parent-managed intensive interventions. *Research in Developmental Disabilities. 22,* 425-447.

Bijou, S. W. (1968). The mentally retarded child. *Psychology Today, 2*(1), 46-51.

Bijou, S. W., & Baer, D. M. (1961). *Child development I: A systematic and empirical theory.* Englewood Cliffs, N J: Prentice Hall.

Bijou, S. W., & Dunitz-Johnson, E. (1981). Interbehavior analysis of developmental retardation. *Psychological Record, 31,* 305-329.

Birnbrauer, J. S., Bijou, S. W., Wolf, M. M., & Kidder, J. D. (1965). Programmed instruction in the classroom. In L. P. Ullmann & L. Krasner (Eds.), *Case studies in behavior modification* (pp. 358-363). New York: Holt, Rinehart, & Winston.

Boeree, C. G. (1998/2000). *Behaviorism.* Accesed at http://www.ship.edu/~cgboeree/beh.html.

Bowman, L. G., Piazza, C. C., Fisher, W. W., Hagopian, L. P., & Kogan, J. S. (1997). Assessment of preference for varied versus constant reinforcers. *Journal of Applied Behavior Analysis, 30,* 451-458.

Bowman, P. W. (1957, May). "Rewards" and "punishments" in an institution for the mentally retarded. *Pineland Hospital Bulletin on Mental Retardation, 1*, 7-13.

Boyd, R. D., & Corley, M. J. (2001). Outcome survey of early intensive behavioral intervention for young children with autism in a community setting, *Autism.* 5, 430-441.

Broden, M., Bruce, C., Mitchell, M. A., Carter, V., & Hall, R. V. (1970). Effects of teacher attention on attending behavior of two boys at adjacent desks. *Journal of Applied Behavior Analysis, 3*, 199-203.

Broden, M., Copeland, G., Beasley, A., & Hall, R. V. (1977). Altering student responses through changes in teacher verbal behavior. Journal of Applied Behavior Analysis, 10, *479-487.*

Burchard, J. D., & Barrera, F. (1972). An analysis of timeout and response cost in a programmed environment. *Journal of Applied Behavior Analysis, 5*, 271-282.

Cameron, M. J., & Kimball, J. W. (1995). Beyond consequences. *Mental Retardation, 33*, 268-270.

Carr, E. G. (1977). The motivation of self-injurious behavior: A review of some hypotheses. *Psychological Bulletin, 84*, 800-816.

Carr, E. G., Dunlap, G., Horner, R. H., Koegel, R. L., Turnbull, A. P., Sailor, W., et al. (2002). Positive behavior support: Evolution of an applied science. *Journal of Positive Behavior Interventions, 4*, 4-16, 20.

Carr, E. G., Horner, R. H., Turnbull, A. P., McLaughlin, D. M., McAtee, M. L., Smith, C. E., et al. (1999a). *Positive behavior support for people with developmental disabilities: A research synthesis.* Washington, DC: American Association on Mental Retardation.

Carr, E. G., Levin, L., McConnachie, G., Carlson, J. I., Kemp, D. C., Smith, C. E., et al. (1999b). Comprehensive multisituational intervention for problem behavior in the community: Long-term maintenance and social validation. *Journal of Positive Behavior Interventions, 1*, 5-25.

Carr, E. G., & Lovaas, O. I. (1983). Contingent electric shock as a treatment for severe behavior problems. In S. Axelrod & J. Apsche (Eds.), *The effects of punishment on human behavior* (pp. 221-245). New York, Academic Press.

Carr, E. G., Dunlap, G., Horner, R. H., Koegel, R. L., Turnbull, A. P., Sailor, W., et al. (2002). Positive behavior support: Evolution of an applied science. *Journal of Positive Behavior Interventions, 4*, 4-16, 20.

Carr, J. E., & Sidener, T. M. (2002). On the relation between applied behavior analysis and positive behavioral support. *The Behavior Analyst, 25*, 245-253.

Chomsky, N. (1959). A review of B. F. Skinner's Verbal Behavior. *Language, 35*(1), 26-58.

Christopherson, E. R., Barnard, S. R., Barnard, J. D., Gleeson, S., & Sykes, B. W. (1981). Home –based treatment of behavior-disordered and developmentally delayed children. In M. J. Begab, H. C. Haywood, & H. L. Garber, (Eds.), *Psychosocial influences in retarded performance: Vol II: Strategies for improving competence* (pp. 257-275). Baltimore, MD: University Park Press.

Cornwell, D., Hobbs, S., & Prytula, R. (1980). Little Albert rides again. *American Psychologist, 35,* 216-217.

Cronin, K. A., & Cuvo, A. J. (1979). Teaching mending skills to mentally retarded adolescents. Journal of Applied Behavior Analysis, 12, 401-406.

Cuvo, A., Veitch, V. D., Trace, M. W., & Konke, J. L. (1978). Teaching change computation to the mentally retarded. *Behavior Modification, 2,* 531-548.

Dixon, M. R. & Hayes, L. J. (1998). Effects of different instructional histories on the resurgence of rule-following. *The Psychological Record, 48,* 275-292.

Dixon, M. R., Hayes, L. J., Binder, L. M., Manthey, S., Sigman, C., & Zdanowski, D. M. (1998). Using a self-control training procedure to increase appropriate behavior. *Journal of Applied Behavior Analysis, 31,* 203-210.

Dunlap, G., Hieneman, M., Knoster, T., Fox, L., Anderson, J., & Albin, R.W. (2000). Essential elements of inservice training in positive behavioral support. *Journal of Positive Behavior Interventions, 2(1),* 22-32.

Favell, J. E., Realon, R. E., & Sutton, K. A. (1996). Measuring and increasing the happiness of people with profound mental retardation and physical handicaps. *Behavioral Interventions, 11,* 47-58.

Fenske, E. C., Zalenski, S., Krantz, P. J., & McClannahan, L. E. (1985). Age at intervention and treatment outcome for autistic children in a comprehensive intervention program. *Analysis and Intervention in Developmental Disabilities, 5,* 49-58.

Ferster, C. B., & Skinner, B. F. (1957). *Schedules of reinforcement.* East Norwalk, CT: Appleton-Century-Crofts.

Fombonne, E. (2001). Is there an epidemic of autism? *Pediatrics, 107,* 411-412.

Foxx, R. M. (2003). The treatment of dangerous behavior. *Behavioral Interventions, 18,* 1-21.

Foxx, R. M. (in press-a). The myth of the nonaversive treatment of severe behavior. In J. W. Jacobson, J. A. Mulick, & R. M. Foxx (Eds.). *Fads: Dubious and improbable treatments for developmental disabilities.* Mahwah, NJ: Lawrence Erlbaum.

Foxx, R. M. (in press-b). The National Institute of Health Consensus Development Conference on the Treatment of Destructive Behaviors, September 1989. In J. W. Jacobson, J. A. Mulick, & R. M. Foxx (Eds.). *Fads: Dubious and improbable treatments for developmental disabilities.* Mahwah, NJ: Lawrence Erlbaum.

Foxx, R. M., & Azrin, N. H. (1973). The elimination of autistic self-stimulatory behavior by overcorrection. *Journal of Applied Behavior Analysis, 6,* 1-14.

Foxx, R. M., & Shapiro, S. T. (1978). The timeout ribbon: A nonexclusionary timeout procedure. *Journal of Applied Behavior Analysis, 11,* 125-136.

Friman, P. C., Hayes, S. C, & Wilson, K. G. (1998). Why behavior analysts should study emotion: The example of anxiety. *Journal of Applied Behavior Analysis, 31,* 137-156.

Fuller, P. R. (1949). Operant conditioning of a vegetative human organism. *American Journal of Psychology, 62,* 587-590.

Gardner, W. (1969). Use of punishment procedures with the severely retarded: A review. *American Journal of Mental Deficiency, 74,* 86-103.

Gerhardt, P., Holmes, D.L., Alessandri, M., & Goodman, M. (1991). Social policy on the use of aversive interventions: Empirical, ethical, and legal considerations. *Journal of Autism and Developmental Disorders, 21,* 265-277.

Girardeau, F. L., & Spradlin, J. F. (1964). Token rewards in a cottage program. *Mental Retardation, 7,* 40-43.

Gold, M. W. (1980). *Did I say that? Articles and commentaries on the Try Another Way system.* Champaign, IL: Research Press.

Green, C. W., Reid, D. H., White, L. K., Halford, R. C., Brittain, D. P., & Gardner, S. M. (1988). Identifying reinforcers for persons with profound handicaps: Staff opinion versus systematic assessment of preferences. *Journal of Applied Behavior Analysis, 21,* 31-43.

Green, G. (2001). Behavior analytic instruction for learners with autism: Advances in stimulus control technology. *Focus on Autism & Other Developmental Disabilities, 16,* 72-85.

Greene, R. J., & Pratt, J. J. (1972). A group contingency for individual misbehaviors in the classroom. *Mental Retardation, 10,* 33-35.

Greenwood, C. R., Carta, J. J., & Atwater, Jane (1991). Ecobehavioral analysis in the classroom: Review and implications. Journal of Behavioral Education, 1, 59-77.

Greenwood C. R., Carta, J. J., Hart, B., Kamps, D., Terry, B., Arreaga-Mayer, C., et al. (1992). Out of the laboratory and into the community: 26 years of applied behavior analysis at the Juniper Gardens Children's Project. *American Psychologist, 47*, 1464-1474.

Gresham, F. M. (1979). Comparison of response cost and timeout in a special education setting. *Journal of Special Education, 13*, 199-208.

Gresham, F. M., & MacMillan, D. L. (1997). Autistic recovery? An analysis and critique of the empirical evidence on the Early Intervention Project. *Behavioral Disorders, 22*, 185-201.

Guralnick, M. J. (1973). Behavior therapy with an acrophobic mentally retarded young adult. *Journal of Behavior Therapy and Experimental Psychiatry, 4*, 263-265.

Hall, R. V., Fox, R., Willard, D., Goldsmith, L., Emerson, M., Owen, M., et al. (1971). The teacher as observer and experimenter in the modification of disputing and talking-out behaviors. *Journal of Applied Behavior Analysis, 4*, 141-149.

Harris, B. (1979). Whatever happened to little Albert? *American Psychologist, 34*, 151-160.

Harris, S. L., & Ersner-Hershfield, R. (1978). Behavioral suppression of seriously disruptive behavior in psychotic and retarded patients: A review of punishment and its alternatives. *Psychological Bulletin, 85*, 1352-1375.

Hart, B., & Risley, T. R. (1981). Grammatical and conceptual growth in the language of psychosocially disadvantaged children: Assessment and intervention. In M. J. Begab, H. C. Haywood, & H. L. Garber (Eds.), *Psychosocial influences in retarded performance: Vol II: Strategies for improving competence* (pp. 181-198). Baltimore, MD: University Park Press.

Hart, B., & Risley, T. R. (1999). *The social world of children learning to talk.* Baltimore, MD: Paul H. Brookes.

Hawkins, R. P., Peterson, R. F., Schweid, E., & Bijou S. W. (1966). Behavior therapy in the home: Amelioration of problem parent-child relations with the parent in a therapeutic role. *Journal of Experimental Child Psychology, 4*, 99-107.

Hayes, S. C., & Hayes, L. J. (1992). Verbal relations and the evolution of behavior analysis. *American Psychologist, 47*, 1383-1395.

Herbert, J. D., Sharp, I. R., & Gaudiano, B. A. (2002). Separating fact from fiction in the etiology and treatment of autism: A scientific review of the evidence. *Scientific Review of Mental Health Practice, 1*(1), 23-43.

Holburn, S. (1997). A renaissance in residential behavior analysis? A historical perspective and a better way to help people with challenging behavior. *The Behavior Analyst, 20*, 61-85.

Holburn, S. (2001). Compatibility of person-centered planning and applied behavior analysis. *The Behavior Analyst, 24*, 271-281.

Holburn, S., & Vietze, P. (1999). Acknowledging barriers in adopting person-centered planning. *Mental Retardation, 37*, 117-124.

Holland, J. G. (1978). Behaviorism: Part of the problem or part of the solution? *Journal of Applied Behavior Analysis, 11*, 163-174.

Hopkins, B. L. (1970). The first twenty years are the hardest. In R. Ulrich, T. Stachnick, & J. Mabry (Eds.), *Control of human behavior: From cure to prevention.* (Vol 2, pp. 358-365). Glenview, IL: Scott, Foresman, & Co.

Homme, L. E., DeBaca, P. C., Divine, J. V., Steinhorst, R., & Rickert, E. J. (1963). Use of the Premack principle in controlling the behavior of school children. *Journal of the Experimental Analysis of Behavior, 6*, 544.

Horner, R. H., & Carr, E. G. (1997). Behavioral support for students with severe disabilities: Functional assessment and comprehensive intervention. *Journal of Special Education, 31*, 84-104.

Horner, R. H., Dunlap, G., Koegel, R. L., Carr, E. G., Sailor, W., Anderson, J. A., et al. (1990). Toward a technology of "nonaversive" behavioral support. *Journal of the Association for Persons with Severe Handicaps, 15*, 125-132.

Iwata, B. A., Dorsey, M. F., Slifer, K. J., Bauman, K. E., & Richman, G. S. (1982). Toward a functional analysis of self-injury. *Analysis and Intervention in Developmental Disabilities, 2*, 3-20.

Jacobson, J. W. (1993). Public policy and the punishment of the powerless. *Child & Adolescent Mental Health Care, 3*, 7-18.

Jacobson, J. W. (2000). Early intensive behavioral intervention: Emergence of a consumer-driven service model. *Behavior Analyst, 23*, 149-171.

Jacobson, J. W., & Mulick, J. A. (2000). System and cost research issues in treatments for people with autistic disorders. *Journal of Autism and Developmental Disorders, 30*, 585-593.

Jastrow, J. (1935). Has psychology failed? *American Scholar, 4*, 261-269.

Johnston, J. M., & Shook, G. L. (2001). A national certification program for behavior analysts. *Behavioral Interventions, 16*, 77-85.

Jones, M. C. (1924). Elimination of children's fears. *Journal of Experimental Psychology, 7*, 82-85.

Kahng, SW., Iwata, B. A., Fischer, S. M., Page, T. J., Treadwell, K. R. H., Williams, D. E., & Smith, R. G. (1998). Temporal distributions of problem behavior based on scatter plot analysis. *Journal of Applied Behavior Analysis, 31*, 593-604.

Kamps, D. M., Barbetta, P. M., Leonard, B. R., & Delquadri, J. (1994). Classwide peer tutoring: An integration strategy to improve reading skills and promote peer interactions among students with autism and general education peers. *Journal of Applied Behavior Analysis, 27*, 49-61.

Kantor, J. R. (1950). *Psychology and logic (Vol. II).* Bloomington, IN: Principia Press.

Kauffman, J. M. , & Hallahan, D. P. (1995). (Eds.). *The illusion of full inclusion: A critique of a current special education bandwagon.* Austin, TX: Pro-Ed.

Kazdin, A. E. (1972). Response cost: The removal of conditioned reinforcers for therapeutic change. *Behavior Therapy, 3*, 533-546.

Kazdin, A. E. (1973). The effect of response cost and aversive stimulation in suppressing punished and nonpunished speech disfluencies. *Behavior Therapy, 4*, 73-82.

Keller, F. S. (1974). Ten years of personalized instruction. *Teaching of Psychology, 1*(1), 4-9.

Keller, F. S., & Schoenfeld, W. N. (1950). *Principles of psychology.* New York: Appleton-Century-Crofts.

Kircher, A. S., Pear, J. J., & Martin, G. L. (1971). Shock as punishment in a picture-naming task with retarded children. *Journal of Applied Behavior Analysis, 4*, 227-233.

Konarski, E. A., Favell, J. E., & Favell J. E. (Eds.). (1997). *Manual for the assessment and treatment of the behavior disorders of people with mental retardation.* Morganton, NC: Western Carolina Center Foundation.

Landau, R. J. (1993). Legislation and regulation in the age of "new" aversives. *Child & Adolescent Mental Health Care, 3*, 19-29.

Lane, H. (1989). *When the mind hears: A history of the deaf.* New York: Vintage Books.

Lerman, D. C., & Vorndran, C. M. (2002). On the status of knowledge for using punishment: Implications for treating behavior disorders. *Journal of Applied Behavior Analysis, 35*, 431-464.

Lindsley, O. R., Skinner, B. F., & Soloman, H. C. (1953). *Study of psychotic behavior*. Studies in Behavior Therapy, Harvard Medical School, Department of Psychiatry, Metropolitan State Hospital, Waltham, MA, Office of Naval Research Contract N5-ori-07662, Status Report IV, 1 June 1953-31 December 1953.

Lindsley, O. R., Skinner, B. F., & Soloman, H. C. (1955). *Study of psychotic behavior*. Behavior Research Laboratory, Harvard Medical School, Department of Psychiatry, Metropolitan State Hospital, Waltham, MA, Office of Naval Research Contract N5-ori-07662, Status Report IV, 1 January 1955-31 August 1955.

Linscheid, T. R., Hartel, F., & Cooley, N. (1993). Are aversive procedures durable? A five year follow-up of three individuals treated with contingent electric shock. *Child & Adolescent Mental Health Care, 3*, 67-76.

Linscheid, T. R., Iwata, B. A., Ricketts, R. W., Williams, D. E., & Griffin, J. C. (1990). Clinical evaluation of the self-injurious behavior inhibiting system (SIBIS). *Journal of Applied Behavior Analysis, 23*, 53-78.

Linscheid, T. R., Pejeau, C., Cohen, S., & Footo-Lenz, M. (1994). Positive side effects in the treatment of SIB using the Self-Injurious Behavior Inhibiting System (SIBIS): Implications for operant and biochemical explanations of SIB. *Research in Developmental Disabilities, 15*, 81-90.

Lovaas, I. (2000, August 2). *Clarifying comments on the UCLA Young Autism Project*. Accessed online at http://www.feat.org/lovaas/full.htm 4/20/03.

Lovaas, O. I. (1987). Behavioral treatment and normal educational and intellectual functioning in young autistic children. *Journal of Consulting and Clinical Psychology. 55*, 3-9.

Lovaas, O. I., Freitag, G., Gold, V. J., & Kassorla, I. C. (1965). Experimental studies in childhood schizophrenia: Analysis of self-destructive behavior. *Journal of Experimental Child Psychology, 2*, 67-84.

Lovaas, O. I., Freitag, G., Kinder, M. I., Rubenstein, B. D. , Schaeffer, B., & Simmons, J. W. (1966). Establishment of social reinforcers in two schizophrenic children on the basis of food. *Journal of Experimental Child Psychology, 4*, 109-125.

Lovaas, O. I., Koegel, R. L., Simmons, J. Q., & Long, J. S. (1973). Some generalization and follow-up measures of autistic children in behavior therapy. *Journal of Applied Behavior Analysis, 6*, 131-165.

Lovaas, O. I., Schaeffer, B., & Simmons, J. Q. (1965). Building social behavior in autistic children by use of electric shock. *Journal of Experimental Research in Personality, 1*, 99-109.

Lovass, O. I., & Simmons, J. Q. (1969). Manipulation of self-destruction in three retarded children. *Journal of Applied Behavior Analysis, 2*, 143-157.

Lovett, H. (1996). *Learning to listen: Positive approaches and people with difficult behavior.* Baltimore, MD: Paul H. Brookes.

MacMillan, D. L., & Forness, S. R. (1973). Behavior modification: Savior or savant? In G. Tarjan, R. K. Eyman, & C. E. Meyers (Eds.), *Sociobehavioral studies in mental retardation: Papers in honor of Harvey F. Dingman* (pp. 186-210). Washington, DC: American Association on Mental Deficiency.

Mahoney M. J. (1989). Scientific psychology and radical behaviorism: Important distinctions based in scientism and objectivism. *American Psychologist, 44*, 1372-1377.

Malott, M. (1999). *Reflections on twenty-five years of ABA: Past, present, and future.* Paper presented at a symposium at the annual meeting of the Association for Behavior Analysis, Chicago, IL.

Marholin, D., O'Toole, K., Touchette, P., Berger, P., & Doyle, D. (1979). "I'll have a Big Mac, large fries, large coke, and apple pie," . . . or teaching adaptive community skills. *Behavior Therapy, 10*, 236-248.

Marquis, D. P. (1941). Learning in the neonate: The modification of behavior under three feeding schedules. *Journal of Experimental Psychology, 29*, 263-282.

Matson, J. L. (1978). Training socially appropriate behaviours to moderately retarded adults: A social learning approach. *Scandinavian Journal of Behaviour Therapy, 7*, 167-175.

Matson J. L. (Ed.). (1994). *Autism in children and adults: Etiology, assessment, and intervention.* Pacific Grove, CA: Brooks/Cole.

Matson, J. L., Benavidez, D. A., Compton, L. S., Paclawskyj, T., & Baglio, C. (1996). Behavioral treatment of autistic persons: A review of research from 1980 to the present. *Research in Developmental Disabilities, 17*, 433-465.

Matson, J. L., & Farrar-Schneider, D. (1993). Common behavioral decelerators (aversives) and their efficacy. *Child and Adolescent Mental Health Care, 3*, 49-64.

Matson, J. L., & Ollendick, T. H. (1976). Elimination of low frequency biting. *Behavior Therapy, 7*, 410-412.

Matson, J. L., & Taras, M. (1989). A 20 year review of punishment and alternative methods to treat problem behaviors in developmentally delayed persons. *Research in Developmental Disabilities, 10*, 85-104.

Maurice, P., & Trudel, G. (1982). Self-injurious behavior prevalence and relationships to environmental events. In J. H. Hollis & C. E. Meyers (Eds.), *Life threatening behavior: Analysis and intervention* (pp. 81-102). Washington, DC: American Association on Mental Deficiency.

McEachin, J. J., Smith, T., & Lovaas, O. I. (1993). Long-term outcome for children with autism who received early intensive behavioral treatment. *American Journal on Mental Retardation. 97*, 359-372.

Miller, M. A., Cuvo, A. J., & Borakove, L. S. (1977). Teaching naming of coin values: Comprehension before production versus production alone. *Journal of Applied Behavior Analysis, 10*, 735-736.

Moore, J. (1984). Conceptual contributions of Kantor's interbehavioral psychology. The Behavior Analyst, 7, 183-187.

Moore, J. (2000). Thinking about thinking and feeling about feeling. *The Behavior Analyst, 23*, 45-56.

Mulick, J. A., & Butter, E. M. (2002). Educational advocacy for children with autism. *Behavioral Interventions, 17*, 57-74.

Mulick, J. A., & Butter, E. (in press). Positive behavior support: A paternalistic utopian delusion. In J. W. Jacobson, J. A. Mulick, & R. M. Foxx (Eds.), *Fads: Dubious and improbable treatments for developmental disabilities*. Mahwah, NJ: Lawrence Erlbaum.

National Institutes of Health. (1989). *Treatment of destructive behaviors in persons with developmental disabilities*. Bethesda, MD: Author.

National Research Council. (2001). *Educating Children with Autism*, Committee on Educational Interventions for Children with Autism, Division of Behavioral and Social Sciences and Education, Washington, D.C.: National Academy Press.

Nelson, J. R., Johnson, A., & Marchand-Martella, N. (1996). Effects of direct instruction, cooperative learning, and independent learning practices on the classroom behavior of students with behavioral disorders: A comparative analysis. *Journal of Emotional and Behavioral Disorders, 4*, 53-62.

New York State Department of Health Early Intervention Program. (1999). *Clinical Practice Guideline: The Guideline Technical Report, Autism/Pervasive Developmental Disorders, Assessment and Intervention for Young Children.* Albany, NY: Author.

Nolley, D., Buttefield, B., Fleming, A., & Muller, P. (1982). Nonaversive treatment of severe self-injurious behavior: Multiple replications with DRO and DRI. In J. H. Hollis & C. E. Meyers (Eds.), *Life threatening behavior: Analysis and intervention* (pp. 161-189). Washington, DC: American Association on Mental Deficiency.

Ollendick, T. H., & Matson, J. L. (1976). An initial investigation into the parameters of overcorrection. *Psychological Reports, 39*(3, Pt 2), 1139-1142.

Page, T. J., Iwata, B. A. & Reid, D. H. (1982). Pyramidal training: A large-scale application with institutional staff. *Journal of Applied Behavior Analysis, 15,* 335-351.

Parsons, M. B., & Reid, D. H. (1995). Training residential supervisors to provide feedback for maintaining staff teaching skills with people who have severe disabilities. *Journal of Applied Behavior Analysis, 28,* 317-322.

Paul, D. B., & Blumenthal, A. L. (1989). On the trail of Little Albert. *Psychological Record, 39,* 547-553.

Pennsylvania Code. (1993, January 15). *§ 2380.151. Definition of restrictive procedures,* 23 Pa.B. 343.

Phillips, E. L., Phillips, E. A., Fixsen, D. L., & Wolf, M. M. (1971). Achievement Place: Modification of the behaviors of pre-delinquent boys within a token economy. *Journal of Applied Behavior Analysis, 4,* 45-59.

Porterfield, J. K., Herbert-Jackson, E., & Risley, T. R. (1976). Contingent observation: An effective and acceptable procedure for reducing disruptive behavior of young children in a group setting. *Journal of Applied Behavior Analysis, 9,* 55-64.

Rachlin, H., & Green, L. (1972). Commitment, choice and self-control. *Journal of the Experimental Analysis of Behavior, 17,* 15-22.

Reid, D. H., & Parsons, M. B. (2000). Organizational behavior management in human service settings. In J. Austin & J. E. Carr (Eds.), *Handbook of applied behavior analysis* (pp. 275-294). Reno, NV: Context Press.

Reid, D. H., Everson, J. M., & Green, C. W. (1999). A systematic evaluation of preferences identified through person-centered planning for people with profound multiple disabilities. *Journal of Applied Behavior Analysis, 32,* 467-477.

Repp, A. C., & Singh, N. N. (Eds.). (1990). *Perspectives on the use of nonaversive and aversive interventions for persons with developmental disabilities.* Sycamore, IL: Sycamore Publishing Co.

Reppucci, N. D. (1977). Implementation issues for the behavior modifier as institutional change agent. *Behavior Therapy, 8,* 594-605.

Reppucci, N. D., & Saunders, J. T. (1974). The social psychology of behavior modification: Problems of implementation in natural settings. *American Psychologist, 29,* 649-660.

Ricketts, R. W., Goza, A. B., & Matese, M. (1992). Effects of naltrexone and SIBIS on self-injury. *Behavioral Residential Treatment, 7,* 315-326.

Rincover, A., Newsom, C. D., & Carr, E. G. (1979). Using sensory extinction procedures in the treatment of compulsivelike behavior of developmentally disabled children. *Journal of Consulting and Clinical Psychology, 47,* 695-701.

Risley, T. (1968). The effects and side effects of punishing the autistic behaviors of a deviant child. *Journal of Applied Behavior Analysis, 1,* 21-34.

Risley, T. R. (1997). Montrose M. Wolf: The origin of the dimensions of applied behavior analysis. *Journal of Applied Behavior Analysis, 30,* 377-381.

Risley, T., & Wolf, M. (1967). Establishing functional speech in echolalic children. *Behaviour Research and Therapy, 5*(2), 73-88.

Rogers-Warren, A., & Warren, S. F. (Eds.). (1977). *Ecological perspectives in behavior analysis.* Baltimore, MD: University Park Press.

RRTC on Positive Behavioral Support. (undated). *Positive behavior support.* Accessed online at http://rrtcpbs.fmhi.usf.edu/pbsinfo.htm.

Sailor, W., Guess, D., Rutherford, G., & Baer, D. M. (1968). Control of tantrum behavior by operant techniques during experimental verbal training. *Journal of Applied Behavior Analysis, 1,* 237-243.

Satcher, D. (1999). *Mental health: A report of the surgeon general.* Bethesda, MD: U.S. Public Health Service.

Schroeder, S. R., Kanoy, R. C., Mulick, J. A., Rojahn, J., Thios, S. J., Stevens, M., et al. (1982). Environmental antecedents which affect management and maintenance of programs for self-injurious behavior. In J. H. Hollis & C. E. Meyers (Eds.), *Life threatening behavior: Analysis and intervention* (pp. 105-159). Washington, DC: American Association on Mental Deficiency.

Schroeder, S. R., Rojahn, J., & Mulick, J. A. (1978). Ecobehavioral organization of developmental day care for the chronically self-injurious. *Journal of Pediatric Psychology, 3*(2), 81-88.

Schwartz, I. S., & Baer, D. M. (1991). Social validity assessments: Is current practice state of the art? *Journal of Applied Behavior Analysis, 24,* 189-204.

Scotti, J. R., Evans, I. M., Meyer, L. H., & Walker, P. (1991). A meta-analysis of intervention research with problem behavior: Treatment validity and standards of practice. *American Journal on Mental Retardation, 96,* 233-256.

Sidman, M., Willson-Morris, M., & Kirk, B. (1986). Matching-to-sample procedures and the development of equivalence relations: The role of naming. *Analysis & Intervention in Developmental Disabilities, 6,* 1-19.

Skinner, B. F. (1938). *The behavior of organisms: An experimental analysis.* Oxford, UK: Appleton-Century.

Skinner, B. F. (1948). *Walden two.* Oxford, UK: Macmillan.

Skinner, B. F. (1953). *Science and human behavior*. Oxford, UK: Macmillan.

Skinner, B. F. (1957). *Verbal behavior*. East Norwalk, CT: Appleton-Century-Crofts.

Skinner, B. F. (1959). *Cumulative record*. East Norwalk, CT: Appleton-Century-Crofts.

Smith, T., Groen, A.D., & Wynn, J.W. (2000). Randomized trial of intensive early intervention for children with pervasive developmental disorder. *American Journal on Mental Retardation, 105*, 269-285.

Striefel, S., Wetherby, B., & Karlan, G. (1978). Developing generalized instruction-following behavior in severely retarded people. In C. E. Meyers (Ed.), *Quality of life in severely and profoundly mentally retarded people:_Research foundations for improvement* (pp. 267-326). Washington, DC. American Association on Mental Deficiency.

Tharp, R. G., & Wetzel, R. J. (1969). *Behavior modification in the natural environment*. New York: Academic.

Thompson, T., Gardner, W. I., & Baumeister, A. A. (1988). Ethical interventions for persons with retardation, autism, and related developmental disorders. In J. A. Stark, F. J. Menolascino, M. H. Albarelli, & V. C. Grey (Eds.), *Mental retardation and mental health* (pp. 213-217). New York: Springer-Verlag.

Touchette, P. E., MacDonald, R. F., & Langer, S. N. (1985). A scatter plot for identifying stimulus control of problem behavior. *Journal of Applied Behavior Analysis, 18*, 343-351.

Trybus, R. J., & Lacks, P. B. (1972). Modification of vocational behavior in a community agency for mentally retarded adolescents. *Rehabilitation Literature, 33*(9) 258-266.

Ullmann, L. P. & Krasner, L. (Eds.). (1965). *Case studies in behavior modification*. New York: Holt, Rinehart, and Winston.

Ullmann, L. P., & Krasner, L. (1969). *A psychological approach to abnormal behavior*. Englewood Cliffs, NJ: Prentice-Hall.

Wacker, D. P., & Berg, W. K. (2002). PBS as a service delivery system. *Journal of Positive Behavior Interventions, 4*, 25-28.

Watson, J. B., & Raynor, P. (1920). Conditioned emotional reactions. *Journal of Experimental Psychology, 3*, 1-4.

Willems, E. P. (1974). Behavioral technology and behavioral ecology. *Journal of Applied Behavior Analysis, 7*, 151-165.

Williams, C. D. (1959). The elimination of tantrum behavior by extinction procedures. *Journal of Abnormal and Social Psychology, 59*, 269.

Wolf, M. M. (1978). Social validity: The case for subjective measurement or how applied behavior analysis is finding its heart. *Journal of Applied Behavior Analysis, 11*, 203-214.

Wolf, M. M., Birnbrauer, J. S., Williams, T., & Lawler, J. (1965). A note on the apparent extinction of the vomiting behavior of a retarded child. In L. P. Ullmann & L. Krasner (Eds.), *Case studies in behavior modification* (pp. 364-366). New York: Holt, Rinehart, & Winston.

Wolf, M. M., Risley, T., & Mees, H. (1964). Application of operant conditioning procedures to the behavior problems of an autistic child. *Behavior Research and Therapy, 1*, 305-312.

Wolpe, J. (1969). *The practice of behavior therapy.* New York: Pergamon Press.

Zimmerman, E. H., & Zimmerman, J. (1962). The alteration of behavior in a special education classroom situation. *Journal of the Experimental Analysis of Behavior, 5*, 59-60.

BEHAVIOR SUPPORT AND INTERVENTION: CURRENT ISSUES AND PRACTICES IN DEVELOPMENTAL DISABILITIES

James K. Luiselli, Ed.D.
The May Institute Inc.

Individuals with developmental disabilities frequently display challenging behaviors such as aggression, self-injury, property destruction, tantrum outbursts, and stereotypy. Problems of this type have numerous and serious consequences: they can cause injury to self and others, are socially stigmatizing, interfere with instruction, compromise educational opportunities, and in some cases, require confinement to a restrictive habilitation setting. For these reasons, intervention research in developmental disabilities has been extensive.

Applied behavior analysis dates to the seminal publication by Baer, Wolf, and Risley (1968) and has been instrumental in formulating, evaluating, and disseminating intervention procedures. Numerous behavioral journals are available to professionals (*Behavioral Interventions, Behavior Modification, Child and Family Behavior Therapy, Journal of Applied Behavior Analysis, Journal of Behavior Therapy and Experimental Psychiatry*) and other multidisciplinary sources regularly publish behavioral intervention research (*American Journal on Mental Retardation, Journal of Autism and Developmental Disorders, Research in Developmental Disabilities*). Although dominated initially by a "technology focused" orientation, the field of applied behavior analysis has evolved substantively over the years, including new thinking about the functional influences on challenging behaviors, the conceptual basis of behavior-change strategies, and the settings where intervention is carried out. This chapter demonstrates where the field has come by discussing contemporary issues in behavior support and intervention.

The chapter begins with a brief historical overview, tracing earlier "generations" of behavioral intervention, and commenting about influences and forces that have shaped current practices. Next, several present intervention trends are highlighted and accompanied by research descriptions and case illustrations. The chapter concludes with a brief summary of future directions.

Historical Overview

The decades of the 1960s and 1970s might be considered the "first generation" of behavioral intervention. Professionals of that era were charged with treating children and adults who had developmental disabilities, engaged in serious challenging behaviors, and were unresponsive to traditional "treatment." In children with autism, for example, Lovaas and colleagues reported improvement in social behavior and elimination of self-injury (Lovaas, Freitag, Gold, & Kassorla, 1965; Lovaas, Schaeffer, & Simmons, 1965). Preliminary applications of token economy systems suggested positive effects on skill acquisition and behavior reduction (Ayllon & Azrin, 1968). These and other studies changed meaningfully the lives of many individuals but did not achieve the research sophistication of present-day standards. It must be remembered, of course, that at that time, applied behavior analysis was at a nascent stage. Thus, interventions usually targeted a single challenging behavior, were implemented by experienced therapists (as opposed to "paraprofessionals"), and were evaluated under simulated conditions. As noted previously, these research efforts were devoted to establishing a "technology" or set of procedures that could be applied to specific challenging behaviors. Functional behavioral assessment, a fundamental feature of contemporary applied behavior analysis (Pelios, Morren, Tesch, & Axelrod, 1999), typically was not conducted formally or seen as a first step toward intervention formulation. Finally, the bulk of intervention methods were consequence-based, often relying on negative (punishment) procedures as the sole treatment focus. To illustrate, many publications appeared that detailed effective intervention using overcorrection, physical restraint, and aversive stimulation (Forehand & Baumeister, 1976).

Around the mid-1980s, the "aversive versus nonaversive debate" gained momentum and was at the heart of many disputes and disagreements among professionals (Repp & Singh, 1990). The dominant concern was that although "aversive" (better explained

as punishment) procedures could be effective in reducing and eliminating challenging behaviors of persons with developmental disabilities, certain limitations could
not be overlooked. Notably, punishment does not teach appropriate behavior or
adaptive skills. Furthermore, the opinion of some practitioners was that individuals
exposed to punishment often demonstrated agitation, extreme emotional reactions,
and escape/avoidance responses, although there is limited research to support or
refute this position. In line with this observation, some professionals, therefore, have
questioned whether punishment was justified. Additional criticisms were that punishment procedures, particularly those that required physical intervention, could be
subject to misapplication and had poor acceptability by practitioners and the lay
public. And lastly, the research supporting punishment as effective behavioral intervention mostly was conducted during brief-duration studies with little attention
paid to long-term (maintenance) outcomes. The other side of the argument is that to
date, only limited research has identified alternative treatments. It should be noted
that the topic of punishment in applied behavior analysis is complex and each of the
issues raised in this cursory discussion have been handled with greater depth elsewhere (Lerman & Vorndran, 2002).

Keeping with this historical perspective, the early 1980s set the tone for "second generation" behavioral intervention. Many developments and influences have to be
considered at this juncture and although it is beyond the scope of this chapter, several
of them are presented briefly. First, the emergence of functional behavioral assessment can be linked to the evaluation methodology described by Iwata, Dorsey, Slifer,
Bauman, and Richman (1982). This approach featured analog assessment in which
purported consequence influences on challenging behaviors were manipulated systematically to isolate source of control over responding and in turn, direct
intervention formulation. The methodology designed by Iwata et al. (1982) was intended to serve as an experimental format for conducting the most rigorous
evaluations. However, indirect and descriptive methods of functional behavioral
assessment subsequently appeared such as the *Motivation Assessment Scale* (Durand
& Crimmins, 1988) and the *Functional Assessment Interview* (O'Neill, Horner, Albin,
Sprague, Story, & Newton, 1997). Geared to practitioners and professionals who
may not have the resources available to conduct an experimental-analog assessment,
these and similar methods are a mainstay of current applied behavior analysis.

A second trend was increased attention toward and understanding of the biological
basis of challenging behaviors (E. G. Carr, 1977; Cataldo & Harris, 1982). Problems
such as severe and chronic self-injury, for example, were shown to be mediated by

physical "causes" (e.g., otitis media, menses, constipation), possibly overlooked when the focus of intervention was exclusively on operant influences. What emerged was a more comprehensive approach to assessment and consideration of behavioral medicine interventions for many persons with developmental disabilities (Luiselli, 1989; Russo & Varni, 1982).

Although the value of positive reinforcement procedures in behavior-reduction intervention has an early history, it wasn't until the 1980s that formal *assessment* of preferences was advocated. The research by Pace, Ivancic, Edwards, Iwata, and Page (1985), for example, demonstrated that stimulus preferences among individuals with profound mental retardation could be identified using objective measurement and that these stimuli then could be tested to verify their reinforcing properties. Additional research at the time concerned ways to enhance the effects of positive reinforcement. As a result, it was learned that positive reinforcement with children who have developmental disabilities is most effective when stimuli are varied routinely (Egel, 1981), preferences are assessed frequently (Mason, McGee, Farmer-Dougan, & Risley, 1989), and the emphasis is on "child-selected" instead of "adult-selected" reinforcer choices (Dyer, Dunlap, & Winterling, 1990).

The final "second generation" influence to be considered is the emergence of the regular education initiative (REI), mainstreaming, and inclusive education (Fuchs & Fuchs, 1994). By the decade of the 1980s, federal and state policies mandated that children who had developmental disabilities had the right to be educated among "non-disabled" peers in their local schools. This requirement meant that many students with a disability would have to have behavior support at school and that the selected interventions would have to be adapted to this context. Therefore, procedures had to be selected because they were acceptable to school personnel (i.e., they had good social validity), were not socially stigmatizing, and conformed to community norms. Furthermore, interventions should capitalize on the social learning opportunities with peers that were, after all, inherent in the school environment. The result was a greater emphasis on preventive, skill-building, and peer-mediated procedures that eventually affected the course of behavioral intervention and support in the area of developmental disabilities as a whole.

Current Intervention Philosophy and Applications

Several areas of intervention research have received recent attention from clinicians and behavior analysts. In what follows, each area is reviewed relative to philosophy and practice.

Antecedent Control. Behavioral intervention based on antecedent control can be considered a preventive therapeutic approach. Broadly defined, antecedent control has the objective of reducing and eliminating challenging behaviors by manipulating conditions and situations that precede these behaviors. Common antecedents would be features of the physical environment (e.g., lighting, groupings), activity schedules, task requirements, and instructions.

Luiselli (1998) presented several advantages of antecedent control as an intervention focus:

(1) Many challenging behaviors are *situation-specific*, meaning they are encountered under select conditions and do not occur otherwise. A teacher, for example, may seek assistance to eliminate a student's tantrum behavior observed only at the conclusion of outdoor recess. Beyond this context, the student never demonstrates a tantrum. If specificity of this type is detected, it suggests that the challenging behavior might be under restricted stimulus control and suggests a manipulation of antecedent variables as intervention.

(2) Although isolating the antecedent influences on challenging behaviors can take time, the possible benefits are notable because frequently, the result is a behavior support plan that is practical and "user friendly." Imagine a situation where an adult with mental retardation reacts negatively when he is given instructions by staff at a supported work environment. There now is sufficient evidence showing that allowing individuals who have developmental disabilities to make life-style choices can impact challenging behaviors effectively (E. G. Carr, Levin, McConnachie, Carlson, Kemp, & Smith, 1994; Sigafoos, 1998). In most cases, establishing choice-making and self-selection protocols are relatively easy to integrate within habilitation settings and do not require extensive staff training.

(3) The practicality of antecedent control intervention also is evident because it can produce permanent behavior-change. Knowing that a particular interaction or circumstance reliably sets the occasion for challenging behavior gives a strong indication that eliminating this source of control could alter responding on a long-term basis. Of course, this strategy assumes that it would be reasonable to manipulate conditions in this way

without compromising learning objectives or sacrificing important elements of a service plan.

(4) The fact that antecedent intervention has a prevention focus is noteworthy when considering individuals who present with the most serious challenging behaviors or themselves are physically resistant and imposing. As an illustration, it would be contraindicated to have staff implement a physical consequence (e.g., overcorrection, restraint) contingent on the aggressive behavior of a large and strong man. That is, rather than have staff wait for this behavior to occur so that a "negative" (and purportedly punishing) consequence can be imposed, an alternative conceptualization would be to alter the probability of its occurrence, thereby eliminating a physical encounter.

A number of antecedent control interventions have been reported in the extant literature. Kennedy and Itkonen (1993) described a 22 year old woman with mental retardation who performed challenging behaviors (arguing, grabbing objects, hitting, self-injury) at school on days she awoke late in the morning. A late wake-up meant she missed breakfast, required assistance from staff, and reacted negatively to prompting. The challenging behaviors were reduced to near-zero levels when an intervention plan was used that allowed the woman to turn off her alarm clock independently, and select a preferred breakfast and clothing if she woke up within 5 minutes of the alarm. In a second application, Kennedy and Itkonen (1993) targeted challenging behaviors (screaming, dropping to the floor, tearing clothes, hitting) of a 20 year old woman who had mental retardation, cerebral palsy, and vision impairment. These problems were encountered when she arrived at school and typically, following a prolonged transportation route along city streets where her bus had to make numerous stops. The bus travel to school was changed to a highway so that delays would be minimized and this manipulation essentially eliminated the challenging behaviors.

Eliminating the conditions that set the occasion for challenging behaviors, as in the previous example of changing a bus transportation route, may not be possible or warranted in certain situations. Similarly, arranging circumstances that can easily promote replacement behaviors sometimes is difficult. An antecedent intervention option in such cases is to identify an already existing source of positive stimulus control and then "fade" or transfer this control to more acceptable "terminal" stimuli. Zarcone, Iwata, Vollmer, Jagtiani, Smith, and Mazaleski (1993) illustrated this approach with three adults who had mental retardation and escape-motivated self-injurious behavior. Instructions from a therapist provoked high-frequency self-injury, during an initial baseline phase and an escape-extinction intervention. The self-injurious behavior of each adult decreased rapidly when instructions were initially eliminated and subsequently introduced gradually ("faded-in") at a rate of one per session if frequency of self-injury was at or less than .50 responses per minute during the previous session.

A study by Thiele, Blew and Luiselli (2001) exemplifies how several antecedent control procedures can be combined into an effective intervention "package." The participant was a 17 year old male who was blind, nonverbal, and diagnosed with severe mental retardation. He displayed intense tantrum behavior comprised of crying, screaming, jumping, and self-injury (striking head and face with hands) during his morning "wake-up" routine at a residential school. Functional behavioral assessment suggested that tantrums were attention-maintained. The resulting intervention plan included several procedures to "pre-empt" the occurrence of a tantrum: (1) a staff person initiated social contact with the student as soon as he awoke each morning and (2) only staff who were "highly preferred" by the student conducted intervention. Figure 1 shows the frequency of tantrums each day in the upstairs bedroom and downstairs living area of the community home where the student lived. These data reveal near elimination of tantrum behavior and positive effects obtained with two staff persons.

Finally, Piazza, Contrucci, Hanley, and Fisher (1997) assessed the destructive behavior (aggression, property destruction) of an 8 year old girl with mental retardation and found that it was occasioned by "direct prompts" during hygiene routines. A "direct prompt" was an instruction from a therapist in the form, "Brush your teeth," and it was combined with physical guidance that was provided contingent on noncompliance. "Nondirective prompts" (e.g., "I wonder how this toothbrush works?"), noncontingent positive reinforcement (praise and tangible items), and withdrawal of physical guidance effectively eliminated the destructive behaviors. This intervention is another example of how more than one antecedent control procedure can be formulated into a multicomponent behavior support plan.

Establishing Operations. Until recently, the concept of establishing operations (EOs) was largely neglected in formulating and implementing behavioral interventions. Michael (1993) defined an EO as "an environmental event, operation, or stimulus condition that affects an organism by momentarily altering (a) the reinforcing effectiveness of other events and (b) the frequency of occurrence of that part of the organism's repertoire to those events as consequences" (p. 192). An EO then, has two functions. First, it has a *reinforce-enhancing* function because it alters the "potency" of particular consequences that have been identified as "reinforcement." And second, it has an *evocative* function because it contemporaneously increases the frequency of behaviors that previously were reinforced. Whereas a discriminative stimulus (Sd) refers to the differential availability of reinforcement, EOs concern the *motivational* influences of stimulus events. Or as stated by Kennedy and Meyer (1998), "EOs are defined as events that alter the value of a reinforcer without altering the schedule of reinforcement or discriminative stimuli associated with reinforcer availability" (p. 331).

From a clinical perspective, the manipulation of EOs can be considered a type of antecedent control intervention. In this regard, McGill (1999) outlined how various sources of reinforcement and establishing operations might influence challenging behaviors. For challenging behaviors that are maintained by *social-positive reinforcement,* specific consequences would be attention and tangible items and the relevant establishing operation would be deprivation of attention and tangible items respectively. Challenging behaviors with *social-negative reinforcement* as a maintaining consequence, would have escape as the specific consequence and aversive interactions (e.g., presentation of instructional "demands") the relevant establishing operation. With challenging behaviors that are maintained by *automatic reinforcement,* the specific consequence would be sensory stimulation and the deprivation of stimulation the relevant establishing operation.

The schema presented by McGill (1999), including clinical implications, is demonstrated in several applied studies. O'Reilly (1995) identified escape-maintained aggression by a 31 year old man who had severe mental retardation and verified that the challenging behavior was more frequent on days when he had less than five hours of sleep the night before. In this case, sleep deprivation was an EO that affected challenging behavior that was negatively reinforced. Similar analyses have identified onset of menses (E. G. Carr & Smith, 1995), allergy symptoms (Kennedy & Meyer, 1996), and otitis media (O'Reilly, 1997) as other "biological" EOs.

In many training and instructional program with persons who have developmental disabilities, tangible items such as food and social consequences such as adult attention are used as positive reinforcement. EOs can function in many ways to increase or decrease the reinforcing effect of consequence events. In a recent study by Zhou, Iwata, and Shore (2002), nine adults with severe mental retardation participated in training sessions that included their most preferred food as positive reinforcement.

Two sessions were scheduled each day, one 30 minutes before the lunch meal (premeal) and one 30 minutes following the lunch meal (postmeal). The response rates of 4 of the 9 adults were higher during the premeal sessions and for the remaining 5 adults, there was no difference. Although these findings were not conclusive, the data suggest that for some individuals, the reinforcing efficacy of food will be strongest if it is incorporated into training activities that precede (instead of follow) daily meals. The EO in this case is a relative state of hunger.

Regarding adult attention as positive reinforcement, O'Reilly (1999) measured challenging behaviors (yelling and head hitting) of a 20 year old man with severe mental retardation during functional analysis analogue sessions. The analysis concluded that the challenging behaviors were maintained by social attention. In a second evaluation phase, the man was exposed either to high levels of attention or no attention for 1 hour immediately before the analogue sessions. Head hitting, but not yelling, was more frequent in the analogue sessions following the no-attention condition. Similar to the results of Zhou et al. (2002), a state of deprivation (absence of social attention) altered the reinforcing effect of behavior-contingent consequences.

As seen in the preceding examples, and as an outcome of related research, *noncontingent reinforcement* (NCR) has gained popularity as a method of behavior-reduction (Tucker, Sigafoos, & Bushell, 1998). NCR requires first, that the source of reinforcement for challenging behavior is identified (e.g., social attention, escape, sensory stimulation) and second, that it be presented on a fixed or variable schedule that is independent of frequency. An individual with attention-maintained challenging behavior, for example, might receive positive comments, praise, and approval from a practitioner every two minutes regardless of how many times the behavior occurs (Hagopian, Fisher, & Legacy, 1994; Mace & Lalli, 1991; Vollmer, Iwata, Zarcone, Smith, & Mazaleski, 1993). Noncontingent access to escape also has been shown to decrease challenging behaviors that are maintained by negative reinforcement (Vollmer, Marcus, & Ringdahl, 1995). And for challenging behaviors that have automatic reinforcement as the source of control, provision of noncontingent alternative stimulation can decrease responding (Kennedy & Souza, 1995; Luiselli, 1994; Piazza et al., 1998). NCR strategies are intended to reduce the motivation to perform challenging behaviors by eliminating or attenuating relative states of deprivation. Furthermore, as compared to behavior-contingent procedures such as the differential reinforcement of other behavior (DRO), NCR may be easier to implement and integrate within habilitation settings (Vollmer et al., 1993).

NCR interventions can be effective but it should be noted that not all professionals agree about terminology (Poling & Normand, 1999; Vollmer, 1999). Positive and negative reinforcement, after all, is defined operationally by its contingent presentation, and functionally by an increase in the frequency of behavior that precedes it. Strictly speaking, one cannot have *non*contingent reinforcement and NCR applications do not produce an increase in measurable behavior. With the goal of maintaining accurate terminology to unsure consistent communication among professionals, it may be more prudent to label NCR according to presentation schedule, as in *fixed time attention* and *fixed time escape*.

Behavioral Momentum. Inconsistent or poor compliance with instructions, requests, and activity demands is a common problem for many persons with developmental disabilities. Persistent noncompliance makes it difficult for sustained learning to occur, causes lengthy delays during transitions, and has been found to covary with challenging behaviors (Cataldo, Ward, Russo, Riordan, & Bennett, 1986; Russo, Cataldo, & Cushing, 1981). A number of compliance training programs have been instituted, based mainly on differential reinforcement of instruction following and physical (graduated) guidance. Unfortunately, for some individuals the contingencies maintaining noncompliance (e.g., avoidance and escape) are stronger than the reinforcement that would be available for alternative behaviors. Guidance procedures have the disadvantage of requiring physical contact that generally, is contraindicated with persons who are extremely uncooperative, forceful, and combative.

Behavioral momentum intervention for noncompliance was introduced by Mace, et al. (1988) in a series of studies with adult men who had moderate to severe mental retardation. As defined by these researchers, "Behavioral momentum refers to the tendency for behavior to persist following a change in environmental conditions-the greater the rate of reinforcement, the greater the behavioral momentum" (p. 123). Using one of the studies to illustrate the application of behavioral momentum, a 36 year old man with severe mental retardation had a low probability of complying with instructions such as "Please put your lunch box away" ("do" commands) and "Please don't leave your lunch box on the table' ("don't" commands). Instructions the man complied with consistently ("high probability") were selected and presented to him sequentially, ending with a "low probability" request. For example, a "high probability" instructional sequence might be: "Give me five" ("high probability")— "Show me your pipe" ("high probability")—"Shake my hand" ("high probability")—"Please put your lunch box away" ("low probability"). The results of

Mace et al. (1988) were that the presentation of a sequence of "high probability" instructions preceding a "low probability' task request either increased compliance or reduce compliance latency and task duration.

Numerous replications and extentions of behavioral momentum as intervention for noncompliance have been reported with children and adults (Duchame & Worling, 1994; Houlihan, Jacobson, & Brandon, 1994; Mace & Belfiore, 1990; Zarcone, Iwata, Mazaleski, & Smith, 1994). There are different interpretations of behavioral momentum, some proposed cogently from an EO perspective (see McGill, 1999), but certainly this strategy has much to offer. One advantage is that it serves as an intervention strategy that is geared specifically to the reduction of noncompliance. Even with persons who are oppositional, they usually will respond compliantly to a subset of instructions that can form a "high probability" instructional sequence. Overtime, it is possible to reduce the number of "high probability' instructions that precede the "low probability" request, making it easier to implement behavioral momentum and possibly, transfer stimulus control from the "high probability" sequence to "low probability" instructions (Ardoin, Martens, & Wolfe, 1999). Further research is warranted to investigate critical parameters associated with behavioral momentum, its effect on challenging behaviors associated with noncompliance, and procedural variations that can be adapted to different habilation settings. Unfortunately, these methods have been used far too infrequently in practice.

Positive Behavior Support. Positive behavior support (PBS) is less a specific strategy than a philosophical stance toward intervention with people who have developmental disabilities. Sugai, Horner, Dunlap et al. (2000) posit that, "PBS is a general term that refers to the application of positive behavioral interventions and systems to achieve socially important behavior change" (p. 133). PBS has its roots in the previously cited "movement" stressing nonaversive treatment (Horner et al., 1990). It bears emphasis, however, that PBS is not a new theory of behavior or a departure from applied behavior analysis but instead, "an application of a behaviorally based systems approach to enhance the capacity of schools, families, and communities to design effective environments that improve the fit or link between research-validated practices and the environments in which teaching and learning occur" (Sugai et al., 2000, p. 133). PBS, in fact, has the theoretical and methodological underpinnings of applied behavior analysis but as qualified by Hieneman and Dunlap (2000), "has expanded its parent discipline to incorporate increased focus on ecological validity (i.e., a commitment to implementation in natural contexts) and accountability defined in terms of meaningful, socially valid outcomes" (p. 161).

The integral features of PSB are (1) functional behavioral assessment, (2) context-derived intervention plans, (3) outcome-focused assessment, and (4) social validity (satisfaction and acceptability) as a measure of efficacy. The critical role of functional behavioral assessment, of course, is to ensure that intervention is matched to controlling influences that both predict and maintain challenging behaviors. Intervention procedures should "fit" the context in which they occur by being practical, normalized, and culturally sensitive. In addition to measuring the direct effect of intervention on primary challenging behaviors, PBS also targets skill acquisition and lifestyle changes that are meaningful, comprehensive, and durable. A systems perspective requires that these outcomes extend across multiple environments that include home, school and community. The skills, values, and endorsements of "stakeholders," or the people who implement intervention, is another important consideration distinguishing PSB.

Proponents of PBS advocate that intervention be conducted in the natural or "real world" settings inhabited by people who have developmental disabilities. Frequently, applied behavior analysis intervention research is performed under the most controlled conditions, by seasoned professionals, in contexts that are contrived, artificial, and simulated. This situation obviously has implications for the generalization and transfer of intervention methods and effects.

The issue of community-referenced PBS has been examined in several ways. Hieneman and Dunlap (2000) surveyed family members, direct service providers, and trainers/consultants to derive factors governing the success of community intervention for children with developmental disabilities. In addition to basic elements such as the characteristics of the children being served, aspects of the challenging behaviors (e.g., history, frequency, intensity), and components of the behavior support plan, the stakeholders endorsed other (possibly overlooked) factors: (1) integrity of plan implementation, (2) organization of the physical environment, (3) "buy in" with the intervention, (4) capacity of care providers, (5) relationship with the children, (6) collaboration among change-agents, (7) intervention philosophy, and (8) community acceptance. Apropos to these findings, it is apparent that at least in the opinion of the people charged with behavioral intervention, success is interpreted from a broad range of interrelated factors.

Kincaid, Knoster, Harrower, Shannon, and Bustamante (2002) measured the impact of PBS with people who had developmental disabilities (preschool age through adulthood) by soliciting behavior and quality of life indicators from parents, teachers, administrators, specialists, and direct/respite care staff from 3 states. Approximately 82% of respondents verified that challenging behaviors were less frequent following training in PBS intervention. The vast majority reported that "the PBS approach was efficient in terms of effectiveness, comfort, consistency of implementation, and interference" (p. 114). Modest improvements were documented for the quality of life measures that encompassed interpersonal relationships, self-determination, social inclusion, personal wellbeing, and emotional health. Although preliminary, these results suggest that PBS models can affect behavior change on multiple levels, as per the subjective ratings and impressions of stakeholders. Future research should include direct-observation measurement, as well as other information-gathering techniques, to yield the most comprehensive and valid assessment of PBS.

Concerning the efficacy of PBS, E. G. Carr, Horner, Turnbull et al. (1999) reviewed pertinent articles published during the period 1985-1996 and reported several principal findings. It was concluded that PBS is a meaningful intervention approach with people who have developmental disabilities and challenging behaviors. PBS was effective in one-half to two-thirds of cases, with increased favorable outcome when intervention was designed from functional behavioral assessment. Results improved further when behavior support was assumed by "typical" change-agents. At the time this review was completed, PBS suffered from infrequent documentation of quality of life indices, long-term maintenance, and the degree of assistance necessary for direct-care providers.

Summary and Conclusions

In a review of intervention research practices published 7 years ago, Scotti, Ujcich, Weigle, Holland, and Kirk (1996) wrote:

> "The time is well past for the behavioral intervention literature to merely focus on demonstrating the effects on circumscribed target behaviors of certain procedures implemented in carefully controlled (and often segregated) settings. Broader effects must not only be assessed, but actively sought. These include not only assessing the effects of intervention on collateral behaviors, but determining changes in lifestyle and quality of life that occur as a result of intervention (e.g., level of independence, choice making, living in typical homes in the community, meaningful employment and social roles, friendships and social networks). Furthermore, enhancing lifestyle

and quality of life should be a crucial intervention component, rather
than simply an outcome of target behavior reduction." (p. 133).

How to respond to these assertions? On one hand, an ever increasing percentage of people with developmental disabilities receive education and habilitative care in community settings, be it public schools, supported employment, or residential living. As discussed in this chapter, delivering intervention in natural environments demands that behavior supports be adapted accordingly: they should enhance skill development, be as robust (multimethod) as possible, appeal to the practitioners who implement them, reflect "positive programming," and have an effect long-term. Hopefully, the selection of intervention approaches reviewed earlier attest to the need for "goodness of fit" when prescribing behavior-reduction procedures for people with developmental disabilities in the settings where they go to school, work, live, and recreate.

The convictions voiced by Scotti et al. (1996) were consistent with new directions in behavioral intervention emerging at the time and subsequently, endorsed by other professionals (E. G. Carr, 1997; Horner, 2000). To a large extent, the evolution of applied behavior analysis conceptualization and implementation relates principally to the doctrine of PBS. For some, the concern is whether PBS is substantively different from applied behavior analysis, is subsumed by it, or simply is another label adopted by some professionals. In a persuasive article, J. E. Carr and Sidener (2002) verified a pronounced increase in journal publications on PBS between 1989-2002. They also examined 8 key characteristics of PBS (person-centered planning, functional assessment, positive strategies, multicomponent intervention, environmental focus, meaningful outcomes, ecological validity, systems-level emphasis) and compared them to the defining characteristics of applied behavior analysis. They concluded, "conceptualizing PBS apart from applied behavior analysis is unsupported by the evidence" (p. 249). The proposed alternative offered by J. E. Carr and Sidener (2002) was that PBS is a model of service delivery within the broader discipline of applied behavior analysis. The "take home" point here is that despite consensus among many professionals, the present status of behavior support and intervention in developmental disabilities reflects diverse theory and practice, an ever growing sophistication, and a breadth of knowledge that continues to expand.

The advantages of assessment-derived, positively oriented, prevention-directed, and multicomponent intervention notwithstanding, there are many areas that require intensified scrutiny and research attention:

(1) There is a need to conduct maintenance evaluations of behavior support that extend months and years beyond the initial phases of intervention. Consider the admonition of Baer, Wolf, and Risley (1968) that effects of intervention which do not endure over time should not be considered effective. More recently, Kennedy (2002) advised that the extended maintenance of behavior-change methods by practitioners be viewed as a criterion for social validity. That is, procedures and arrangements that are acceptable are the ones which will be implemented with integrity and sustained long-term. The requirement, it seems, is to study how maintenance can be facilitated and to have post-intervention evaluation an expectation for journal publication.

(2) Although notable examples have occurred (E. G. Carr & Carlson, 1993), there are too few studies that have incorporated rigorous experimental designs to evaluate multicomponent interventions applied in community settings. Conducting sophisticated research outside the most controlled environments can be an arduous task but is necessary to advance clinical practice and inform professionals. Some of this research may require adjustments to traditional applied behavior analysis experimental methodology (Hersen & Barlow, 1984) or novel data-based evaluation strategies.

(3) The dominant dependent measure reported in intervention research has been the frequency of challenging behaviors. Behavior reduction should be a primary consideration but taken in isolation, is insufficient to judge efficacy. We should expect instead that a more valid appraisal of the strength of behavior support would be evidence of concomitant acquisition of functional skills, increased learning opportunities, broadened exposure to social networks, and enhanced emotional satisfaction.

(4) Practitioners would benefit from more research about effective intervention for the *most serious* challenging behaviors (Foxx, 2003). Alluding to a point made earlier, individuals who present with extreme and treatment-resistant problems are those most likely to receive restrictive intervention, usually within inpatient settings. However, as presented by Bird and Luiselli (2000), people with developmental disabilities who have "at risk" challenging behaviors and protracted histories of invasive treatment can sometimes be supported at the community level in response to a "lifestyle" management orientation that addresses environmental, skill building, positive reinforcement, personal choice-making, and quality of life domains. Unfortunately, poorly regulated pharmacological management (or "chemical restraint") is the most frequent outcome for these individuals, and lack or staff and adequate staff training are often the problem.

In summary, more than 4 decades of research have been devoted to behavior support and intervention in developmental disabilities. The contributions of applied behavior analysis have been extensive, producing many innovative methods, which have been replicated, refined, and disseminated. This chapter had the purpose of highlighting the current status of behavior support and intervention by looking at historical roots, influential trends, specific procedures, and philosophies. It can be concluded that principles of applied behavior analysis remain the foundation of contemporary behavioral intervention. Of significance is the adoption of systems-wide models of behavior support, which are geared toward "real world" settings, and implemented by relevant stakeholders. In many ways, we are at yet another "generation" of intervention research and practice, one that promises further advances in comprehensive, ethical, and socially relevant behavior support of people with developmental disabilities.

References

Ardoin, S. P., Martens, B. K., & Wolfe, L. A. (1999). Using high-probability instruction sequences with fading to increase student compliance during transitions. *Journal of Applied Behavior Analysis, 32,* 339-351.

Ayllon, T., & Azrin, N. H. (1968). *The token economy: A motivational system for therapy and ehabilitation.* New York: Appleton-Century-Crofts.

Baer, D. M., Wolf, M. M., & Risley, T. R. (1968). Some current dimensions of applied behavior analysis. *Journal of Applied Behavior Analysis, 1,* 91-97.

Bird, F. L., & Luiselli, J. K. (2000). Positive behavioral support of adults with developmental disabilities: Assessment of long-term adjustment and habilitation following restrictive treatment histories. *Journal of Behavior Therapy and Experimental Psychiatry, 31,* 5-19.

Carr, E. G. (1977). The motivation of self-injurious behavior: A review of some hypotheses. *Psychological Bulletin, 84,* 800-816.

Carr, E. G. (1997). The evolution of applied behavior analysis into positive behavior support. *Journal of The Association for Persons with Severe Handicaps, 22,* 208-209.

Carr, E. G., & Carlson, J. I. (1993). Reduction of severe problem behaviors in the community using a multicomponent treatment approach. *Journal of Applied Behavior Analysis, 26,* 157-172.

Carr, E. G., Horner, R. H., Turnbull, A. P., Marquis, J. G., Magito-McLaughlin, D., & McAltee, M. L. (1999). *Positive behavior support as an approach for dealing with problem behavior in people with developmental disabilities: A research synthesis.* Washington, DC: American Association on Mental Retardation.

Carr, E. G., Levin, L., McConnachie, G., Carlson, J. I., Kemp, D. C., & Smith, C. E. (1994). *Communication-based intervention for problem behavior: A user's guide for producing positive change.* Baltimore, MD: Paul H. Brookes Publishing.

Carr, E. G., & Smith, C. E. (1995). Biological setting events for self-injury. *Mental Retardation and Developmental Disabilities Research Reviews, 1,* 94-98.

Carr, J. E., & Sidener, T. M. (2002). On the relation between applied behavior analysis and positive behavior support. *The Behavior Analyst, 25,* 245-253.

Cataldo, M. F., & Harris, J. C. (1982). The biological basis for self-injury in the mentally retarded. *Analysis and Intervention in Developmental Disabilities, 2,* 21-39.

Cataldo, M. F., Ward, E. M., Russo, D. C., Riordan, M., & Bennett, D. (1986). Compliance and correlated problem behavior in children: Effects of contingent and noncontingent reinforcement. *Analysis and Intervention in Developmental Disabilities, 6,* 265-282.

Ducharme, J. M., & Worling, D. E. (1994). Behavioral momentum and stimulus fading in the acquisition and maintenance of child compliance in the home. *Journal of Applied Behavior Analysis, 27,* 639-647.

Durand, V. M., & Crimmins, D. B. (1988). Identifying the variables maintaining self-injurious behavior. *Journal of Autism and Developmental Disorders, 18,* 99-117.

Dyer, K, Dunlap, G., & Winterling, V. (1990). Effects of choice making on the serious problem behaviors of students with severe handicaps. *Journal of Applied Behavior Analysis, 23,* 515-524.

Egel, A. L. (1981). Reinforcer variation: Implications for motivating developmentally disabled children. *Journal of Applied Behavior Analysis, 14,* 345-350.

Forehand, R., & Baumeister, A. A. (1976). Deceleration of aberrant behavior among retarded individuals. In M. Hersen, R. M. Eisler, & P. M. Miller (Eds.), *Progress in behavior modification-volume 2* (pp. 223-278). New York: Academic Press.

Foxx, R. M. (2003). The treatment of dangerous behavior. *Behavioral Interventions, 18,* 1-21.

Fuchs, D., & Fuchs, L. S. (1994). Inclusive schools movement and the radicalization of special education reform. *Exceptional Children, 60,* 294-309.

Hagopian, L. P., Fisher, W. W., & Legacy, S. M. (1994). Schedule effects of noncontingent reinforcement on attention-maintained destructive behavior of identical quadruplets. *Journal of Applied Behavior Analysis, 27,* 317-325.

Hersen, M., & Barlow, D. H. (1984). *Single case experimental designs: Strategies for studying behavior change.* New York: Pergamon.

Hieneman, M., & Dunlap, G. (2000). Factors affecting the outcomes of community-based behavioral support: I. Identification and description of factor categories. *Journal of Positive Behavior Interventions, 2,* 161-169.

Horner, R. H. (2000). Positive behavior support. *Focus on Autism and Other Developmental Disabilities, 15,* 97-105.

Horner, R. H., Dunlap, G., Koegel, R. L., Carr, E. G., Sailor, W., Anderson, J., et al. (1990). Toward a technology of nonaversive behavioral support. *Journal of Thee Association for Persons with Severe Handicaps, 15,* 125-132.

Houlihan, D., Jacobson, L., & Brandon, P. K. (1994). Replication of high-probability request sequence with varied interprompt times in a preschool setting. *Journal of Applied Behavior Analysis, 27,* 737-738.

Iwata, B. A., Dorsey, M. F., Slifer, K. J., Bauman, K. E., & Richman, G. S. (1982). Toward a functional analysis of self-injury. *Analysis and Intervention in Developmental Disabilities, 2,* 1-20.

Kennedy, C. H. (2002). The maintenance of behavior change as an indicator of social validity. *Behavior Modification, 26,* 594-604.

Kennedy, C. H., & Itkonen, T. (1993). Effects of setting events on the problem behaviors of students with severe disabilities. *Journal of Applied Behavior Analysis, 26,* 321-327.

Kennedy, C. H., & Meyer, K. A. (1996). Sleep deprivation, allergy symptoms, and negatively reinforced behavior. *Journal of Applied Behavior Analysis, 29,* 133-135.

Kennedy, C. H., & Meyer, K. A. (1998). Establishing operations and the motivation of challenging behavior. In J. K. Luiselli & M. J. Cameron (Eds.), *Antecedent control: Innovative approaches to behavior support* (pp. 329-346). Baltimore, MD: Paul H. Brookes Publishing.

Kennedy, C. H., & Souza, G. (1995). Functional analysis and treatment of eye poking. *Journal of Applied Behavior Analysis, 28,* 27-37.

Kincaid, D., Knoster, T., Harrower, J. K., Shannon, P., & Bustamante, S. (2002). Measuring the impact of positive behavior support. *Journal of Positive Behavior Interventions, 4,* 109-117.

Lerman, D. C., & Vorndran, C. M. (2002). On the status of knowledge for using punishment: Implications for treating behavior disorders. *Journal of Applied Behavior Analysis, 35,* 431-464.

Lovaas, Frietag, Gold, & Kassorla, I. C. (1965). Experimental studies in childhood schizophrenia: Analysis of self-destructive behavior. *Journal of Experimental Child Psychology, 2,* 67-84.

Lovaas, O. I., Schaeffer, B., & Simmons, J. Q. (1965). Building social behavior in autistic children by use of electric shock. *Journal of Experimental Research in Personality, 1,* 99-109.

Luiselli J. K. (1989) (Ed.). *Behavioral medicine and developmental disabilities.* New York: Springer-Verlag.

Luiselli, J. K. (1994). Effects of contingent and noncontingent reinforcement on stereotypic behaviors in a child with posttraumatic neurological impairment. *Journal of Behavior Therapy & Experimental Psychiatry, 25,* 325-330.

Luiselli, J. K. (1998). Intervention conceptualization and formulation. In J. K. Luiselli & M. J. Cameron (Eds.), *Antecedent control: Innovative approaches to behavior support* (pp. 29-44). Baltimore, MD: Paul H. Brookes Publishing.

Mace, F. C., & Belfiore, P. (1990). Behavioral momentum in the treatment of escape-motivated stereotypy. *Journal of Applied Behavior Analysis, 23,* 507-514.

Mace, F. C., Hock, M. L., Lalli, J. S., West, B. J., Belfiore, P., Pinter, E., et al. (1988). Behavioral momentum in the treatment of noncompliance. *Journal of Applied Behavior Analysis, 21,* 123-141.

Mace, F. C., & Lalli, J. S. (1991). Linking descriptive and experimental analyses in the treatment of bizarre speech. *Journal of Applied Behavior Analysis, 24,* 553-562.

Mason, S. A., Mcgee, G. G., Farmer-Dougan, V., & Risley, T. R. (1989). A practical strategy for ongoing reinforcer assessment. *Journal of Applied Behavior Analysis, 22,* 171-179.

McGill, P. (1999). Establishing operations: Implications for the assessment, treatment, and prevention of problem behavior. *Journal of Applied Behavior Analysis, 32,* 393-418.

Michael, J. L. (1993). Establishing operations. *The Behavior Analyst, 16,* 191-206.

O'Neill, R. E., Horner, R. H., Albin, R. W., Sprague, J. R., Storey, K., & Newton, J. S. (1997). *Functional assessment and program development for problem behavior: A practical handbook.* Pacific Grove, CA: Brookes/Cole.

O'Reilly, M. F. (1995). Functional analysis and treatment of escape-maintained aggression correlated with sleep deprivation. *Journal of Applied Behavior Analysis, 28,* 225-226.

O'Reilly, M. F. (1997). Functional analysis of episodic self-injury correlated with recurrent otitis media. *Journal of Applied Behavior Analysis, 30,* 165-167.

O'Reilly, M. F. (1999). Effects of pre-session attention on the frequency of attention-maintained behavior. *Journal of Applied Behavior Analysis, 32,* 371-374.

Pace, G. M., Ivancic, M. T., Edwards, G. L., Iwata, B. A., & Page, T. J. (1985). Assessment of stimulus preference and reinforcer value with profoundly retarded individuals. *Journal of Applied Behavior Analysis, 18,* 249-255.

Pelios, L., Morren, J., Tesch, D., & Axelrod, S. (1999). The impact of functional analysis methodology on treatment choice for self-injurious and aggressive behavior. *Journal of Applied Behavior Analysis, 32,* 185-195.

Piazza, C. C., Contrucci, S. A., Halney, G. P., & Fisher, W. W. (1997). Non-directive prompting and noncontingent reinforcement in the treatment of destructive behavior during hygiene routines. *Journal of Applied Behavior Analysis, 30,* 705-708.

Piazza, C. C., Fisher, W. W., Hanley, G. P., LeBlanc, L. A., Worsdell, A. S., Lindauer, S. E., & Keeney, K. M. (1998). Treatment of pica through multiple analysis of its reinforcing functions. *Journal of Applied Behavior Analysis, 31,* 165-189.

Poling, A., & Normand, M. (1999). Noncontingent reinforcement: An inappropriate description of time-based schedules that reduce behavior. *Journal of Applied Behavior Analysis, 32,* 237-238.

Repp, A. C., & Singh, N. N. (1990). *Perspectives on the use of nonaversivee and aversive interventions for persons with developmental disabilities.* Sycamore, IL: Sycamore Publishing.

Russo, D. C., Cataldo, M. F., & Cushing, P. J. (1981). Compliance training and behavioral covariation in the treatment of multiple behavior problems. *Journal of Applied Behavior Analysis, 14,* 209-222.

Russo, D. C., & Varni, J. W. (1982). *Behavioral pediatrics: Research and practice.* New York: Plenum.

Scotti, J. R., Ujcich, K. J., Weigle, K. L., Holland, C. M., & Kirk, K. S. (1996). Interventions with challenging behavior of persons with developmental disabilities: A review of current research practices. *Journal of The Association for Persons with Severe Handicaps, 21,* 123-134.

Sigafoos, J. (1998). Choice making and personal selection strategies. In J. K. Luiselli & M. J. Cameron (Eds.), *Antecedent control: Innovative approaches to behavior support* (pp. 187-221). Baltimore, MD: Paul H. Brookes Publishing.

Sugai, G., Horner, R. H., Dunlap, G., Hieneman, M., Lewis, T. J., Nelson, et al. (2000). Applying positive behavior support and functional behavioral assessment in schools. *Journal of Positive Behavior Interventions, 2,* 131-143.

Thiele, T., Blew, P., & Luiselli, J. K. (2001). Antecedent control of slee-awakening disruption. *Research in Developmental Disabilities, 22,* 399-406.

Tucker, M., Sigafoos, J., & Bushell, H. (1998). Use of noncontingent reinforcement in the treatment of challenging behavior: A review and clinical guide. *Behavior Modification, 22,* 529-547.

Vollmer, T. R. (1999). Noncontingent reinforcement: Some additional comments. *Journal of Applied Behavior Analysis, 32,* 239-240.

Vollmer, T. R., Iwata, B. A., Zarcone, J. R., Smith, R. G., & Mazaleski, J. L. (1993). The role of attention in the treatment of attention-maintained self-injurious behavior: Noncontingent reinforcement and differential reinforcement of other behavior. *Journal of Applied Behavior Analysis, 26,* 9-21.

Vollmer, T. R., Marcus, B., & Ringdahl, J. (1995). Noncontingent escape as treatment for self-injurious behavior maintained by negative reinforcement. *Journal of Applied Behavior nalysis, 28,* 15-26.

Zarcone, J. R., Iwata, B. A., Vollmer, T. A., Jagtiani, S., Smith, R. G., & Mazaleski, J. L. (1993). Extinction of self-injurious escape behavior with and without instructional fading. *Journal of Applied Behavior Analysis, 26,* 353-360.

Zarcone, J. R., Iwata, B. A., Mazaleski, J. L., & Smith, R. G. (1994). Momentum and extinction effects on self-injurious escape behavior and noncompliance. *Journal of Applied Behavior Analysis, 27,* 649-658

Zhou, L., Iwata, B. A., & Shore, B. A. (2002). Reinforcing efficacy of food on performance during pre- and post-meal sessions. *Journal of Applied Behavior Analysis, 35,* 411-414.

Figure 1.
Frequency of tantrums displayed by a 17 year old with severe mental retardation.
Intervention was implemented during his wake-up routine at a residential school. From:
Thiele, T., Blew, P., & Luiselli, J. K. (2001). Antecedent control of sleep-awakening disruption.
Research in Developmental Disabilities, 22, 399-406.

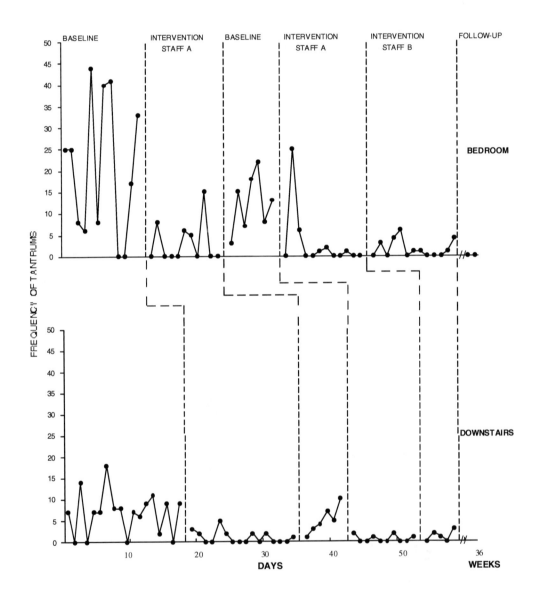

3

MODELS OF SERVICE PROVISION

Jay W. Bamburg, Ph.D., Brandi B. Smiroldo, Ph.D.,
and Stephen J. Anderson, Ph.D.
Hammond Developmental Center

As in most fields of study and service, delivery of psychological and behavioral healthcare has evolved over time. Current research and practice in this area has changed dramatically since the early days of psychological treatment and reflects advances in both science and human understanding. In previous times, some groups of people routinely received either inferior or limited services, or no services at all, based on prevailing social and cultural values (Gearhart & Litton, 1975; Blatt & Kaplan, 1966; Kanner, 1964). One such group is people with developmental disabilities, particularly those with more global difficulties, or mental retardation.

This chapter reviews models of service provision from three perspectives. First, we will revisit historical models of service provision to put recent advancements in perspective. Second, we will review how such advancements have resulted in the current model and address strengths and weaknesses of current options. Finally, we will describe how both continued advancements and development in noted areas as well as the authors' experiences might shape future service provision for individuals with developmental disabilities.

Where We Started

The Age of Institutionalization

Prior to the mid nineteenth century, individuals with developmental disabilities were typically cared for in home settings with no additional services and supports provided formally by public or private agencies. Between roughly 1840 and 1860, small facilities came into existence, focusing on developing basic training in work and functional life skills (Scheerenberger, 1983). These small centers sprang up in the U.S. and western Europe in numerous locations and demonstrated significant progress in teaching persons with mental retardation. These early successes were met with an increasing momentum to help many other persons with comparable disabilities. State colonies or homes were established, but the demand for services far outpaced the capacity of the service delivery system. Soon after 1860, states began building institutional settings, which expanded and flourished until roughly the middle twentieth century (Scheerenberger, 1983).

There was ample support for institutions at this time, for several reasons. First, few people had expertise in meeting the needs of persons with mental retardation. Available knowledge fell primarily under the rubric of medicine. Administrators of facilities were typically physicians, and their influence was reflected in not only diagnostics and treatment, but also composition of early professional organizations. Second, economic realities of the late nineteenth and early twentieth century made it difficult for families to support a person with mental retardation. Many persons with mental retardation were not thought to be able to contribute to their own care in a substantive way. Third, a combination of unfamiliarity and popular misconceptions, perpetrated through inaccurate publications, led to a social stigma associated with mental retardation. Fourth, most medical professionals encouraged families to send family members with disabilities to institutions, genuinely believing that this was their best opportunity for help or care. Fifth, advances in medical technology resulted in more individuals with significant disabilities surviving birth and living longer lives. Finally, community misperceptions of the time centered around the idea that these individuals were "deviant" and best kept away from the mainstream of society.

The institutions (i.e., state colonies, state schools, developmental centers) were large and understaffed with regard to both direct support professionals and professional staff (Blatt & Kaplan, 1966). Professional staff comprised mostly physicians or other medical care. Other professionals with expertise in learning-based approaches were neither involved nor available at this time. Institutions were typically located away from population centers, with agricultural endeavors consuming much of the individuals' daily time and energy.

Prior to 1960, service provision within institutions for individuals with developmental disabilities centered on a custodial care model (Scheerenberger, 1983). Those who could be trained worked in primarily agricultural efforts to help provide for their own support. Yet, training techniques were unsophisticated and limited in scope. Training was often by rote, and teaching strategies for persons with moderate to profound disabilities were limited at best. The institutional model reflected the limited knowledge and understanding of its time: it emphasized meeting people's basic needs such as clothing, food, health and safety but went no farther. Though such basic care is necessary to attaining good outcomes and quality of life, it is certainly not sufficient to achieve them. Treatment provided within such settings was rudimentary and focused on current medical thinking (Scheerenberger, 1983). Behavioral challenges were addressed through such arcane techniques as "insulin shock therapy," (a procedure involving rolling a person up in a wet sheet and injecting them with enough insulin to induce a diabetic coma) or "fever therapy" (artificially inducing a fever by putting people in steam cabinets or hot baths, to alleviate presumed syphilis-based 'madness'). By comparison, the development of pharmacologic agents, beginning with chlorpromazine (Thorazine™) in the mid 1950s, was greeted as a welcome and humanitarian treatment. Neuroleptic medications resulted in many individuals being sedated to remain calm and cooperative.

The state of service provision within institutional (congregate living) settings did not develop on its own. On the contrary, treatment and living conditions in institutional settings reflected prevailing social views of individuals with developmental disabilities, as well as the crudeness of treatment and service options at that time (Whitman, Scibak, & Reid, 1983). As societal views changed and science and clinical practice improved, so did conditions in institutional settings. Conditions in other settings at this time in history are generally not discussed because families generally had no other options for assistance in supporting people with disabilities.

The 1960s brought revolutionary developments to the field of developmental disabilities. Advancing behavioral technology resulted in recognition on the part of some professionals that individuals with developmental disabilities could in fact learn and acquire meaningful skills which could positively impact their life choices (Azrin & Foxx, 1971; Bensberg, Colwell, & Cassel, 1965). These techniques were initially used primarily with persons with mild to moderate levels of mental retardation. (Further development was required to adapt comparable teaching strategies for persons with severe disabilities.) As behavioral technology progressed, the focus of service provision shifted from custodial care to habilitation and skills training. Subsequent advances in behavioral technology had two significant effects: First, learning-based approaches were shown to lead to positive outcomes. Second, such progress in learning led to increasing awareness that people with disabilities were in fact people first. These advances not only resulted in dramatic change in institutions, but also heralded the beginning of the end of the age of institutions. Social and political factors were also changing during this time; these changes provided an impetus for further technological, clinical, and scientific advances (Scheerenberger, 1983). The following section discusses these issues in more detail.

The Evolution of Service Provision Models

Clinical/Scientific Factors

The field of mental retardation has impacted advancements in the psychology field in general. Such advancements have likewise resulted in changes in the focus and effectiveness of service provision for individuals with mental retardation.

The earliest child clinics and psychology journals focused mostly on service provision and treatment for persons with mental retardation (Scheerenberger, 1983). These early efforts provided the impetus for other clinics and journals to address children's needs, including those with disabilities. To date, numerous journals exist that are either tailored specifically to issues in supporting individuals with developmental disabilities or have a large percentage of research devoted to the topics. Examples include *Research in Developmental Disabilities, Mental Retardation, The American Journal on Mental Retardation, Journal of Intellectual Disability Research, Journal on Autism and Developmental Disabilities, Journal of Positive Behavioral Interventions,* and *Behavior Modification.* Additionally, national organizations have formed to improve services for individuals with developmental disabilities. The American Association on Mental Retardation and the National Association on Dual Diagnosis (Mental Health/Mental Retardation) are both organizations whose target audience is individuals with developmental disabilities, their families/supporters, and professionals who provide services for these individuals. The Association for Applied Behavior Analysis and the Association on Positive Behavioral Support are in large part dedicated to research and technology that improves services for this group of individuals.

Interfacing with the advancements in clinics and journals is the Behavior Analysis movement. The Behavior Analysis movement has resulted in several advancements and contributions to the field of psychology in general and the area of mental retardation in particular. Skinner's operant research marked the beginnings of a scientific focus on the analysis of individual behavior (Kratochwill & Bijou, 1987; Matson &

Coe, 1992). The tools of traditional psychological practice were of only limited benefit in addressing the needs of persons with developmental disabilities; thus, habilitation and treatment services for individuals with developmental disabilities was greatly enhanced by the work of Skinner and those who followed (Manikam, 1989). Insight-oriented methodologies gave way to skill acquisition protocols as practitioners began to appreciate the distinction between performance deficits and skill deficits. Successful methods were developed to improve areas such as daily living activities, socialization and interaction with others, and community/survival skills. These methods significantly enhanced the independence of the individuals being served (Azrin & Amrstrong, 1973; Azrin & Foxx, 1971; Bensberg et al., 1965).

All scientific advancements occur within and are shaped by the larger social context of the times. Thus, professionals must constantly strive to improve service options in innovative ways that mirror the values of the larger community. A number of social and political factors shape services for people with developmental disabilities. We next address issues that have been particularly influential in this area.

Social and Political Factors

The social reform movement called to attention the plight of people in institutions. Efforts to enact more just laws to support the needs of persons with mental retardation resulted in heightened awareness and a shift from arcane to more humanitarian efforts. While public consciousness was raised, improvements in day to day life for persons with mental retardation would not take place until some years later.

The 1930s saw the advent of the advocacy movement for individuals with developmental disabilities (Fiedler & Antonak, 1991; Scheerenberger, 1983). Its infancy was marked by a small movement facilitated mostly by families of individuals with developmental disabilities. The movement progressed so that by the 1950s a nationwide organization, the Association for Retarded Citizens (ARC), was formed. Numerous societal factors converged to create an environment that supported the organization of the ARC. These included a lack of community services, bad institutional conditions, the gaining of the platform at the White House Conference on Children and Youth and the potential for getting federal money for programs (Fiedler & Antonak, 1991). The ARC is based in family support and information sharing. The organization has had a significant impact on the legal and political landscape regarding individuals with developmental disabilities (Fiedler & Antonak, 1991; Scheerenberger, 1983). Following the success of the ARC, various other organizations and support groups have formed to advocate for individuals with developmental disabilities. The advocacy movement continues today with a greater emphasis on self-advocacy and self-determination. At present, most states have protection and advocacy groups/boards that provide aid and legal support to individuals with developmental disabilities. The advocacy movement has expanded also in its recruitment of non-family members into its fold which supports the integration of individuals with developmental disabilities into the larger community.

As a natural offshoot of advocacy the normalization movement made its first impact in the United States in the late 1960s and early 1970s (Nirje, 1969; Wolfensberger, 1980). Normalization proposed and enumerated an ideology of supporting individuals with mental retardation. The movement advocated for both an ideology and a process of both developing capacity and improving individuals' functioning in community settings. The normalization movement advocated moving persons with mental retardation into communities. Initial efforts focused on individuals who have more skills and fewer noted difficulties (typically those functioning within the milder ranges of mental retardation). The movement sought to remove restrictions on persons with mental retardation by eliminating institutional placement.

The mainstreaming movement extended normalization into the classroom and significantly impacted service delivery for persons with developmental disabilities within the school setting. Dunn (1968) questioned the justifiability of self-contained classes for "educable mentally retarded pupils," there was an accelerating movement to avoid placing handicapped learners in self-contained classes. The most idealized definition of mainstreaming involved the temporal, instructional, and social integration of children with developmental disabilities with other peers, based on an ongoing, individually determined, educational planning and programming process. The process called for clarification of responsibility among regular and special education administrative, instructional, and supportive personnel. The movement involves more than simple placement of persons with developmental disabilities in regular education programs; it also involves the development of an instructional plan that serves not only to identify academic needs, but also to indicate both the curriculum and the teaching methods needed to achieve identified objectives (Kaufman, Gottlieb, Agard, & Kukic, 1975). This movement was influential in the treatment of students with developmental disabilities, as mainstreaming appeared in Public Law 94-142 (1975) under the auspices of least restrictive educational environment.

Despite social and political advances, there was limited recognition and protection of the civil rights of persons with mental retardation before 1970. Though institutions remained the mainstay of treatment options in many areas, overcrowded and inadequate habilitation was the rule. Organizations such as the United Nations have addressed the condition, stating that persons with mental retardation have a right to proper medical care, physical therapy, and to such education, training, rehabilitation, and guidance, as would enable them to develop their abilities and maximum potential. This notion was advanced in April, 1972 (*Wyatt v. Stickney*), when the Supreme Court held that because the only constitutional justification for civilly committing a person with mental retardation to an institution is habilitation, "it follows ineluctably that once committed such a person is possessed with an inviolable constitutional right to habilitation." *Wyatt* also stated that "no person shall be admitted to an institution unless a prior determination has been made that residence in the institution is the least restrictive placement available." After *Wyatt*, similar class action suits were brought in a number of states.

Public Law 96-247 (1980) established the Civil Rights of Institutionalized Persons Act (CRIPA) and authorized the Attorney General of the US to initiate "action for redress in cases involving deprivation of rights of institutionalized persons secured or protected by the Constitution or laws of the United States. This legislation does not seek to define standards, but rather, outlines the means by which the federal government investigates constitutional violations in institutions. In conducting reviews of state facilities, the Department of Justice relies on the procedures outlined in CRIPA and the issues established in *Youngberg v. Romeo* (1982) decision for the legal basis of investigations.

On June 18, 1982, the Supreme Court issued a ruling in the case of *Youngberg v. Romeo* that established the constitutional rights of persons with mental retardation. The majority opinion addressed liberty interest, freedom from unnecessary restraint, and the right to habilitation (Ellis, 1982) and indicated that it was unconstitutional to confine persons involuntarily in unsafe conditions. Though these decisions dramatically altered the legal landscape, corresponding changes in both living conditions and service provision occurred much more slowly.

Emerging from the civil rights litigation concerning persons with mental retardation came a focus on downsizing institutions and moving individuals to a less restrictive living environment. The movement, coined deinstitutionalization, was a logical outgrowth of the normalization movement and its efforts to ensure that individuals with mental retardation were integrated into the larger community. The deinstitutionalization movement gained its impetus from a series of landmark legal decisions such as *Pennhurst(1977)* and, more recently, *L. C. v. Olmstead (1997)*. In *Pennhurst*, Pennsylvania law recognized the legal right to the provision of habilitative services in a least restrictive setting. Twenty years later, as the debate concerning the issue continued, *Olmstead* continued to recognize this right, but also emphasized the importance of an individual's choice in determining residential location. Though the argument continues, the clear trend in most states is towards a greater focus on community based services.

Most states recognize the need for movement toward more community-based settings and smaller institutions. Service provision models currently include a variety of living options including family based living, extended family living (e.g., foster care), supported independent living, community/group home placement, Intermediate Care Facilities, and placement in specialized units in psychiatric hospitals. Though a wide array of choices is nominally available, most individuals face a limited menu of actual residential choices. Unfortunately, the movement towards community-based services has seen a dichotomy develop between inpatient/institutional and community/family based services. The fragmentation of these services has led to a polarization of policy, philosophy, and funding for people with developmental disabilities. Services rarely overlap and coordination between agencies for optimal service provision is rare.

The Clinical Realm meets Society

In the last decade, the previously mentioned sociopolitical factors have affected clinical and scientific endeavors in the field of psychology. Most professionals who daily address the challenges of serving individuals with developmental disabilities recognize the interplay between the sociopolitical issues (or larger ecological context) and individualized clinical and intervention decisions. Now both philosophically and scientifically, psychologists and other healthcare providers focus on integrating the two areas with regard to improving services and developing both treatment and support options (Koegel, Koegel, & Dunlap, 1996).

Positive Behavior Support (PBS) practices draw on advances in applied behavior analysis and expand the philosophy to incorporate contextual and societal quality of life issues for each individual (Koegel, Koegel, & Dunlap, 1996). PBS focuses on building and increasing an individual's strengths and modifying environmental factors, and seeks to render problem behavior inefficient and ineffective. The Positive Behavior Supports model focuses on developing a quality life, and views most problem behavior as a means of communicating displeasure with an unsatisfying lifestyle.

Goals in a Positive Behavior Supports model are based in person centered values. The model recognizes that while person centered values cannot replace empirical work, these values must inform and shape empirical work (Carr et al., 2002). The Positive Behavioral Supports model focuses on developing quality of life for the individual rather than focusing narrowly on challenging behavior.

We next address current service provision models. Later sections of this chapter will focus on future models of service provision. Descriptions in these sections draw heavily on the philosophy of Positive Behavior Supports.

Current Service Models

While many states differ in funding sources and what they call facilities, most provide similar types of services and settings for persons with developmental disabilities. Settings include home-based, foster-parent or extended family living, community-based supported independent living, group homes (private and ICF-MR), developmental centers (private and ICF-MR), mental health facilities, and various types of court enforced incarceration. Though providing a wide array of services and supports, the current delivery of services in most states falls short of accepted standards of care for people with developmental disabilities. A number of issues bring about the failures within current models of service delivery. Variables contributing to diminished services are discussed below and include financial issues, segmented service provision, and inadequate provision of services by professionals.

One factor contributing to failures in current service delivery models is inadequate funding. Funding issues occur at an individual, an agency, and a systems level. Individuals living in community based settings often cannot receive adequate supervision or professional services because of limited dollars allotted to the individual and/or provider agency. In many instances the funding sources do not adequately reimburse for needed specialized services (i.e., psychological and psychiatric care). This factor is also true for families with disabled loved ones in the home. Many states distribute limited funds to these families, either assuming that family dollars, with limited input from other sources, will cover costs associated with in-home care, or simply due to a lack of sufficient available funds. In most states large and small residential providers, private providers, and home placements compete for dollars from the same "small" pool of money. Each of these placements is normally successful in garnering limited funds, but most lament that more funds are needed. The end result of this system of operations is that most placements are under-funded and insufficient services and care are provided.

A second variable that contributes to the failure of the current systems of service provision is a lack of continuity in services. The problem appears at both local and state levels in a number of situations. First, community providers are often placed in situations in which specialized consultation, care, or placement is required for stabilization of medical, psychiatric, or other emergency situations. Often adequate professionals, psychiatric beds, or temporary inpatient placement are difficult or impossible to obtain. The result is decreased care and quality of life for the individual in question. Larger residential centers encounter similar problems. A primary difficulty in many states is securing adequate community placements, with appropriate resources, to support those wishing to transition into a community living situation. In general, funds are low, beds are full, and effective professionals are difficult to find. The result is a slow-down in the process of moving people from larger settings to smaller, community based placements. The same is true for acute psychiatric care or infirmary care to promote healing. Without access to these settings, it often becomes the job of the residential center to house individuals that are in need of acute care in different settings; thus services are provided in settings that are not the most suitable for promoting stabilization or healing.

Breakdowns in service provision related to organizational structure are multi-layered in many states. Most states have, at a minimum, three different agencies for the provision of mental health services: a branch for developmental disabilities, a branch for mental health, and a branch for addictive disorders. These branches all compete for funding and operate on tight budgets. Now, the system is presented with large groups of people who are dually diagnosed (mental illness and developmentally disabled), and some of these individuals are also struggling with substance abuse difficulties. Whose responsibility does the individual become? Where are they placed? Who pays for care? Unfortunately, there is no single answer to these questions. If a developmental disability is present, the responsibility typically falls on the agency governing developmental disabilities to provide placement and care. However, when adequate professionals are not available, other agencies must be accessed for consultation and treatment. The agencies often play a shell game with the care of the individual in question, shuffling placements and treatment with a primary goal of cutting cost and secondary goal of providing care. [This method of case management is simply not acceptable.] Additionally, most states also have a fragmented system between developmental center (institutional based) settings and community based settings. This fragmentation often does not allow for the collaboration across service settings that would be needed to provide more normalized services within a wide array of settings allowing for individualized service and support needs. Within and across state organizations boundaries are often drawn that eliminate the ability for a smooth flow between various branches of the service and support system.

The final variable impacting service provision models is a lack of trained and knowledgeable professionals to provide services in various settings. Few schools train professionals to provide for the needs of persons with mental retardation. Thus, the population is underserved due to a lack of population-specific training. By definition, roughly 3-5% of the population could be diagnosed with mental retardation (American Psychiatric Association, 2000). Additionally, this group of individuals generally experiences other concomitant difficulties such as increased prevalence of both behavioral challenges and mental health symptoms (Borthwick-Duffy, 1994). Less than 3% of graduate training centers in psychology actually offer training, supervision and experience in providing services to individuals with developmental disabilities (Logan, Lott, & Mayville, 2000). Due to this training deficiency, a paucity of resources exists for supporting these individuals. In addition, many practitioners have no interest in providing services for persons with disabilities, making quality services in many settings even more difficult to obtain.

The previous section has listed factors which, from our experience, render current systems of service delivery ineffective. So how do systems optimize both dollars and care? We feel that what is needed is a system that provides supports, services, and treatment in a variety of settings. To this end, we recommend a Regional Service Center.

The Future of Services: Regional Service Centers

A practical model for service provision in the near future involves the concept of Regional service centers. By definition, regional service centers provide a range of social, psychiatric/psychological, and medical services to identify and/or address identified needs. While several states have facilities that they refer to as regional centers, no generally accepted model for a regional center exists. Examples of states using a regional center model include California, Mississippi, Ohio, and New Mexico. These centers provide an array of services, including case management, psychological/ psychiatric assessment, support services, treatment planning, and staff training.

This model presumes a reallocation of some resources currently located in developmental centers to regional service centers. The regional service center can provide multiple layers of supports, depending on individuals' identified needs. There are a number of reasons for the shift to this model of service delivery. First, many states lack the funding to garner the needed resources in multiple settings. In the best cases, when the funds are available, there is a paucity of expertise (as noted previously) to provide needed services to people with developmental disabilities. Rural areas typically have proportionately fewer skilled professionals than population centers, making the task of finding quality service delivery even more challenging. A regional service center could allocate in-house resources to support a range of consumer needs, regardless of residential placement. The regional service center could also serve a consultative role to other community-based professionals, resulting in an expansion of community capacity to provide needed services. Third, crisis situations often result in people with developmental disabilities being routed to hospital emergency rooms, psychiatric hospitals, developmental centers, or jails. A much better alternative placement would be respite and acute care services provided by the regional service centers. This approach would facilitate appropriate assessment and treatment, timely stabilization of crises, and hasten the individual's return home. The center would also replace disjointed state systems that pit community versus residential services in a never-ending fight for funding. By unifying systems into a single entity, states can improve communication, decrease administrative costs, and focus more resources on providing much-needed supports for individuals with developmental disabilities. Such a merger would also provide a clearer vision, a more unified philosophy of service, and a better continuity of care across service settings.

Regardless of a persons' residence, the regional service center would be available for all individuals with developmental disabilities within a particular area. The center would provide a variety of services including the following: a) direct services such as positive behavior support, psychiatric care, specialized medical and therapeutic services; b) specialty consultation; c) staff training; d) respite care; e) acute psychiatric or medical care; and f) crisis support. The services would be available to all persons with developmental disabilities. Below is a proposed outline for a breakdown of services.

The Regional Center as a Safety Net

People with developmental disabilities currently live and receive services in a variety of community based and residential settings. The regional center would offer a variety of services to these individuals regardless of where they live. First, the regional center would serve as a multi-layered, crisis support center for persons living in community based settings. The first layer would involve telephone consultation from an appropriately trained professional to the community based provider or caregiver. If problems persist, the crisis support model would involve an in-home visit in which the situation would be assessed and recommendations rendered to best address the person's needs. Finally, and as a rare last resort, the regional center would provide acute care placement for people who cannot be stabilized in their current setting. These services will be discussed in more detail below.

Persons in community based settings often require respite care to allow caregivers the opportunity to attend to significant matters. The regional center could be one option for providing respite services to allow individuals a safe, stimulating environment while caregivers must attend to other matters. Finally, regional centers would also provide both community and school-based consultations and expertise when available services have not satisfactorily addressed presenting problems. This service would be a liaison to the community-based provider; a second opinion rendered from experienced, highly qualified professionals.

The goal in this instance is to utilize expertise in the regional center to optimize services for consumers living in the community. The regional center would provide these services for persons living in the community with a goal of safe, quick stabilization while avoiding extended hospitalizations, nursing home placements, incarcerations, or other restrictive placements.

The Regional Center as Secondary Support

 The second goal of the regional center would be providing direct services for persons living at home or in other settings. Depending on the location of the service provider, regular or specialized services may not readily be accessible without significant travel. The regional center would facilitate delivery of appropriate expertise to persons who otherwise might be denied needed supports. The question of cost and payment for these services has been raised in a number of forums; however, current waiver systems, and state, and federal regulations have established an accepted fee schedule for direct services and consultation. Individuals in need of services would have the choice of using their funding to pay for services provided through the regional center.

As with individuals who receive all services in the community, persons receiving partial services from community providers would have access to learning opportunities, crisis support, respite services, acute psychiatric, medical, and behavioral care, specialty and/or ongoing consultation, and access to infirmary based medical services to promote stabilization, healing, and expedite a return home. Services provided by the regional center would be limited only by the expertise within the particular center. Thus, the regional center would likely provide specialized medical consultation, psychiatric care, behavioral assessment and consultation, staff training, and other services as dictated by individual need. This goal of the regional center would be to provide services in areas where services are not readily available, or to provide services that are difficult to obtain; thus, filling in gaps in community service provision.

The Regional Center as a Total Service Provider

The third goal of the regional center is to provide complete services for persons that otherwise would not be readily served in community based settings. This step would still include community provider involvement, as the current waiver system in most states dictates that case management be provided by an entity other than the primary provider. However, with the exception of case management, the center would provide all required services for the individual to live a valued, outcome-based life in a community setting. The supports to be provided would be completely dictated by each individual. The individual would benefit from a large number of learning/experiential opportunities in the community; however, in those cases in which other existing community based alternatives were not the most viable option, learning and educational opportunities within the community setting would be made available with the regional center as the provider. Services would include, but are not limited to, medical, psychiatric, psychological, habilitative, physical therapy, occupational therapy, speech/language therapy, and other support services. The long-term goal of this facet of the regional center would be to support people in a way that allows them to succeed in the most appropriate community placement, normally with family or private providers. Rather than living in congregate settings while waiting for either community opportunities or for more significant barriers to be addressed and overcome, the individuals would be supported by the regional service center in their preferred community living option.

The Regional Center as an Inpatient Setting

The final goal of the regional center is to serve as an inpatient setting for four basic groups of people with developmental disabilities: 1) individuals with significant medical, behavioral, or psychiatric issues that render them a danger to self or others in the community; 2) people in need of respite care for 7-21 days; 3) people in need of medical, psychiatric, or behavioral stabilization to expedite return to a less restrictive setting; and 4) people requiring infirmary-based medical services for convalescence, with the goal of medical stabilization and return to a less restrictive setting.

A few facts are critical in discussing the rationale for some inpatient setting options. First, the vast majority of current residents of developmental centers are either profoundly handicapped with multiple physical and/or medical difficulties or have been ordered by the court to reside in developmental centers due to failed community placements in conjunction with criminal activity. Second, many psychiatric beds in the United States are filled with persons with developmental disabilities that have not been successfully supported in regular, community based placements. Next, jails and prisons around the United State house a large number of individuals with developmental disabilities (Denkowski & Denkowski, 1985). Some of these individuals could be better served in the structured, support-rich environment offered by inpatient care in the regional center. Finally, and perhaps most importantly, most private service providers actively avoid placements involving individuals with medical, legal, behavioral, or psychiatric challenges. Persons in these groups create unwanted liability and a strain on already challenged financial and human resources.

The number of persons with developmental disabilities, and the extent of disability that can be adequately supported in a variety of living settings, has been a significant debate in the literature for the past 20 years (Reiss, McKinney, & Napolitan, 1990; Smull & Harrsion, 1992). We feel that the regional center model best addresses the support needs of all people with developmental disabilities. Individuals with developmental disabilities are a diverse group of people with varied preferences, goals, and needs. Our goal as service providers is to help shape a system that seeks to provide easy and reliable access to effective services and supports with the appropriate expertise available across a range of settings so that individuals with developmental disabilities and their families are able to make informed decisions about their service and support needs. This endeavor is not one that can be addressed with a one-size fits all mentality. The regional service center would allow individuals with developmental disabilities, their families and friends, and professionals with expertise in a variety of areas and from a variety of organizations to work collaboratively with the larger community to provide the most appropriate services and supports in the most appropriate setting for each individual while constantly striving to:

a) increase options for community-based living and service provision

b) Train and educate more professionals who can provide services and supports so that access across settings is increased

c) Form a network of support and information sharing across all stakeholders in this endeavor and most importantly,

d) Provide opportunities and support to individuals with developmental disabilities so that each person is able to enjoy a rich array of life experiences

If we can accomplish such lofty goals we will emerge with a community that is stronger and more successful through the joining and collaboration of all of its members.

References

American Psychiatric Association (2000). *Diagnostic and statistical manual of mental disorders (4ᵗʰ ed., text revision)*. Washington, DC: Author.

Azrin, N .H. & Armstrong, P. M. (1973). The mini-meal: A method for teaching eating skills to the profoundly retarded. *Mental Retardation, 11,* 9-11.

Azrin, N. H. & Foxx, R. M. (1971). A rapid method of toilet training the institutionalized retarded. *Journal of Applied Behavior Analysis, 4,* 89-99.

Bensberg, G. J., Colwell, C. N., & Cassel, R. H. (1965). Teaching the profoundly retarded self-help activities by behavior shaping techniques. *American Journal on Mental Deficiency, 69,* 674-679.

Blatt, B. & Kaplan, F. (1966). *Christmas in Purgatory.* Boston: Allyn & Bacon.

Borthwick-Duffy, S. (1994). Epidemiology and prevalence of psychopathology in people with mental retardation. *Journal of Consulting and Clinical Psychology, 62,_*17-27.

Carr, E. G., Dunlap, G., Horner, R. H., Koegel, R. L., Turnbull, A. P., Sailor, W., et al. (2002). Positive behavior support: Evolution of an applied science. *Journal of Positive Behavior Interventions, 4,* 4-16.

Denkowski, G. C. & Denkowski, K. M. (1985). The mentally retarded offender in the state prison system: Identification, prevalence, adjustment, and rehabilitation. *Criminal Justice and Behavior, 12,* 53-70.

Dunn, L. M. (1968). Special education for the mildly retarded: Is much of it justifiable? *Exceptional Children, 35,* 5-22.

Ellis, J. W. (1982). The Supreme Court and institutions: A comment on Youngberg v. Romeo. *Mental Retardation, 20,* 197.

Fiedler, C. R. & Antonak, R. F. (1991). Advocacy. In J. L. Matson & J. A. Mulick (eds.), *Handbook of Mental Retardation.* New York: Pergamon Press.

Gearhart, B. & Litton, F. (1975). *The trainable retarded.* St. Louis: Mosby.

Kanner, Leo. (1964). *A History of the Care and Study of the Mentally Retarded.* Springfield, IL: Charles C. Thomas.

Kaufman, M. J., Gottleib, J., Agard, J. A., & Kukic, M. B. (1975). Mainstreaming: Toward an explication of the construct. In E. L. Meyen, G. A. Vergason, & R. J. Whelan (Eds.), *Alternatives for Teaching Exceptional Children* (pp. 35-54). Denver: Love Publishing.

Koegel, L. K., Koegel, R. L., & Dunlap, G. (1996). *Positive Behavioral Support.* Baltimore: Brookes Publ.

Kratochwill, T. R. & Bijou, S. W. (1987). The impact of behaviorism on educational psychology. In J. A. Glover & R. R. Ronning (Eds.), *Historical foundations of educational psychology.* New York: Plenum Press.

L.C. v. Olmstead. 98-356. (Georgia, 1997).

Logan, J. R., Lott, J. D., & Mayville, E. A. (2000). *Top researchers and institutions in mental retardation: 1979-1999.*

Manikam, R. (1989). Treatment overview and description of psychotherapy. In J. L. Matson (Ed.), *Chronic schizophrenia and adult autism.* New York: Springer.

Matson, J. L. & Coe, D. A. (1992). Applied Behavior Analysis: Its impact on the treatment of mentally retarded emotionally disturbed people. *Research in Developmental Disabilities, 13,* 171-189.

Nirje, B. (1969). The normalization principle: Implications and comments. *Journal of Mental Subnormality, 16,* 62-70.

Pennhurst State School and Hospital v. Haldeman. Pennsylvania, 1977.

Public Law 94-142. (1975*). Education of All Handicapped Children Act (IDEA).*

Public Law 96-247. (1980). *Advancement of the Civil Rights for Institutionalized Persons Act (CRIPA).*

Reiss, S., McKinney, B., & Napolitan, J. T. (1990). Three new mental retardation service models: Implications for behavior modification. In J. L. Matson (Ed.), *Handbook of Behavior Modification with the Mentally Retarded (2nd ed.).* New York: Plenum Press.

Scheerenberger, R. C. (1983). *A History of Mental Retardation.* Baltimore: Brookes Publ.

Smull, M. W. & Harrison, S. B. (1992). *Supporting People with Severe Retardation in the Community.* Alexandria, VA: National Association of State Mental Retardation Program Directors.

Whitman, T. L., Scibak, J., & Reid, D. (1983). *Behavior Modification with the Mentally Retarded: Treatment and Research Perspectives.* New York: Academic Press.

Wolfensburger, W. (1980). A brief overview of the principle of normalization. In R. J. Flynn & K. G. Nitch (Eds.), *Normalization, Social Integration, and Community Services.* Baltimore: University Press.

Wyatt v. Stickney. 325 F. Supp. 781. (Alabama, 1970).

Youngberg v. Romeo. 457 U.S 307. (1982).

4

TRAINING AND SUPERVISING DIRECT SUPPORT PERSONNEL TO CARRY OUT BEHAVIORAL PROCEDURES

Dennis H. Reid
Carolina Behavior Analysis and Support Center
Morganton, North Carolina

Since the late 1960s, numerous aspects of the quality of life among people with developmental disabilities have been enhanced through behavioral research and application. Behavioral interventions have been shown repeatedly to reduce challenging behavior, promote skill development, and generally increase life enjoyment. The contributions of behavioral research and application in developmental disabilities are well reflected throughout other chapters in this text.

In most situations, behavioral procedures are maximally effective with individuals who have developmental disabilities when applied within typical environments in which those individuals live, work, and play. To effectively reduce challenging behavior, for example, behavioral procedures typically must be applied in every environment in which a given individual is likely to display the behavior of concern. Similarly, procedures designed to teach adaptive skills are usually most effective when the procedures are carried out in the environments in which individuals would normally use the skills.

Because behavioral procedures are most effective when used in the day-to-day environments in which individuals with disabilities spend their time, the procedures usually must be applied by direct support personnel who routinely interact with the individuals in those settings. Such personnel include residential direct service staff, teacher assistants, job coaches, sheltered workshop staff, and personal assistants. The important role of direct support personnel in the effective application of behavioral procedures has been noted repeatedly (Hastings & Brown, 2000; Reid, Parsons, & Green, 1989a). In short, if direct support personnel do not apply behavioral procedures in a proficient manner, then many individuals with developmental disabilities will not experience the benefits of the existing behavioral technology (cf. Neef, 1995).

Although the importance of proficient application of behavioral procedures by direct support personnel is well established, it is also well recognized that most persons who enter direct support positions have minimal or no formal preparation regarding behavioral interventions (Burch, Reiss, & Bailey, 1987; Reid & Parsons, 2002, chap.1). Consequently, a critical component in the application of behavioral procedures to improve the life of people with developmental disabilities is training support personnel how to use respective procedures. Direct service staff cannot be expected to proficiently apply behavioral procedures if they have not had opportunities to receive training in behavioral applications.

Recognition of the importance of training staff in the use of behavioral procedures has resulted in a considerable amount of applied research on staff training strategies. Such research has lead to the development of a highly effective technology for training direct service personnel to carry out behavioral procedures with individuals who have disabilities. The research has also indicated though that staff training in and of itself is not sufficient for ensuring support personnel implement behavioral procedures in a proficient and effective manner (Smith, Parker, Taubman, & Lovaas, 1992). Rather, on-the-job support and supervision is usually needed to ensure that staff proficiently apply their newly learned behavioral skills on a day-to-day basis (Harchik & Campbell, 1998; Sturmey, 1998).

The significance of on-the-job supervision of staffs= implementation of behavioral procedures is perhaps best illustrated when effective supervision is not provided. Many well designed behavior plans have failed to reduce challenging behavior or enhance skill development not because the plans were poorly designed, but because the plans were not carried out in the manner in which they were intended. One of the most common frustrations among clinicians and other authors of behavior support plans is the lack of adequate implementation of the plans by direct service personnel (Reid & Parsons, 2002, chap. 1). In turn, when direct service staff fail to adequately carry out respective behavior plans, there has been a failure to provide appropriate support and supervision of the staffs= program duties (cf. Hastings & Brown, 2000). Although there are many ways in which supervision can break down in typical service settings, the end result is the same: without adequate supervision of staffs= program implementation, behavior plans frequently will not be applied in the desired manner.

In essence, the benefits of behavioral procedures for enhancing quality of life among many people with developmental disabilities will be realized only to the degree that their support personnel are adequately trained and supervised in the proficient application of those procedures. As noted earlier, there has been a substantial amount of research on means of training important work skills to direct service staff. There has likewise been a significant amount of research on methods of supervising the daily work performance of direct service personnel. It is the purpose of this chapter to describe implications of that research in terms of currently recommended practices for training and supervising support personnel in applying behavioral procedures with people who have developmental disabilities.

Empirical Basis of Recommended Practices for Training and Supervising Direct Support Personnel to Carry Out Behavioral Procedures

The technology of behavior change procedures for reducing undesirable behavior and promoting desirable behavior among people with developmental disabilities has its basis in applied behavior analysis (Baer, Wolf, & Risley, 1968; 1987). A characteristic of behavior change procedures derived from applied behavior analysis is that the procedures are *evidenced-based*. That is, the procedures have been developed from applied research that empirically supports the efficacy of the procedures, and the principles upon which they are based. The emphasis on evidence-based procedures is likewise relevant when considering strategies to train and supervise support staff in the application of behavioral procedures.

The significance of relying on an empirically substantiated, evidence-based foundation for deriving means of training and supervising the work performance of direct service personnel B in this case, performance related to application of behavior change procedures with their consumers who have developmental disabilities B cannot be overstated. The human services are replete with approaches to staff training and supervision that have no scientific basis to support their utility. Rather, many strategies used in a training or supervisory capacity are based on temporary management fads espoused in the popular media, folklore, and guess work. Such approaches rarely have significant effects in regard to impacting the quality of staff work performance (Sturmey, 1998).

The focus of this chapter is on training and supervising the work performance of direct service personnel using strategies that have an evidence base in applied research to support their efficacy. The specific body of research that forms the basis of the recommended practices to be discussed has been referred to in several ways, including *organizational behavior management* (Sturmey, 1998), *performance management* (Daniels, 1994), and *behavioral outcome management* (Everson & Reid, 1999). Despite the somewhat varying labels, the research stems from well established principles of behavior as applied to staff performance in the work place, and conforms to the empirically substantiated practices within the more general field of applied behavior analysis (Reid, Parsons, & Green, 1989b).

The body of research upon which the practices to be described are based is far too comprehensive to summarize in-depth here. Rather, only selected references to key sources will be presented. For a more complete description of the background research, the interested reader is referred to Table 1, which presents several texts that describe behaviorally based approaches to staff training and supervision. Additionally, Table 2 presents a number of articles and chapters that review or summarize research in this area.

Recommended Practices for Training Staff to Carry Out Behavioral Procedures

Proficient application of behavioral procedures requires two types of skills (Reid et al., 2003). The first type, *verbal skills*, involves in essence an understanding of what and how certain procedures will be used. The second type, *performance skills*, involves being able to apply or perform the procedures proficiently during the day-to-day job.

Distinguishing between verbal and performance skills is more than an academic exercise. In particular, it is important to distinguish between the two sets of skills because each set requires somewhat different types of strategies for training purposes (see Gardner, 1972, for an early, classic demonstration of the differential effects of the two types of training strategies on verbal versus performance skills). Verbal skills generally require verbally based training strategies involving spoken and/or written instructions (Reid & Parsons, 2000). In contrast, performance skills typically must include more performance-based strategies such as demonstration or modeling

(Mansdorf & Burstein, 1986) and performance practice (Stoddard, McIlvane, McDonagh, & Kledaras, 1986).

An additional reason to distinguish between the two types of skills involved in learning to apply behavioral procedures relates to how training is often conducted with direct support personnel. Many training approaches involve primarily or exclusively verbally-based training strategies. A common training strategy, for example, when a clinician desires to train staff how to implement a new behavior development or support plan with a respective individual centers on a meeting with the staff. During the meeting, the clinician describes the procedures constituting the plan and perhaps a rationale for the plan, and allows staff to ask questions about the procedures. A written copy of the plan may also be given to the staff. Because this process relies on verbal training strategies (i.e., spoken and written instructions), it may be sufficient for teaching staff a basic understanding of the procedures in terms of being able to describe the procedures. However, such a process is not likely to ensure that staff will be able to actually carry out the procedures.

From the perspective of implementing behavioral procedures to help reduce challenging behavior or increase adaptive behavior among individuals with developmental disabilities, it is critical that staff be able to carry out the procedures proficiently on a day-to-day basis. Hence, the typical training strategy just described that focuses on verbal strategies rarely represents a satisfactory training approach. Rather, training must also emphasize performance-based strategies. The discussion here will focus on training strategies that emphasize performance-based approaches but also include components for training relevant verbal skills.

A Step-By-Step Protocol of Recommended Practices for Training Staff to Carry Out Behavioral Procedures

The technology for training staff derived from applied research is well represented in a basic, step-by-step protocol for training how to carry out behavioral procedures. The protocol, which represents a synthesis of currently recommended practices in staff training endeavors, is summarized in Table 3 (see Parsons & Reid, 1995; Sturmey, 1998, for elaboration on the training protocol and its research-based development). The training process presented in Table 3 can be used to train staff how to implement procedures to prevent or reduce challenging behavior, as well as how to apply teaching strategies and increase desired behavior among people with developmental disabilities.

Training staff to carry out a behavioral procedure, or set of procedures constituting a behavior-reduction or teaching plan, begins (**Step 1**) with the staff trainer verbally describing the procedures. The description should include a review of the rationale regarding why the procedures need to be implemented. As will be discussed in the next section on supervising staffs= day-to-day application of a behavior plan, in large part the rationale should already be apparent to staff if they have been appropriately involved in the development of the plan.

Following the verbal description, each staff trainee should be provided with a written description of the intended procedures (**Step 2**). The written description should be a very concise summary of what staff should do to carry out the procedures. More comprehensive descriptions of behavior reduction or teaching procedures (e.g., a formally written behavior support plan) can be left for staff to review at their convenience. Contrary to common practice in a number of agencies, the comprehensive, formal program should not constitute the written instructions provided to staff for training purposes. Formal programs that contain information such as background history of a given individual, summaries of previously attempted procedures, medication regimes, etc., make it difficult for staff to quickly view a set of procedures and identify exactly what they need to do in a given circumstance.

Whereas the two steps just summarized involve verbal training strategies, the remaining steps in the recommended approach for training direct service personnel focus on performance strategies. Specifically, **Step 3** involves the staff trainer demonstrating how to conduct the procedures. In most cases, the demonstration can occur in a role-play situation (Jones & Eimers, 1975) in which a staff member plays the role of the individual consumer with whom the procedures will be used, and the trainer demonstrates how to conduct the procedures with that individual. In some cases, the procedures can actually be demonstrated in vivo (Templeman, Fredericks, Bunse, & Moses, 1983) with the individual for whom the procedures are intended. However, in the latter situation, safeguards are necessary to ensure that the dignity and privacy of the individual can be protected and that the demonstration does not risk promoting various types of problem behavior by the individual. Immediately following the procedural demonstration, whether in a role-play or in-vivo situation, each staff trainee should practice performing the procedures in the same manner that the staff trainer just demonstrated (**Step 4**).

Step 5 of the training process involves the staff trainer carefully observing each staff member practice performing the procedures and providing feedback based on the observed proficiency of each trainee=s performance. The feedback should include supportive statements for procedural components performed adequately by a respective staff member and as needed, corrective feedback regarding components of the procedures that were not performed adequately (the following chapter sections provide a more in-depth discussion on how to provide supportive and corrective feedback). Finally, **Step 6** involves repeating the preceding two steps involving trainee practice with trainer feedback until each staff trainee is observed to proficiently perform all aspects of the procedures. This latter step represents a *competency-based* component (Burch et al., 1987; Shore, Iwata, Vollmer, Lerman, & Zarcone, 1995) to the teaching process.

The final, competency-based step in the training process is critical to the overall success of a training endeavor. Training should never be considered complete until the staff trainer observes each trainee perform the designated behavioral procedures competently. It is only in this manner that a staff trainer can be assured that staff truly have the skills to carry out the procedures proficiently. Although ensuring staff know how to carry out behavioral procedures does not ensure that they will perform the procedures adequately during the daily job routine as indicated previously, if staff do not know how to perform the procedures it is certain that the procedures will not be carried out adequately as part of staffs= regular job duties.

An underlying premise for effectively implementing the staff training protocol just described is that the person responsible for conducting the training be knowledgeable in the behavioral procedures and skilled in performing the procedures; the staff trainer must be skilled in what s/he is training to staff (Reid & Parsons, 2002, chap. 7). Although such a premise may appear obvious, it is emphasized here because the premise often is not reflected in common practice. For example, in a number of community residential settings such as group homes, a psychologist or behavior specialist may send a written copy of a behavior support plan to the group home manager and expect the manager to train staff how to implement the plan. In such a case, the manager often is not very well versed in the plan=s procedures and may have uncertainties regarding how specific components of the plan should be carried out. To avoid such a situation, it is usually necessary that clinicians who develop behavior plans be directly involved to at least some degree in the staff training process.

Recommended Practices for Supervising Staff in Carrying Out Behavioral Procedures

Similar to the development of an evidence-based technology for training work skills to direct service staff, a considerable amount of applied research has lead to a technology for supervising staffs= day-to-day performance of those skills (see Tables 1 and 2). As also similar to staff training endeavors, there are now several well-established, component steps that constitute an effective approach to staff supervision. However, relative to the strategies for training staff, application of the component steps for supervision are more complex. The complexity is due to the need for a supervisor to alter which supervisory steps are followed based on the existing adequacy of staff performance, and how staff respond to the supervisor=s actions. The complexity is also due to the existence of a wider array of specific strategies for carrying out the component steps. Such variety allows for a degree of choice on the part of the supervisor or author of a behavior plan regarding how to work with staff, based in part on how staff respond to respective supervisory strategies as well as how comfortable and skilled a supervisor or author is with using various strategies. Before implementing the key steps to staff supervision though, certain pre-requisites are usually necessary to enhance the likelihood that supervision will be successful.

Pre-Requisites to Effective Supervision

One critical pre-requisite to successful supervision of staffs= implementation of behavior plans has already been discussed, that of ensuring staff are adequately trained in the target procedures. Three other important pre-requisites that have not been discussed to this point include: (1) involvement of staff in the development of behavior plans, (2) clarification of who is responsible for supervising staffs= performance related to carrying out behavior plans and, (3) establishment of an environment that promotes efficacious implementation of behavior plans.

In considering the basic pre-requisites for effective supervision, an underlying premise of successful supervision also warrants attention. Specifically, concern must be directed to not only ensuring that whatever supervisory strategies employed are effective in terms of improving or maintaining staff proficiency in carrying out behavior plans, but also to staff *acceptance* of the strategies. The importance of staff acceptance on the success of supervisory strategies has been well discussed (see Parsons, 1998, for a review). Such discussion will not be repeated here except to emphasize that if supervisory strategies are not well accepted by staff, the strategies are not likely to serve their intended purpose of beneficially impacting staff performance. Staff discontent with what their supervisors do can result in a number of deleterious effects on the impact of supervisory actions, all of which detract from the overall proficiency with which supports and services are provided by direct service personnel. The following discussion focuses on supervisory strategies that tend to be both effective *and* acceptable to staff.

Involving staff in the development of behavior plans. Whenever the need for a behavior plan becomes apparent for an individual who has a developmental disability, it is recommended that the clinician responsible for developing the plan involve staff in the development process. The importance of obtaining staff input in the development of a behavior plan is generally well established in terms of establishing plans of high quality and ecological validity (Knoster, 2000). For our purposes here however, involving staff in the development of a behavior plan is advantageous from a supervisory perspective. Such involvement can increase the likelihood that staff will be responsive to implementing the plan once developed.

Involving staff in the development of procedures that the staff will be expected to perform as part of their daily work routine represents a *participative management* approach to supervision (Reid et al., 1989b, chap. 4). Participative management can increase staff acceptance of the procedures that they are expected to carry out (Phillips, 1998; Peck, Killen, & Baumgart, 1989), in this case behavior change procedures to be implemented with their consumers or clients. As just noted, staff acceptance of supervisory actions can be critical to the overall success of supervisory strategies.

Identifying responsibility for staff supervision. Before strategies can be effectively applied to ensure proficient staff performance in carrying out behavior plans, it must be determined who will implement the supervisory strategies (Reid & Parsons, 2002, chap.2). With many aspects of the daily work performance of direct service staff, it is readily apparent that staffs= immediate supervisor is responsible for ensuring proficient job performance. In regard to carrying out behavior plans though, the responsibility is not always readily apparent.

 In most agencies providing supports and services for people with developmental disabilities, personnel who develop behavior plans (e.g., psychologists, behavior analysts) have minimal or no supervisory authority over direct service staff. Relatedly, in many agencies such as community residential settings, personnel who develop behavior plans for staff to carry out may not be present in staffs= work site on a daily or even weekly basis. When clinicians have no direct authority over staff and/or are not frequently present in staffs= work area, it is difficult for those persons to supervise staff performance in carrying out behavior plans designed by the professionals. In such situations, supervisory responsibility for program implementation duties must be shared with staffs= immediate supervisor (Reid & Parsons, 2002, chap. 2).

When professionals who develop behavior plans must rely on someone else such as the staff supervisor to actively supervise staffs= program implementation, that aspect of ensuring implementation proficiency should be openly discussed prior to expecting staff to carry out the plans. The author of the behavior plan should discuss with the supervisor what needs to be done to ensure proficient implementation of the plan and who is to be responsible for each supervisory aspect. As indicated in subsequent sections, such aspects include who is going to monitor staff performance, implement supportive action, and correct nonproficient performance.

If supervisory responsibilities are not clearly delineated, then often there is minimal supervision specifically directed to staffs= implementation of behavior plans. As a result, staff proficiency in carrying out such plans is likely to be inconsistent at best. It should also be noted though that when delineating specific supervisory roles and actions, authors of behavior plans should never be totally excluded from the supervisory process. Authors of behavior plans should help in monitoring staff implementation performance as well as provision of supportive and corrective feedback as needed (again, see later chapter sections). Participating in supervision of staff performance as a means of ensuring program implementation integrity is an important B and required B part of the professional responsibilities of clinicians who design behavior plans (cf. Risley & Reid, 1995).

Evaluation of environmental adequacy. Prior to developing a behavior plan to be implemented with one of an agency=s clients, the professional expected to develop the plan should evaluate the adequacy of the routine environment of the individual. The quality of environments in which people with developmental disabilities spend their time varies significantly. Some environments include high quality features that reduce the likelihood that formal behavior plans will be needed to reduce challenging behavior, and increase the likelihood that if such plans are necessary, they will be effective. In contrast, other environments actually tend to promote various types of challenging behavior, as well as reduce the probability that behavior plans will significantly reduce the behavior.

It is beyond the scope of this chapter to thoroughly describe environmental features that should exist in agencies providing supports and services for people with developmental disabilities. A number of other sources provide detailed discussions about desired environmental characteristics (e.g., Holburn & Vietze, 2002; Landesman & Vietze, 1987). The point of concern here is that authors of behavior plans should evaluate the adequacy of the environments in which staff will be expected to carry out the plans. If the environments appear problematic in terms of making it unlikely that certain plans can be effective, then it makes little sense to expect staff to carry out the plans. Relatedly, if there are insufficient numbers of staff to adequately carry out respective behavior plans, then efforts directed to supervising staff implementation proficiency will be futile. In these types of situations, professionals charged with developing behavior plans should bring concerns about the adequacy of the overall environment to the attention of appropriate agency executives prior to placing demands on staff related to implementing the plans (Risley & Reid, 1995).

Basic Components of Effective Supervision of Staff Implementation of Behavioral Procedures

Although there are many different strategies involved in effectively supervising staff implementation of behavior plans, each strategy basically relates to at least one of three primary components (Harchik & Campbell, 1998; Sturmey, 1998): (1) objectively and systematically monitoring staff implementation performance, (2) providing support for proficient performance, and (3) correcting nonproficient performance.

Monitoring staff implementation of behavior plans. The importance of systematically monitoring or observing behaviors that are targeted to be changed is well accepted when applying behavioral procedures with people who have developmental disabilities. Although perhaps not as well recognized when considering staff implementation of those procedures, monitoring staff implementation performance is no less important. Systematically monitoring staff performance in carrying out behavior plans is the only way to obtain accurate information about the degree to which the plans are being implemented as intended. In turn, accurate information about staff proficiency in carrying out behavior plans forms the basis for all other supervisory actions for promoting proficient performance and correcting nonproficient performance.

Monitoring staff work performance associated with carrying out behavior plans can be conducted using the same types of monitoring systems used to systematically observe the behavior of consumers who are the recipients of the plans. Because there are numerous descriptions of behavioral monitoring systems (see in particular Thompson, Felce, & Symons, 2000), the various systems will not be reviewed here. Rather, the most common types of systems relevant for monitoring staff implementation of behavior plans will be presented.

Essentially, there are two aspects of staff performance associated with carrying out behavior plans that warrant attention from a monitoring perspective. First, monitoring is needed to determine if staff carry out a respective plan when the plan is intended to be implemented. Second, monitoring is necessary to evaluate when plans are carried out, the degree to which the plans are implemented correctly. For the former purpose, an *event-recording* monitoring system can be used in which the implementation is simply recorded as having occurred or not (Williams, Vittorio, & Hausherr, 2002). For the latter purpose, monitoring with a *performance checklist* is usually recommended (Lattimore, Stephens, Favell, & Risley, 1984; Risley & Favell, 1979). A performance checklist essentially task analyzes program implementation of a given behavior plan into specific actions that staff must follow to carry out the plan. When monitoring actual implementation, each action on the checklist is recorded as being performed correctly (i.e., the way the action is described on the checklist) or incorrectly (either performed in a manner other than how the action is described on the checklist or not performed at all). Following completion of the checklist after observing a staff member carry out a behavior plan, a percentage of actions performed correctly can be determined. Such a percentage typically represents a useful indication of the performance proficiency of a staff person in carrying out the behavior plan (e.g., Parsons, Reid, & Green, 1996).

Monitoring with the use of performance checklists is most useful if it can be predicted when a staff person will implement a behavior plan such that the observer B usually the author of the plan or the staff person=s supervisor B can be present to monitor the staff member=s performance. For example, behavior plans that involve teaching a particular skill to an individual often are carried out on a relatively predictable schedule such as during a specific type of situation that occurs during generally consistent time periods. Using a checklist to monitor staff implementation of a behavior plan to reduce challenging behavior can be more difficult. The need to use a given behavior reduction plan usually is based in large part on when the challenging behavior is exhibited by an individual, and such behavior is not always predictable. In the latter situation, authors of plans and staff supervisors typically will need to attempt to observe staff implementation of behavior reduction plans at time periods when the problem behavior of concern is most likely expected to occur.

An alternative monitoring approach for behavior reduction plans that increases the likelihood of observing at a time when various components of the plans should be implemented is with a monitoring system that incorporates features of *interval* monitoring (McGimsey, Greene, & Lutzker, 1995) and checklists. With this type of monitoring system (see Reid & Parsons, 2002, chap. 9, for a detailed example) a given individual who has a behavior reduction plan in place is observed continuously along with the staff who interact with the individual for a set time period, such as 10 or 20 minutes. The time period is broken down into smaller intervals such as 1-minute periods. Within each 1-minute period, each action that represents part of a plan (drawn from the checklist) that could be implemented during the interval is recorded along with whether the responsible staff person carried out that action and whether the action was carried out correctly. Many behavior reduction plans include a variety of components that can be carried out at different time periods such as certain actions designed to prevent problem behavior (e.g., providing positive attention at specified time intervals if problem behavior is not occurring) as well as actions to perform when the problem behavior occurs. Consistent use of this type of monitoring system often will provide a sufficiently accurate representation of staff proficiency in carrying out various aspects of behavior reduction plans.

Although monitoring systems can be used to obtain information on staff proficiency in implementing behavior plans in much the same way as monitoring systems designed to evaluate changes in the behavior of an individual who is the recipient of a behavior plan, there are also some special concerns when monitoring staff performance. One such concern is staff *reactivity* to having their work performance observed (Phillips, 1998). Reactivity refers to staff changing their performance when they are aware that the performance is being observed; in this case performing more proficiently when being observed. Reactivity can be problematic because information obtained from a monitoring session will not be reflective of how staff typically implement a behavior plan (i.e., when not being observed).

Although reactivity can be a concern with almost any monitoring system, from a supervisory standpoint reactivity can be beneficial. The ultimate goal in supervision is for staff to perform in a proficient manner, and if reactivity to having one=s performance observed serves to improve performance then that effect should be capitalized on by supervisors and clinicians. Staff should be made aware that their performance in carrying out behavior plans will be observed and the observations should occur frequently. In one sense, the more frequently staff implement a behavior plan proficiently B even if due at least in part to reactivity to having their performance observed

B the more practice staff have in implementing the plan correctly. Consequently, the more likely it becomes that staff will continue to carry out the plan appropriately. In contrast, if clinicians or supervisors suspect that certain staff are carrying out a given plan correctly *only* when being observed, then such reactivity often can be overcome and a more accurate evaluation of staff performance can be accomplished by not only observing frequently, but doing so on an unpredictable schedule (cf. Fleming & Sulzer-Azaroff, 1992).

An issue related to staff reactivity to having their performance observed by a supervisor or clinician is the frequency with which the supervisor and clinician are present in staff's work site. If supervisors and clinicians are to frequently observe staff performance as a means of dealing with reactivity, they must be frequently present in staff's work area. Frequent presence of clinicians and supervisors also serves other beneficial functions from a supervisory stand point. In short, generally the more frequently a supervisor and clinician are present in staffs= work area, the more likely it is that staff will perform their duties associated with behavior plans in a proficient manner (Reid & Parsons, 2002, chap.3).

Frequent presence of a clinician and supervisor is one of the most critical variables affecting staff proficiency in carrying out behavior plans. Such presence can serve the purpose of prompting appropriate staff performance as well as reinforcing proficient program implementation (see later section on supportive supervisory activities). Every clinician should strive to be present in the work site of staff as frequently as possible, and work with supervisors to promote their frequent presence as well.

A final concern with monitoring systems particularly relevant with staff performance pertains to staff acceptance of the monitoring process. As indicated previously, success in working with staff to promote proficient application of behavior plans can be seriously affected by the degree to which supervisory practices are accepted by staff. Staff acceptance is especially a concern when monitoring their work performance. Systematic monitoring of work performance frequently is not well received by staff (Reid & Parsons, 1995a). There are a several reasons why staff tend to dislike having their performance observed, although most of the reasons often pertain to negative experiences staff have had with previous monitoring procedures or misinterpretations regarding the reasons for the monitoring.

Because of the discontent monitoring can engender among staff, special attention is warranted by clinicians and supervisors regarding how their monitoring practices are received by staff. In many situations, staff dislike of monitoring practices can be avoided or reduced by following several key steps. First, staff should be informed prior to formal monitoring of their performance why monitoring is necessary, focusing on the need to observe first hand how plans are being implemented and individual responses to the plans. Second, staff should be made aware precisely what is being monitored and how the monitoring will be accomplished. Awareness of the focus and process of monitoring can prevent misconceptions staff may develop regarding the purpose of the monitoring. Third, feedback — and particularly positive feedback — should be provided as quickly as possible after each monitoring activity such that staff are informed of the outcome of the monitoring (which again can help prevent misconceptions from developing). Fourth, common courtesy should be practiced when conducting observations of staffs= implementation of behavior plans, such as by politely greeting staff when entering their work area for monitoring purposes and when leaving the work area. More detailed discussions on how monitoring can be conducted in a manner that minimizes staff discontent are provided elsewhere (Reid & Parsons, 1995b, chap. 3). Most importantly though, problems with staff discontent with monitoring can be avoided if monitoring is conducted in conjunction with an overall supportive approach to supervision.

Supporting proficient implementation of behavior plans. Proficient implementation of behavior plans should not be taken for granted by clinicians or supervisors (cf. Sturmey, 1998). Rather, deliberate actions should be taken to support staffs= proficient program implementation. On a general level, such actions involve: (1) setting the occasion for staff to carry out behavior plans proficiently and (2) responding to proficient performance in a way that maintains such performance as well as promotes increased performance proficiency if necessary. Setting the occasion for desired performance involves actions already discussed: using participative management strategies in the development of behavior plans, ensuring staff are well informed about the content of plans and well trained to implement the plans, and monitoring staffs= program implementation in a manner that is acceptable to staff.

From a behavioral perspective, responding to competent implementation of behavior plans in a way that maintains skillful performance and/or fosters increased competence centers on the consequences clinicians and supervisors provide for staff performance. There are numerous ways consequences can be provided to support proficient staff performance in carrying out behavior plans. For organizational purposes the various ways can be considered as primarily representing two general types of consequences. One type involves explicit presentation of feedback while the other focuses on consequences other than feedback.

Providing feedback to staff regarding their program implementation performance, and particularly positive feedback, is generally considered a readily available and cost efficient means of supporting proficient work performance among staff (Balcazar, Hopkins, & Suarez, 1986). In the purest sense, feedback involves providing information to staff regarding their observed performance (Ford, 1980). In a supportive, supervisory capacity, feedback involves providing information about observed performance along with expressions of approval for the performance (i.e., positive feedback). Positive feedback is arguably the most potent means clinicians and supervisors have for supporting and maintaining proficient staff performance in carrying out behavior plans (see next chapter section for a protocol for presenting feedback).

Feedback can be presented both formally and informally. Formal feedback refers to feedback presented during specially scheduled meetings with staff with the explicit purpose of reviewing a staff person=s work performance. Informal feedback involves feedback presented during the ongoing job routine of staff, often in an impromptu manner. A general rule of thumb is that informal feedback should be presented very frequently as part of a clinician=s and supervisor=s routine interactions with staff, and formal feedback should be presented periodically as a supplement to informal feedback.

Feedback can also be presented both verbally (i.e., spoken) and in written format (e.g., informal notes, computer messages, memoranda, and letters). In a manner somewhat analogous to informal and formal feedback, it is generally recommended that verbal feedback be presented most frequently and supplemented with periodic written feedback. Reliance on verbal versus written feedback can also be based in part on personal preferences of respective clinicians and supervisors as well as preferences of individual staff.

Consequences other than feedback have also been used to improve and maintain proficient work performance among direct service staff. Such consequences are used by supervisors and clinicians in attempts to reinforce targeted staff work behavior. A wide variety of consequences have been used to reinforce various aspects of staff work performance in human service settings including, for example, contingent monetary bonuses (Arco, 1993), more flexible or desired work schedules (Iwata, Bailey, Brown, Foshee, & Alpern, 1976), and being relieved of nonpreferred work duties (Shoemaker & Reid, 1980). Although presentation of these types of consequences usually includes some type of feedback regarding staff performance, the reinforcing value of the consequences is presumed to be due primarily to the desired objects or privileges obtained.

Despite the reinforcing effects on staff work behavior of the types of consequences just exemplified, their application in a supportive supervisory capacity can be problematic. Such consequences often require extra financial resources for an agency and can involve significant time investments to arrange to be provided. Relatedly, these types of consequences frequently can be presented to one or only a small group of staff at a time even if the performance of many staff merits positive support (Daniels, 1994, chap. 9). Hence, for supporting proficient implementation of behavior plans by direct service personnel, it is generally recommended that supportive management strategies focus on the use of positive feedback. Other types of consequences can be used to periodically supplement the more routine provision of feedback.

Correcting nonproficient implementation of behavior plans. If the pre-requisites for successful supervision are established and the component steps for supportive management are routinely practiced as just summarized, then problems with how behavior plans are implemented are likely to be minimized. Nevertheless, concerns over staff performance in this area are still likely to occur from time to time. When such concerns do arise, they must be resolved. Resolution of problems with staff proficiency in carrying out behavior plans often can be achieved through a corrective management approach.

Like supportive management strategies, the most readily available and cost efficient means of corrective management involves the use of performance feedback. However, whereas the primary intent of feedback used in a supportive management capacity is to maintain staff performance adequacy, the intent of feedback from a corrective perspective is to change aspects of how staff are performing. The essence of corrective feedback involves informing staff that some aspect of their implementation of a behavior plan is not satisfactory, and specifically what should be done to improve the performance.

Feedback provided within a corrective management capacity can be applied in the same formats as feedback used within supportive management approaches (i.e., verbal, written, formal, and informal formats). The same general recommendations for how to use the different feedback formats as discussed earlier with supportive feedback pertain to corrective feedback as well. That is, corrective feedback generally should be provided most frequently in a spoken and informal manner, based on when problems with staff proficiency in carrying out a given behavior plan first become apparent. If necessary to bring about further improvement in staff performance, the informal, verbal feedback should be supplemented with more formal and written feedback.

Although the recommended means of providing supportive and corrective feedback are similar as just noted, there are also some special concerns for using feedback in a corrective capacity with staff performance. Most notably, from the perspective of the recipient of the feedback (i.e., the staff person whose performance is of concern), there are some inherently negative aspects of receiving corrective feedback. By its nature, corrective feedback entails informing a staff person that some aspect of his/her performance is not satisfactory. Additionally, whether accurate or not, in a number of cases the staff person may view potential threats to his/her job security or pay status when corrective feedback is provided. Because of the negative aspects inherent in receiving corrective feedback, special concerns are warranted among clinicians and supervisors regarding staff acceptance of their corrective feedback.

Several ways exist to minimize negative reactions by staff to receiving corrective feedback concerning their implementation of behavior plans. Most importantly, clinicians and supervisors should provide positive feedback within a supportive management capacity much more frequently than corrective feedback. Also, presentation of corrective feedback can be embedded within presentations of positive feedback. Table 4 presents a protocol for embedding corrective feedback within delivery of positive feedback.

Steps 1 and 2 in the feedback protocol in Table 4, as well as Step 7, represent the positive aspects of an overall approach to providing corrective feedback. Steps 3 and 4 pertain to corrective feedback directly, and Steps 5 and 6 indirectly by helping to ensure the staff person understands the concerns and can prepare for the next time feedback will be provided. This protocol for providing feedback has been shown to correct nonproficient aspects of staff work behavior and to be generally well received by human service staff (Parsons & Reid, 1995; Parsons et al., 1996).

Another concern with corrective management that relates to staff acceptance of the process pertains to the private versus public nature of providing corrective feedback. Corrective management strategies should be presented in a private manner whenever possible such that only the staff person whose behavior is of concern is immediately aware of the feedback. Corrective feedback should not be provided to a staff person in a manner that other staff in the work place can listen to or observe (i.e., corrective feedback should not be presented to a staff person in a public manner). Staff frequently report that one of the most unpleasant and undesired supervisory activities involves providing negative information about a staff person=s performance in the presence of other staff members (Parsons, Reid, & Crow, in press).

Summary and Future Directions

As emphasized repeatedly throughout this chapter, staff training and supervisory strategies are most likely to be successful if the strategies have been developed through applied research that establishes the efficacy of the strategies. The recommended practices for training and supervising staff implementation of behavior plans discussed to this point have their basis in a rather impressive body of scientific research. As such, the practices can represent valuable tools for clinicians and supervisors who work with human service staff to ensure behavior plans are carried out in a proficient manner. Nevertheless, continued research is warranted to further improve means of working with human service personnel to ensure that supports and services for people who have developmental disabilities are provided in the best manner possible.

In light of the currently available, evidence-based technology for training and supervising the work performance of direct support staff, an apparent need for continued research is better dissemination and adoption of the technology within human service settings. Empirically substantiated, behaviorally based strategies for working with staff are appropriately practiced in relatively few human service agencies, or are practiced only in a small part of agency operations (Babcocket al., 1998; Sturmey, 1998). Precisely why the strategies are not employed on a more widespread basis is not entirely clear and warrants the attention of investigators. Perhaps one reason is that though effective, behavioral approaches to staff training and supervision can be somewhat time consuming and labor intensive (Phillips, 1998). Research is warranted to further refine the approaches to enhance the efficiency with which they can be successfully applied. Research is likewise warranted to train supervisors in the knowledge and skills for applying the existing technology of staff training and supervision (Sturmey & Stiles, 1996). If more supervisors in human service settings become skilled in applying effective staff training and supervisory strategies, then staff proficiency in applying behavioral procedures can be enhanced. In turn, more agency consumers with developmental disabilities can experience the therapeutic value of behavioral applications as illustrated throughout other chapters in this text.

References

Alvero, A. M., Bucklin, B. R., & Austin, J. (2001). An objective review of the effectiveness and essential characteristics of performance feedback in organizational settings (1985-1998). *Journal of Organizational Behavior Management, 21(1)*, 3-29.

Arco, L. (1993). A case for researching performance pay in human service management. *Journal of Organizational Behavior Management, 14(1)*, 117-136.

Arco, L., & Birnbrauer, J. S. (1990). Performance feedback and maintenance of staff behavior in residential settings. *Behavioral Residential Treatment, 5*, 207-217.

Babcock, R. A., Fleming, R. K., & Oliver, J. R. (1998). OBM and quality improvement systems. *Journal of Organizational Behavior Management, 18(2/3)*, 33-59.

Baer, D. M.., Wolf, M. M., & Risley, T. R. (1968). Some current dimensions of applied behavior analysis. *Journal of Applied Behavior Analysis, 1*, 91-97.

Baer, D. M., Wolf, M. M., & Risley, T. R. (1987). Some still-current dimensions of applied behavior analysis. *Journal of Applied Behavior Analysis, 20*, 313-327.

Balcazar, F., Hopkins, B. L., & Suarez, Y. (1986). A critical, objective review of performance feedback. *Journal of Organizational Behavior Management, 7(3/4)*, 65-89.

Burch, M. R., Reiss, M. L., & Bailey, J. S. (1987). A competency based "hands-on" training package for direct care staff. *Journal of The Association for Persons with Severe Handicaps, 12*, 67-71.

Christian, W. P., Hannah, G. T., & Glahn, T. J. (Eds.). (1984). *Programming effective human services: Strategies for institutional change and client transition.* New York: McGraw-Hill.

Daniels, A. C. (1994). *Bringing out the best in people: How to apply the astonishing power of positive reinforcement.* New York: McGraw-Hill.

Demchak, M. A. (1987). A review of behavioral staff training in special education settings. *Education and Training in Mental Retardation, 22*, 205-217.

Everson, J. M., & Reid, D. H. (1999). *Person-centered planning and outcome management: Maximizing organizational effectiveness in supporting quality lifestyles among people with disabilities.* Morganton, NC: Habilitative Management Consultants.

Fleming, R., & Sulzer-Azaroff, B. (1992). Reciprocal peer management: Improving staff instruction in a vocational training program. *Journal of Applied Behavior Analysis, 25*, 611-620.

Ford, J. E. (1980). A classification system for feedback procedures. *Journal of Organizational Behavior Management, 2(3),* 183-191.

Gardner, J. M. (1972). Teaching behavior modification to nonprofessionals. *Journal of Applied Behavior Analysis, 5,* 517-521.

Gardner, J. M. (1973). Training the trainers: A review of research on teaching behavior modification. In R. D. Rubin, J. P. Brady, & J. D. Henderson (Eds.), *Advances in behavior therapy Vol. 4* (pp. 145-158). New York: Academic Press.

Harchik, A. E., & Campbell, A. R. (1998). Supporting people with developmental disabilities in their homes in the community: The role of organizational behavior management. *Journal of Organizational Behavior Management, 18,* 2/3, 83-101.

Harchik, A. E., Sherman, J. A., Hopkins, B. L., Strouse, M. C., & Sheldon, J. B. (1989). Use of behavioral techniques by paraprofessional staff: A review and proposal. *Behavioral Residential Treatment, 4,* 331-357.

Hastings, R. P., & Brown, T. (2000). Functional assessment and challenging behaviors: Some future directions. *Journal of The Association for Persons with Severe Handicaps, 25,* 229-240.

Holburn, S., & Vietze, P. M. (Eds.) (2002). *Person-centered planning: Research, practice, and future directions.* Baltimore: Paul H. Brookes.

Iwata, B. A., Bailey, J. S., Brown, K. M., Foshee, T. J., & Alpern, M. (1976). A performance-based lottery to improve residential care and training by institutional staff. *Journal of Applied Behavior Analysis, 9,* 417-431.

Jahr, E. (1998). Current issues in staff training. *Research in Developmental Disabilities, 19,* 73-87.

Jones, F. H., & Eimers, R. C. (1975). Role playing to train elementary teachers to use a classroom management "skill package". *Journal of Applied Behavior Analysis, 8,* 421-433.

Knoster, T. P. (2000). Practical application of functional behavioral assessment in schools. *Journal of The Association for Persons with Severe Handicaps, 25,* 201-211.

Landesman, S., & Vietze, P. (Eds.) (1987). *Living environments and mental retardation.* Washington, DC: American Association on Mental Retardation.

Lattimore, J., Stephens, T. E., Favell, J. E., & Risley, T. R. (1984). Increasing direct care staff compliance to individualized physical therapy body positioning prescriptions: Prescriptive checklists. *Mental Retardation, 22,* 79-84.

Mansdorf, I. J., & Burstein, Y. (1986). Case manager: A clinical tool for training residential treatment staff. *Behavioral Residential Treatment, 1,* 155-167.

McGimsey, J. F., Greene, B. F., & Lutzker, J. R. (1995). Competence in aspects of behavioral treatment and consultation: Implications for service delivery and graduate training. *Journal of Applied Behavior Analysis, 28,* 301-315.

Miller, L. M. (1978). *Behavior management: The new science of managing people at work.* New York: John Wiley & Sons.

Neef, N. A. (1995). Research on training trainers in program implementation: An introduction and future directions. *Journal of Applied Behavior Analysis, 28,* 297-299.

Parsons, M. B. (1998). A review of procedural acceptability in organizational behavior management. *Journal of Organizational Behavior Management, 18,* 2/3, 173-190.

Parsons, M. B., & Reid, D. H. (1995). Training residential supervisors to provide feedback for maintaining staff teaching skills with people who have severe disabilities. *Journal of Applied Behavior Analysis, 28,* 317-322.

Parsons, M. B., Reid, D. H., & Green, C. W. (1996). Training basic teaching skills to community and institutional support staff for people with severe disabilities: A one-day program. *Research in Developmental Disabilities, 17,* 467-485.

Parsons, M. B., Reid, D. H., & Crow, R. E. (in press). The best and worst ways to motivate staff in community agencies: A brief survey of supervisors. *Mental Retardation.*

Peck, C. A., Killen, C. C., & Baumgart, D. (1989). Increasing implementation of special education instruction in mainstream preschools: Direct and generalized effects of nondirective consultation. *Journal of Applied Behavior Analysis, 22,* 197-210.

Phillips, J. F. (1998). Applications and contributions of organizational behavior management in schools and day treatment settings. *Journal of Organizational Behavior Management, 18,* 2/3, 103-129.

Prue, D. M., & Fairbank, J. A. (1981). Performance feedback in organizational behavior management: A review. *Journal of Organizational Behavior Management, 3(1),* 1-16.

Reid, D. H. (Ed.). (1998). *Organizational behavior management and developmental disabilities services: Accomplishments and future directions.* New York: Haworth Press.

Reid, D. H., & Parsons, M. B. (1995a). Comparing choice and questionnaire measures of the acceptability of a staff training procedure. *Journal of Applied Behavior Analysis, 28,* 95-96.

Reid, D. H., & Parsons, M. B. (1995b). *Motivating human service staff: Supervisory strategies for maximizing work effort and work enjoyment.* Morganton, NC: Habilitative Management Consultants.

Reid, D. H., & Parsons, M. B. (2000). Organizational behavior management in human service settings. In J. Austin & J. E. Carr (Eds.), *Handbook of applied behavior analysis* (pp. 275-294). Reno, NV: Context Press.

Reid, D. H., & Parsons, M. B. (2002). *Working with staff to overcome challenging behavior among people who have severe disabilities: A guide for getting support plans carried out.* Morganton, NC: Habilitative Management Consultants.

Reid, D. H., Parsons, M. B., & Green, C. W. (1989a). Treating aberrant behavior through effective staff management: A developing technology. In E. Cipani (Ed.), *The treatment of severe behavior disorders: Behavior analysis approaches* (pp. 175-190). Washington, DC: American Association on Mental Retardation.

Reid, D. H., Parsons, M. B., & Green, C. W. (1989b). *Staff management in human services: Behavioral research and application.* Springfield, IL: Charles C. Thomas.

Reid, D. H., Rotholz, D. A., Parsons, M. B., Morris, L., Braswell, B. A., Green, C. W., et al. (2003). Training human service supervisors in aspects of PBS: Evaluation of a statewide, performance-based program. *Journal of Positive Behavior Interventions, 5,* 35-46.

Reid, D. H., & Whitman, T. L. (1983). Behavioral staff management in institutions: A critical review of effectiveness and acceptability. *Analysis and Intervention in Developmental Disabilities, 3,* 131-149.

Risley, T. R., & Favell, J. (1979). Constructing a living environment in an institution. In L. A. Hamerlynck (Ed.), *Behavioral systems for the developmentally disabled: II: Institutional, clinic, and community environments* (pp. 3-24). New York: Brunner/Mazel.

Risley, T. R., & Reid, D. H. (1995). Management and organizational issues in the delivery of psychological services for people with mental retardation. In J. W. Jacobson & J. A. Mulick (Eds.), *Manual of diagnosis and professional practice in mental retardation* (pp. 383-392). Washington, DC: American Psychological Association.

Shoemaker, J., & Reid, D.H. (1980). Decreasing chronic absenteeism among institutional staff: Effects of a low-cost attendance program. *Journal of Organizational Behavior Management, 2 (4),* 317-328.

Shore, B. A., Iwata, B. A., Vollmer, T. R., Lerman, D. C., & Zarcone, J. R. (1995). Pyramidal staff training in the extension of treatment for severe behavior disorders. *Journal of Applied Behavior Analysis, 28,* 323-332.

Smith, T., Parker, T., Taubman, M., & Lovaas, O. I. (1992). Transfer of staff training from workshops to group homes: A failure to generalize across settings. *Research in Developmental Disabilities, 13,* 57-71.

Stoddard, L. T., McIlvane, W. J., McDonagh, E. C., & Kledaras, J. B. (1986). The use of picture programs in teaching direct care staff. *Applied Research in Mental Retardation, 7,* 349-358.

Sturmey, P. (1998). Overview of the relationship between organizational behavior management and developmental disabilities. *Journal of Organizational Behavior Management, 18,* 2/3, 7-32.

Sturmey, P., & Stiles, L. A. (1996). Training needs of shift supervisors in a residential facility for persons with developmental disabilities: Shift supervisor's and middle manager's perceptions. *Behavioral Interventions, 11,* 141-146.

Templeman, T. P., Fredericks, H. D. B., Bunse, C., & Moses, C. (1983). Teaching research in-service training model. *Education and Training of the Mentally Retarded, 18,* 245-252.

Thompson, T., Felce, D., & Symons, F. J. (Eds.). (2000). *Behavioral observation: Technology and applications in developmental disabilities.* Baltimore: Paul H. Brookes.

Wetzel, R. J., & Hoschoer, R. L. (1984). *Residential teaching communities: Program development and staff training for developmentally disabled persons.* Glenview IL: Scott, Foresman and Company.

Williams, W. L., Vittorio, T. D., & Hauserr, L. (2002). A description and extension of a human services management model. *Journal of Organizational Behavior Management, 22(1),* 47-71.

Table 1
**Books on Evidenced-Based, Behaviorally Oriented Approaches
to Staff Training and Supervision**

Title	Reference
Behavior management: The new science of managing people at work	(Miller, 1978)
Programming effective human services: Strategies for institutional change and client transition	(Christian, Hannah, & Glahn, 1984)
Residential teaching communities: Program development and staff training for developmentally disabled persons	(Wetzel & Hoschoer, 1984)
Staff management in human services: Behavioral research and application	(Reid, Parsons, & Green, 1989b)
Bringing out the best in people: How to apply the astonishing power of positive reinforcement	(Daniels, 1994)
Motivating human service staff: Supervisory strategies for maximizing work effort & enjoyment	(Reid & Parsons, 1995b)
Organizational behavior management and developmental disabilities services: Accomplishments and future directions	(Reid, 1998)
Working with staff to overcome challenging behavior among people who have severe disabilities: A guide for getting support plans carried out	(Reid & Parsons, 2002)

Table 2
Selected articles and book chapters that review and/or describe evidenced-based, behavioral approaches to staff training and supervision in the human services

Title	Reference
Training the trainers: A review of research on teaching behavior modification	(Gardner, 1973)
Performance feedback in organizational behavior management: A review	(Prue & Fairbank, 1981)
Behavioral staff management in institutions: A critical review of effectiveness and acceptability	(Reid & Whitman, 1983)
A critical, objective review of performance feedback	(Balcazar, Hopkins, & Suarez, 1986)
A review of behavioral staff training in special education settings	(Demchak, 1987)
Use of behavioral techniques by paraprofessional staff	*(Harchik, Sherman, Hopkins, Strouse, & Sheldon, 1989)*
Performance feedback and maintenance of staff behavior in residential settings	(Arco & Birnbrauer, 1990)
Current issues in staff training	(Jahr, 1998)
Organizational behavior management in human service settings	(Reid & Parsons, 2000)
An objective review of effectiveness and essential characteristics of performance feedback in organizational settings	(Alvero, Bucklin, & Austin, 2001)

Table 3
Protocol for a performance- and competency-based strategy for training staff how to carry out behavior plans

Training step	Trainer action
1	Describe each procedure to be carried out
2	Provide each staff trainee with a concise, written summary of each procedure to be carried out
3	Physically demonstrate how to carry out each procedure typically in a role-play situation)
4	Have each trainee practice carrying out the procedure
5	Observe each trainee=s practice and provide supportive and corrective feedback
6	Repeat Steps 4 and 5 until each trainee demonstrates competence in performing each procedure to be carried out

Table 4
Protocol for Providing Supportive and Corrective Feedback to Staff Regarding Observed Performance in Carrying Out a Behavior Plan

Feedback step	Supervisor (or clinician) action
1	Begin feedback session with a positive statement regarding the staff person's overall performance
2	Specify procedures within the behavior plan that the staff person carried out correctly
3	Specify procedures within the behavior plan that the staff person carried out incorrectly (if applicable)
4	Specify precisely how to correctly perform the procedures carried out incorrectly by the staff person (if applicable)
5	Ask the staff person if anything needs clarification regarding the feedback presented or if s/he has any questions
6	Inform the staff person when his/her performance in carrying out the plan will be observed again
7	End the feedback session with an overall positive or encouraging statement regarding the staff person=s performance in carrying out the plan

Functional Analysis of Maladaptive Behaviors: Current Status and Future Directions

Peter Sturmey Ph.D. & Haven Bernstein
Department of Psychology Queens College and The Graduate Center,
City University of New York

A functional analysis is said to be the hallmark of behavior analysis. The approach is enshrined in the methods of research papers that investigate the causes of both adaptive and maladaptive behavior. Functional analysis is also a cornerstone of professional practice and is the basis of behavioral interventions which teach appropriate behaviors and reduce maladaptive behaviors. More broadly, functional analysis is also the basic method of investigation in behavior analysis, a natural history approach to the science of behaviors which, some have claimed, is a distinct paradigm or school of psychology (Chiesa, 1994).

There are many kinds of behaviorism. Radical behaviorism is a philosophy of science that informs research and practice in this area (Skinner, 1969: p. 221.) This theory is distinguished on two grounds from other kinds of psychology. First, it has considerable internal consistency concerning the kinds of data collected, their methods of interpretation and the kinds of causes of behavior that may be considered. Second, it rejects classical hypothetico-deductive science, group designs and inferential statistics. Instead functional analysis is characterized by the intense study of a small number of individual organisms, systematic replication of observations, and the gradual evolution principles and laws derived by induction, rather than hypothesis testing (Chiesa, 1994: p. 7). The functional analysis of the behavior of individual organisms is used to identify these principles and laws of behavior.

Definitions of functional analysis

Skinner (1953) examined the question 'why do organisms behave?' He forwarded the notion that the traditional question of cause and effect should be abandoned: it should be replaced by a descriptive, functional relationship between an independent variable and a dependent variable. In this approach there is no search for the causes of behavior, rather there is a search for a description of the variables of which behavior is a function. Skinner noted that there are many popular notions of the causes of behavior such as astrology and numerology. Within some kinds of science, neural causes, such as brain damage, and other inner psychic causes—a person's personality, mind, ideas, impulses, appetite and instincts—are commonly said to be causes of behavior. Skinner rejected these causes. He did so because they are unobservable, mentalistic, and evoke unobservable variables as the causes of behavior. Instead, Skinner proposed that the causes of behavior are located in the environment around the organism and in its history. For example, in order to explain—or develop a functional analysis of—the behavior of drinking, we must identify the environmental variables that can change the probability of drinking. By manipulating these independent variables we can discover functional relationships between them and the probability of drinking. Thus, we could manipulate the time since water was last drunk, the room temperature, or ingestion of salt and then measure the probability of drinking.

 This approach is conceptually parallel to a field of mathematics that is also called functional analysis and that describes the relationship of functions. Hence, in many behavioral functional analyses we may be interested in parametric manipulation of some measurable dimension of the environment, such as rate of non-contingent presentation of water or force required to operate a lever, and observing the shape of the function that emerges. The possible relationships between independent and dependent variables are many. They could be linear, quadratic, 'U'-shaped, inverted 'U'-shaped and may only be observed within certain limited values of the independent variable (Haynes, 1988; Haynes & O'Brien, 1990). A functional analysis may be incomplete. Demonstration of a functional relationship between one independent variable and a dependent variable does not preclude other functional analyses or refinements of the known functional analysis.

Skinner goes on to refine the notion of functional analysis defining functional analysis as "The external variables of which behavior is a function provide for what may be called a causal or functional analysis. We undertake to predict and control the be-

havior of the individual organism" (p. 35). (This latter issue of prediction and control of behavior has been philosophically and ideologically unpalatable to many,
including many ideologues and advocates in the mental retardation community.)
Skinner's (1953) Science and human behavior provided a utopian vision of behavior
analysis. Behavior analysis had largely not been applied to human behavior. Nevertheless, he proposed that it should be extended to explain and change the behavior of
both individual human organisms in such diverse arenas as education, work, clinical
problems, language, social behavior, and also to explain and change society at large,
including the government, law, and even to designing entire cultures.

Skinner's work influenced the development of applied behavior analysis and the notion of functional analysis. Baer, Wolf and Risley (1968) defined functional analysis
as follows: "… the analysis of a behavior … requires a believable demonstration of
the events that can be responsible for the occurrence or non-occurrence of a behavior
… an ability of an experimenter to turn the behavior on and off … "(p. 93-94).
Haynes and O'Brien (1990) refined this notion further. They noted that practitioners were only interested in certain kinds of independent variables that might be the
cause of behavior. Some variables, such as age, gender, and physical characteristics,
cannot be manipulated: they cannot be independent variables. Likewise, practitioners are generally interested in large, rather than subtle, effects. They are only
interested in those independent variables that they can control. Hence, they wrote
that a functional analysis is " … the identification of important, controllable, causal,
functional relationships applicable to a specified set of target behaviors for an individual client … " (p. 654).

Functional analysis can be applied to any observable behavior. Over the years it has
become a dominant methodology to understand and treat maladaptive behaviors in
people with mental retardation (Sturmey, 1995). Functional analysis has also been
applied to a wide range of clinical problems, such as depression, anxiety, schizophrenia, problems of old age (Sturmey, 1996) and to non-human animals (e.g., Ferguson
& Rosalez-Ruiz, 2001). It has been applied to a very wide range of behaviors, including adaptive behaviors, skills and typical development. For example, Poulson,
Kyparissos, Andreatos, Kymissis and Parnes (2002) conducted a functional analysis
of generalized imitation in typically developing 12- to 14-month-old infants. They
observed that acquisition of generalized imitation was not a function of the presence
of a model alone; rather it was a function of the presence of a model and reinforcement of generalized imitation. Similarly, Fields, Reeve, Matneja, Varelas, Belanich,
Fitzer, and Shamoun (2002) conducted a functional analysis of the acquisition of

perceptual classes in students. (A perceptual class of stimuli is a set of different stimuli that all evoke the same response. For example, many line drawings, photographs and auditory stimuli might all evoke the word "mother", even though the stimuli are physically very different). They demonstrated that learning novel classes of perceptual stimuli in students was directly related to the number of domains and the number of stimuli used during training. These two examples show that functional analysis can be used as a framework to describe functional relationships in a variety of adaptive behaviors in typical infants and young adults.

Other uses of the term

The term 'functional analysis' has been used in a variety of other ways (Sturmey, 1996). For example, many practitioners use the conceptual framework of functional analysis, but they do not directly manipulate independent variables (Desrochers, Hile, & Williams-Moseley, 1997; O'Neil, Horner, Albin, Storey & Sprague, 1999). Instead, they simply describe the observed correlation between environmental events and behavior. In some cases correlation between environmental variables and behavior is not even observed: they are hypothesized from interview data. Such approaches may have great practical value, but do not constitute a functional analysis. In order to distinguish them from true functional analyses they are referred to as functional assessments or descriptive analyses.

Within the legal framework of the *Individuals with Disabilities Education Act* (IDEA, 1997) the term functional behavioral assessment (FBA)is used. IDEA required that prior to any behavioral intervention that an FBA is conduced. An FBA may include experimental manipulation of an independent variable, but typically uses non-experimental methods. Lawyers, advocates and the courts decide what constitutes an adequate FBA. Hence, FBA is a legal term.

A variety of approaches to case formulation have become popular within clinical psychology (Sturmey, 1996; Tarrier, Wells, & Haddock, 2000). Case formulations share some features with functional analysis. For example, an attempt is made to identify the idiographic causes of each person behavior and base individualized treatment upon that information. However, there are several fundamental differences between these approaches. Case formulations usually incorporate a variety of non-observable variables, such as cognitions and attributions, do not use observational data, do not define independent variables operationally and do not experimentally evaluate the relationship between independent and dependent variables. Hence, these approaches have only a loose conceptual association with functional analysis.

The use of the term 'functional analysis' is restricted and has specific, narrow uses, although it is used loosely in a variety of other ways. When reading the literature the reader is cautioned to be aware of the way in which the particular author uses the term.

Methods of Functional Assessment

Current behavioral methods of intervening with maladaptive behaviors typically involve treatments based on the function of the behavior, rather than its topography. There are a variety of methods used for this purpose, including interviews, questionnaires, naturalistic observations, and the experimental analysis of behavior.

Desrochers et al. (1997) conducted a survey of the methods used by a large sample of practitioners to determine the functions of maladaptive behaviors in people with mental retardation. They found that interviews, ABC analyses, and checklists were most commonly used. Respondents ranked ABC checklists as being the most informative, and interviews were ranked second. These assessment techniques are the least rigorous, but take less time and skill to conduct than experimental methods. Since there are numerous environmental variables that can maintain behavior, assessment methods such as interviews, questionnaires, and observations may be necessary to identify the variables to be manipulated during a functional analysis. Indirect methods may only show correlations between variables and behavior, but they are a starting point at generating hypotheses as to the function of a problem behavior.

Interviews

An interviewer must enquire about the form of the behavior, its antecedents, consequences and establishing operations in order to determine the function of a behavior. Practitioners are encouraged to ask where, when, and how often the behavior occurs (O'Neil et al., 1999; Sturmey, 1996). Interviews can be used to obtain information about the client and the problem behavior from parents, staff, teachers, or anyone who knows the client well. Interviews should enquire about environmental antecedents and consequences, daily schedules, abilities, activities, staff, medications, medical problems, sleep patterns and more (Desrochers et al., 1997). McGill, Teer, Rye and Hughes (2003) developed a structured interview to assess the impact of setting events on behavior. An interview can also be used to collect information about a behavior's history, although the quality of such data is often unknown. Examples of structured interviews designed specifically for functional assessment include the Functional Assessment Interview (O'Neill et al., 1999), Functional Assessment Checklist for Teachers and Staff (March & Horner, (2002) and the Student Guided Functional Assessment Interview (Reed, Thomas, Sprague & Horner, 1997).

Interviews are commonly used: Desrochers et al. (1997) reported that 95% of practitioners reported using interviews to assess the function of maladaptive behaviors. Yet, relatively little is known about their contribution to a functional analysis. An informant must be able to discriminate the environment and the client's behavior in ways that are not intuitive. They must have the language to understand and respond to the interviewer's questions. The interviewer must have sufficient skill and training to be able to competently pose questions, and to interpret and analyze information gleaned; this requires specific training (Iwata, Wong, Riordan, Lau, 1982; Miltenberger & Fuqua, 1985; Miltenberger & Veltum, 1988).

Questionnaires

Information can also be obtained through questionnaires (Sturmey, 1994a). Examples that focus primarily on consequences include the Questions About Behavioral Function scale (QABF) (Matson & Vollmer, 1995), Motivation Assessment Scale (Durand & Crimmons, 1988), and the Stereotypy Analysis (Pyles, Riordan, & Bailey, 1997), which was developed to analyze the functions of stereotypy. Other instruments are broader in content and have also addressed antecedents and establishing operations. Examples include the Functional Analysis Checklist (Van Houten, Rolider, & Ikowitz, et al, 1989), which identifies a very wide range of environmental events that might be related to the target behavior and the Detailed Behavior Report (Groden & Lantz, 2001). These questionnaires provide guidelines for identifying variables maintaining problem behavior and can be readily administered to third parties, such as staff, professionals and family members.

One example of these questionnaires that has been researched extensively is the QABF. The QABF is a 25-item questionnaire including five subscales representing environmental variables found to typically maintain behavior (Applegate, Matson & Cherry, 1999). The five variables are attention, escape, tangible, nonsocial, and physical. Paclawskyj, Matson, Rush, Smalls and Vollmer (2000) reported that the QABF has acceptable test-retest and inter-rater reliability, as well as high internal consistency.

Several studies have also indicated the construct validity and clinical utility of the QABF. Dawson, Matson, and Cherry (1998) used the QABF and found that the variable maintaining problem behavior was more highly correlated with the topography of the behavior than with a particular diagnosis. They found that aggression was more likely to be a function of attention, that stereotypy was more likely to be automatically reinforced, and that there was no simple relationship between self-injury and behavioral function. Paclawskyj, Matson, Rush, Smalls and Vollmer (2001) showed that the QABF had good concurrent validity with the Motivation Assessment Scale. They also showed that the QABF was able to identify functions when analogue baselines failed to do so for low frequency / high intensity behaviors. Matson, Mayville and Lott (2002) reported further evidence of concurrent validity by showing the behavioral function as measured on the QABF was correlated with measures of social behavior in 100 persons with severe and profound mental retardation. Finally, Matson, Bamburg, Cherry and Paclawskyj (1999) demonstrated the clinical utility of the QABF in a treatment outcome study. In this study behavioral functions were identified in 84% of 398 persons with mental retardation. Further, behavioral interventions based on hypotheses derived from the QABF were more effective in reducing target behaviors than treatment as usual. Thus, there is considerable evidence that the QABF is reliable, valid and clinically useful.

There have been many concerns over the lack of reliability and validity of these questionnaires (Paclawskyj et al., 2000; Sigafoos, Kerr, & Roberts, 1994; Sturmey, 1994a, 1995, 2001). For example, Sigafoos et al. (1994) used the MAS to identify variables maintaining aggressive behavior and found low inter-rater reliability. A number of methods of calculating reliability between two raters fell short of the generally accepted standard. Poor inter-rater reliability was also found using the Functional Analysis Checklist (Sturmey, 2001). The Functional Analysis Checklist contained many items and most items on the checklist were typically not scored. When they were, the other rater rarely agreed with the first observer. Future research should continue to attend to the reliability of psychometric instruments in this area.

Naturalistic Direct Observation

Unstructured observations. In addition to interviews and questionnaires, direct observations can provide information regarding the function of a behavior. This can take a number of different forms (Sturmey, 1996). Merely observing the target behavior, or its precursors, may give rise to hypotheses concerning the function of the behavior. Careful observation of the stimuli to which the client approaches or avoids and observation of stimuli that staff or parents are reluctant to present may give valuable clues as to the function of the target behavior. For example, observation of whether a client approaches or avoids other people or objects, might give evidence for or against behavior maintained by positive reinforcement. Observation of client response to the presentation of educational, work or household tasks, the situations and people associated with these tasks might give evidence for or against behavior reinforced by escape from certain stimuli. Observation of indifference to environmental events, high rates of a target behavior at all times, or only when no alternative activity is available might give evidence for or against behavior that is reinforced by its consequences. Observation of the client's behavioral repertoire may also give clues as to the function of the target behavior. Observation of adaptive behaviors that might serve the same function as the target behavior might also give clues as to the function of the target behavior and may provide information useful when designing interventions. For example, a clinician might observe a sequence of behaviors in which a weak and ineffective adaptive communication response is followed by a strong and effective maladaptive behavior. This observation might give rise to clues as to the function of the target behavior and may aide the therapist in identifying replacement behaviors.

Analysis of baseline graphs may also be a useful source of hypotheses. Often the occurrence of a target behavior is very situation specific. The pattern of the distribution of responses over time may be a fruitful source of hypotheses concerning the variables that control the target behavior.

Scatter plots. Touchette, MacDonald and Langer (1985) noted that simple line graphs that average data over times of day may obscure important variation associated with time of day and location. Touchette et al. (1985) developed a scatter plot in which data are plotted in a two-by-two matrix by day and time of day. If there are patterns in which unusually high rates of behavior occur at certain times and unusually low rates of behavior occur at other times, then this may give clues related to the stimulus control of the target behavior. For example, observation of high rates of a target behavior associated with work suggests escape from demands. (Although other functions are possible, it would be wise to go observe further at work to see what happens there).

Scatter plots are used quite commonly (Desroshers et al., 1997), yet there is little research evaluating their utility. Kahng et al. (1998) analyzed scatter plots from 20 individuals living in four residential facilities. They selected 15 scatter plots with 30 days of data that met minimum reliability criteria and found upon visual inspection that <u>no</u> reliable patterns of responding were apparent. Using control charts, a statistical methodology for identifying trends and outlying data points in time series data, they found that 12 of 15 scatter plots indicated some form of stimulus control. Since there is relatively little data on the utility of scatter plots, no general conclusions were drawn at that time.

Analysis of conditional probabilities. A more sophisticated approach to the analysis of observational data is that which uses conditional probabilities. In this approach, the overall probability of the target behavior is calculated. Deviations from this overall probability are then explored in relation to environmental events. For example, Emerson et al. (1996) conducted a lag sequential analysis of the maladaptive behaviors of three children with mental retardation. They observed a variety of maladaptive behaviors, and their associated antecedent and consequential environmental events. The unconditional probability of Vicky climbing on adults was .016. However, when demands were placed on her this rose over 50% to .025. During social proximity to an adult and during social contact, both of which did not involve demands, the conditional probability of the target behavior fell by approximately one third to .010 in both cases. These deviations from the unconditional probability were all statistically significant.

Summary. There are a wide variety of descriptive methods used to identify the functions of maladaptive behaviors. Many practitioners freely use several methods within the assessment of an individual client's behavior. These methods are generally easy to use, as they only require relatively simple skills, such as interviewing, or graphing data. This factor may well be one of the reasons that these methods are widely used (Desrochers et al., 1997). However, descriptive assessments suffer from some significant limitations. First, they are correlational and necessarily involve confounded data. Merely knowing that a maladaptive behavior is more likely to occur after a staff member asks a client to engage in work, does not establish that escape from tasks is the consequence maintaining the maladaptive behavior. For example, alternative explanations such as escape other variables correlated with presentation of a demand, such as escape from social interaction, noise, crowding or some other person at work can not be excluded on the basis of correlational data. Because of the necessarily confounded nature of data from descriptive analyses, these methods cannot lead to sure conclusions about the function of a target behavior. Functional analysis methods can answer these questions.

Functional Analysis methods

The development of functional analysis methods was much influenced by the Carr's (1977) review of the functions of self-injury. He concluded that self-injury could be maintained by three broad classes of environmental events: positive reinforcement, such as attention or tangibles, negative reinforcement, such as the removal of educational or work demands, and the sensory or automatic consequences of the behavior (Carr, 1977). Carr then conducted a number of seminal studies demonstrating functional relationships between a variety of environmental events, such as escape from demands (Carr, Newsom & Binkoff, 1980), and lack of such as relationship leading to the hypothesis that the maladaptive behaviors were maintained by automatic reinforcement (Rincover, Newsom & Carr, 1979). These studies developed experimental conditions that could be used to identify the functions of maladaptive behaviors experimentally.

This methodology was then systematized into an assessment methodology known as analog baselines (Iwata, Dorsey, Slifer, Bauman & Richman, 1982 / 1994.) Typical analog baseline conditions involve systematically placing the participant in experimental conditions that may mimic the environmental conditions existing in the natural environment that may control the maladaptive behavior. Experimental control is demonstrated using a multi-element design. Commonly used conditions include attention, academic demands, alone and unstructured play. In the attention condition toys are available to the participant, while the therapist works nearby. The therapist does not interact with the participant, except for making statements of disapproval and physical touch contingent upon the target behavior. In the academic demand condition the therapist present educational or work activities appropriate for each participant and requests that the participant engage in these activities. If the participant engages in the target behavior the demands and therapist are removed for 30-s. In the alone condition the participant is placed alone in a room without access to any materials. Finally, in the unstructured play condition the participant is placed in a room with free access to toys. The therapist made periodic initiations and praises the participant for appropriate behavior, while the target behavior is ignored. Higher rates of the occurrence of the maladaptive behavior in one, but not the other, condition is taken as evidence for the function of the maladaptive behavior.

Analog baselines have been used to identify the function of a wide range of maladaptive behaviors such as self-injury, aggression, pica, inappropriate verbal behaviors, stereotypies etc. Researchers have developed additional experimental conditions, such as access to tangible item (Hanley, Iwata & McCord, 2003). They have also refined the most commonly used conditions, and have developed variants method- ologies that require less time (Sturmey, 1995, 1996; Vollmer & Smith, 1996) such as a variety of brief probe methods that can be conducted in the natural environment (Aikman, Garbutt & Furness, 2003; Sigafoos & Saggers, 1995).

More recently, attention has been paid to idiosyncratic functions of problem behav- ior. Carr, Yarbrough, and Langdon (1997) used interviews, naturalistic observation and analog baselines to determine the functions of aggression, self-injury and other problem behaviors in two adolescents and a young adult with autism and mental retardation. These standardized methods yielded ambiguous or only partial results. For example, in the case of Sam the authors observed a modest increase in the fre- quency of problem behavior during demand sessions compared to attention sessions. However, they also noted that Sam had access to small objects such as wristbands during this analysis. When the authors ran the conditions again and precluded access to wristbands there was a much higher frequency of problem behavior during the demand compared to the attention condition. However, during the attention condi- tion Sam now held small balls. Thus, the authors observed an unplanned confound. In the final experiment an analysis of the potential idiosyncratic variables controll- ling variables was performed by comparing Sam's frequency of problem behavior during the attention condition during the presence or small or large balls. The au- thors found that when Sam had access to small balls that the frequency of problem behavior was near zero, but when he had access to large balls the frequency of prob- lem behavior was very large. The authors concluded that Sam's problem behavior was controlled by idiosyncratic variables not included in the analog baselines. Simi- lar analyses of the problem behavior of two other participants revealed that one person's problem behavior was controlled by the presence of puzzles, rather than books and a second person's problem behavior was controlled by the presence of specific magazines, rather than books. Hence, idiosyncratic variables not included in standard functional assessment and analysis methods controlled the behavior of in- terest..

Other examples of idiosyncratic variables come from the analysis of establishing operations that may mediate the effects of the current environment. For example, O'Reilly (1995) used attention, escape from demand, alone, and leisure conditions in order to identify the variable maintaining SIB in a man diagnosed with moderate mental retardation. Occurrences of SIB were undifferentiated in each of the condi- tions. In addition to the analogue baseline, scatter plot data revealed that SIB only occurred only when the man had been placed in respite care the previous night, regardless of the analogue condition. Use of an additional analog measuring SIB during days following respite care and days not following respite care confirmed these results. Horner, Day' and Day (1997) also used an analysis of establishing operations to design idiographic interventions for a variety of problem behaviors.

These studies suggest that it is important that practitioners should not rely excessively on standardized methods of assessment. Clinicians should carefully attend to integrating the results of both descriptive and experimental analyses. There may sometimes be variables that are not included in standard assessments that might be crucial in understanding the causes of problem behavior and that may have critical implications for the design of treatment plans

Another clinically important problem is that there is a proportion of clients for whom the function of their maladaptive behavior can not be determined. Sturmey (1994b) reported a case in which several descriptive and experimental methods were used to identify the functions of self-injury. All methods failed to identify a function. During the extensive assessment period the client continued to engage in high rates self-injurious behavior. Perhaps in some cases, some form of intervention, such as high density non-contingent reinforcement or some differential reinforcement of alternate behavior, could be put in place as assessment of the functions of the target behavior proceeds. Dura (1991) reported similar problems and was able to effectively eliminate aggression in an 11-year-old girl with profound mental retardation and multiple disabilities using differential reinforcement of other behavior and contingent restraint, despite the absence of knowledge of the functions of the girl's aggression.

Convergent validity

As various methods of assessing the functions of maladaptive behavior have been refined, the question has been posed as to whether or not different methods produce the same results (Sturmey, 1995). Given the widespread use of non-experimental methods (Desrochers et al., 1997), it would be desirable that these methods produce the same results as more expensive, labor intense experimental methods. Durand and Crimmins (1988) compared the results of the MAS with those obtained from analog baselines in eight children with developmental disabilities who self-injured. They found that the MAS identified a single function for each of the 8 children and the rate of self-injury was highest in the analog condition that corresponded to the function identified on the MAS. However, the results of the analog baselines conditions were presented as bar charts reflecting the average rate of the behavior in each condition. The authors did not present individual multi-element graphs for each subject making it impossible to judge whether or not experimental control of self-injury occurred in the analog conditions. They also reported a correlation of .99 between the MAS rankings and rates of self-injury in the analog conditions. The authors concluded that the MAS and analog baselines produced the same results.

Cunningham and O'Neill (2000) compared the results of interviews, rating scales, observations, and experimental functional analyses in three children with autism. First, teachers were asked to give their opinion as to why each child engaged in the problem behavior. Next, teachers generated hypotheses based on the Functional Assessment Interview (O'Neill et al., 1999). Third, the teachers completed the MAS. The teachers also conducted direct observations recording antecedent and conse-quent events. Finally, each child was exposed to a series of conditions by the experimenter in which environmental variables that may have been maintaining the target behavior were manipulated. Consistency in identifying the functions of mal-adaptive behaviors was noted across different methods of assessment, perhaps because the same teachers conducted most of the assessments. Thus, like Durand and Crimmins, these authors found evidence of good convergent validity.

Paclawskyj et al. (2001) examined the convergent validity of the QABF, the MAS, and analog baselines in 13 participants, mostly with profound mental retardation. The consumers were referred for assessment of the function of self-injury, aggression, tantrums and stereotypy. Similar results were found across the two questionnaires, but neither corresponded well with results obtained through analog baselines. The QABF and analog baselines produced the same result in 56% of the cases, the MAS and analog baselines produced the same results in 44% of the cases, and the QABF and MAS produced the same results in 62% of the cases. Hence, agreement between the three methods was modest. Additionally, analog baselines produced undifferen-tiated results in 3 of 13 participants because of the low rates of the target behaviors. Correlations between the QABF and MAS were statistically significant in only 5 of 16 correlations. Thus, there was modest and unacceptably low convergent validity be-tween the methods, even between the QABF and MAS. This finding strongly suggests that the results may be influenced by the methods used. Subsequent research has gone on to identify variables that might account for these divergent findings.

A possible explanation for the divergent results of these studies comes from Yarborough and Carr (2000) who compared the convergent validity of interviews using the Functional Assessment Interview Form (O'Neill et al., 1999) and experimental analyses of behavior for high and low frequency target behaviors. The participants were three adolescents with mental retardation. The authors found very good agreement between informant based functional assessments and experimental analyses of behavior, but only for high frequency target behaviors. Convergent validity was very poor for low frequency target behaviors. They concluded that there was good convergent validity between interview and analog baseline methods, but only for high frequency behaviors. They suggested that factors such as increased opportunity to observe the high frequency target behaviors and environment, the simplicity of the situation and the apparent high strength of reinforcers for high frequency target behaviors might all contribute the reliability of identifying the function of high frequency target behaviors.

Reed et al. (1997) conducted an interesting study using interview methods in which the results from teacher and student interviews were compared. Seven of the 10 students who participated had no categorical label, two were classified as having Attention Deficit Hyperactivity Disorder (ADHD) and one was classified as having ADHD and Severe Emotional Disabilities. Some aspects of the interview were moderately reliable such as identifying the type and number of target behaviors. Other aspects of the interviews, such as identifying the settings events and the implied treatment strategies, were very unreliable. Thus this study reported little convergent validity between two sets of interviewees.

Studies on the validity of the various methods of assessing the functions of maladaptive behaviors have produced divergent results. Some have found very close convergence between different methodologies and others have produced poor convergent validity. Yarborough and Carr's (2000) study suggests that perhaps the rate of the target behavior may be an important mediating variable, although no replication studies of this observation have yet been published. Other relevant factors, which may be important, such as training observers and reporters to accurately discriminate and report functions and the skills of clinicians interpreting divergent information, have yet to be explored.

Training in Functional Assessments

Early research in functional analysis focused on basic research and demonstration. As the notions of functional analysis moves from small-scale demonstration to being incorporated into practice and legislation, the issues of dissemination, staff training and support come to the fore. This section reviews research in training and dissemination of skills related to functional analysis.

Training in functional assessment skills

Interviewing. Interviewing is a component of descriptive analyses and a number of papers have addressed training professionals in the behavioral interviewing skills. Miltenberger and Fuqua (1985) used modeling rehearsal and feedback to teach behavioral interviewing skills to four graduate students. Clinician behavior was measured by developing a task analysis of the elements of a clinical interview and observing student behavior during simulated interviews. The students rapidly learned the skills, and expert raters rated their interview highly. Miltenberger and Veltum (1988) extended this finding in an analog study by evaluating the relative contribution of different components of the package to the acquisition of clinician interview skills in two studies. In the first study they demonstrated that undergraduate students learned interviewing skills using instructions, audio and video models. In their second study written materials alone were only effective in changing the interviewing skills of only two of six participants. The subsequent addition of modeling and feedback each contributed to an improvement in clinician interviewing skill. Iwata et al., (1982) reported similar results.

Conducting reinforcer assessments. In order to teach skills to individuals with disabilities, staff must be able to identify appropriate reinforcers for each individual client. Thus, identifying stimuli that function as reinforcers is an important component of a functional assessment and also an important component of developing an intervention based on assessment results. Lavie and Sturmey (2002) taught three staff members to conduct a paired-stimulus preference assessment (Fisher, Piazza, Bowman, Hagopian, Owens, & Slevin, 1992). The purpose of such a preference assessment was to identify items most preferred by the client and serve simultaneously as the most potent reinforcers. The procedure involved presenting two stimuli to the client at a time in all possible combinations. Data was taken as to which stimulus the client approached during each trial. Staff training consisted of a brief description of the procedure, a checklist describing each of the steps, a verbal description of the steps on the checklist, demonstration of the procedure using a videotape model, completion of the procedure, and feedback based on performance. Staff members successfully learned to carry out the preference assessment in about 80 minutes.

Efficient training procedures are very important in clinical settings. Research should examine the efficient training of both reinforcer assessment and other skills   necessary to treat individuals with disabilities effectively. For example, Lavie and Sturmey (2002) taught staff to conduct stimulus preference assessments, but did not teach them how to interpret or apply the data collected during the preference assessment. Future research should build on this study to identify and teach clusters of functional professional skills.

Training to conduct analog baselines. Iwata, Wallace et al. (2000) used written materials, videotapes instruction, a written quiz, rehearsal and feedback to teach conducting analog baselines to undergraduate students. These methods were shown to be effective in teaching functional assessment skills to undergraduates. Moore, Edwards, Sterling-Turner, Riley, DuBard, and McGeorge (2002) also trained two regular first and fourth grade teachers and one, fifth grade inclusion teacher functional analysis methodology. All three teachers had limited exposure to behavior-analytic procedures. Initially, teachers were provided with written and verbal information regarding analog conditions used during a functional analysis and presented with questions about the information. Next, simulated analog conditions were arranged with a graduate student playing the role of the client. The analog conditions included attention and demand. During all conditions the graduate student who role played the client emitted the same number of target responses, non-target problem responses, and appropriate responses. Data were taken on teacher performance. Observers recorded correct presentation of trials, appropriate use of prompts and physical guidance, implementation of escape contingent upon the target behavior, and teacher praise during the demand condition. They also recorded correct initiation of the condition, delivery of disapproval contingent upon the target behavior, and ignoring appropriate and non-targeted problem behavior during the attention condition. Feedback was provided for the teachers following each simulated condition. After training all three teachers implemented functional analyses conditions correctly.

In order for parents to conduct functional assessments of the behavior of their children, parents must be able to operationally define behavior and identify antecedents and consequences (McNeill, Watson, Henington & Meeks, 2002). Therefore, McNeill et al. (2002) developed a training package to teach parents to identify functions of problem behavior, develop treatment plans, and teach appropriate behavior. The training package included questionnaires used to identify problem behavior and its possible causes, instructions on how to operationally define behavior, identify antecedents and consequences, use reinforcement to increase appropriate behavior, and use various methods of differential reinforcement to decrease inappropriate behavior. Based on post-tests completed by the parents, it was concluded that four sessions may be sufficient to identify functions of inappropriate behavior and design treatment plans.

Training staff to implement interventions. To make practical use of functional assessment methods in clinical, school, and home settings, staff, teachers and parents must be trained in the use of such methods and the treatments derived from them. Behavior-reduction programs involve more intricate procedures than behavior-acquisition programs, and inappropriate behavior can sometimes impair the ability of staff to deal with the client (Shore, Iwata, Vollmer, Lerman, & Zarcone, 1995). While inconsistent use of appropriate techniques during behavior acquisition programs may still lead to some acquisition of skills, inconsistent use of appropriate techniques during behavior-reduction programs may intensify or prolong the occurrence of problem behavior. Shore et al. (1995) used a pyramidal technique of staff training in which supervisors were trained to collect data and review and implement treatment procedures, and teach the treatment procedures to direct-care workers. In order to validate the intervention and to demonstrate a functional relationship between direct care staff and client behavior, data were collected on both clients and direct-care workers' behavior. Following training by supervisors who had previously been trained on data collection, program implementation, and staff training, direct-care workers improved in their implementation of antecedent responses, consequences for inappropriate behavior, and consequences for appropriate behavior.

Reid et al. (2003) evaluated a state-wide program to disseminate positive behavioral support (PBS). The program incorporated training supervisors to promote PBS practices among their staff. In order for PBS to be implemented, both supervisors and staff must be trained. Supervisors must also be able to train new staff since turnover rates are sometimes high among direct-care staff. Successful training involves mastery of the knowledge and skills taught during training, generalization of the knowledge and skills to the workplace, and acceptance of the training program by participants. Some of the skills taught during training include defining behavior, identifying antecedents and consequences, teaching functional skills, and recording and analyzing data as well as knowledge of positive and negative reinforcement, methods of functional assessment, and problem solving. It is often insufficient to teach these skills using paper and pencils techniques or role playing. Trainers and supervisors must be able to observe the application of knowledge and skills in true clinical situations (Sawka, McCurdy & Mannella, 2002).

Future Directions

Clearly, functional analysis will continue to be an active area of future research (Hanley et al., 2003) and an important and expanding aspect of professional practice. Areas of future interest may include expansion of areas of application, refinement of independent variables and their relationships to maladaptive behaviors, clarification of the relationship between basic and applied research, early intervention, and staff training and dissemination.

Expansion and refinement of variables

Functional analysis methods have been applied most frequently to high rate SIB and, to a lesser extent, to other maladaptive behaviors in people with mental retardation. Often these assessments have taken place in analog settings, such as experimental rooms in university laboratories or in assessment rooms in inpatient units. More recently several researchers have implemented functional analyses in naturalistic settings such as clients' family homes (O'Reilly, 1995), school settings (Sasso et al., 1992) outpatient clinics (Derby et al., 1992; Vollmer, Northup, Ringdahl, LeBlanc, & Chauvin, 1996; Wacker et al., 1994). The range of independent variables included in a functional analysis has expanded. Sleep deprivation (O'Reilly, 1995), ear infections (O'Reilly, 1997), prior social interaction (O'Reilly, Lancioni, & Emerson, 1999), transitions from one activity to another (McCord, Thompson & Iwata, 2001), social proximity (Oliver et al., 2001), escape from noise (McCord et al., 2001) and idiosyncratic variables (Carr et al., 1997) have all been investigated. Establishing operations (Michael, 1982) have received greater attention (Iwata, Smith & Michael, 2000; McGill, 1999). Researchers have also addressed establishing operations, such as respite care (O'Reilly, 1996), background noise, mood (Carr, Magito, McLaughlin, Giacobbe-Grieco, & Smith, 2003), premenstrual distress (Carr, Smith, Giacin, Whelan, & Pancari, 2003), as well as the interactions between drugs and behavioral processes (Northup, et al., 1997).

Over time there has also been a progressive refinement of independent variables that have been evaluated within functional analysis. One example has been the progressive dissection of access to attention as a reinforcer. For example, Richman and Hagopian (1999) were unable to identify the function of two children's destructive behavior using regular analog baselines. However, based on interview information from staff they were able to identify specific types of attention that might be reinforcing for staff. Subsequent analyses were able to show that access to specific forms of attention reinforced destructive behavior. Thus, what was formerly a single independent variable might be analyzed in various ways. "Attention" might be given at various voice volumes, from various distances, with various contents (DeLeon, Arnold, Rodriguez-Catter, & Uy, 2003), and accompanied by a variety of different kinds of non-verbal behavior from the other person. The effectiveness of attention as a consequence may be affected by the availability of other consequences such as reprimands (Piazza, Bowman, Contrucci, Delia, Adelinis, & Goh, 1999). Sturmey, Lee, Reyer and Robek (2003) developed a modified stimulus preference assessment method to identify client preference for different staff members, thereby opening up the possibility of investigating the effects of access to individual staff members as an independent variable in future investigations of attention. Similar trends may be observed in the progressive dissection of differing aspects of escape (Smith, Iwata, Goh & Shore, 1995) and automatic reinforcement functions (Vollmer, 1994).

Another important trend has been the expansion of application of functional analysis to new problems and new populations. Functional analysis has been applied to treat a variety of mental health issues in people with mental retardation, such as phobias, depression, anxiety disorders, anger management problems and bizarre psychotic speech (Sturmey, Reyer, Lee, & Robek, in press). These methods have been applied to a wide range of clinical populations outside of mental retardation, including a wide range of mental health problems, in children, adolescents, adults and seniors (Sturmey, 1996, 2003). Currently research into the functional analysis of Attention Deficit Hyperactivity Disorder (e.g., Bicard & Neef, 2002; Northup et al., 1997), children with language delays (Vollmer et al., 1996), psychoses and seniors (Buchanan & Fisher, 2002; Heard, & Watson, 1999) appear to be very active and important areas of research.

Positive Behavioral Support

As noted above, PBS has become a very active area of practice and research, especially within special education. The recent initiation of the *Journal of Positive Behavioral Interventions* and publication of a substantial literature attest to the vigor of this field. PBS is characterized by a commitment to non-aversive interventions, skills building, environmental redesign, functional analysis and community-based intervention. Proponents of this approach also take a broad perspective on measuring outcomes across the person's entire life, including client satisfaction and adaptation, rather than merely assessing reduction in a target behavior. PBS will likely continue to be an important extention of the literature on functional analysis

Early intervention

Early work in behavior analysis paid considerable attention to infant and child development (Bijou, 1976; Bijou & Bear, 1961, 1965, 1967) and work in this area has continued (e.g., Poulson et al,. 2002). Recently there has been increased attention paid to early intervention and functional analysis, especially related to autism (New York Department of Health, 1999a, 1999b, 1999c). This renewed interest in behavior analytic approaches to infancy and early childhood has stimulated interest in descriptive research related to the development of maladaptive behaviors. Stereotypies are very common in infants and young children with developmental disabilities, including those enrolled in early intervention (Berkson, Tuma & Sherman, 2001; Kroeker, Unis, Sackett, 2002) where perhaps only 1 in 20 show SIB. As in typically developing children (Thelen, 1979, 1981), these behaviors often reduce over time (Berkson, 2002), although a significant minority of children continue to show high levels of these behaviors, which may be intense. The relationship of stereotypies and SIB displayed in infancy and early childhood to later clinically significant problems is not known due to the lack of longitudinal studies. However, some have speculated that they may be related and therefore early intervention to prevent or ameliorate later clinically significant problems may be possible. For example, lack of mobility (Murphy, Hall, Oliver, & Kissi-Debra, 1999; Smith & Van Houten, 1996) and in some cases lack of social contact (Hall, Oliver & Murphy, 2001a, 2001b) are correlated with the development of abnormal motor behaviors. Kurtz et al. (2003) used analog baselines to a series of 30 young children who showed a variety of forms of self-injury. The chidlren were all aged under 5 years (mean age of 2 years and 9 months) and self-injury began on average at 17 months. Most, but not all, had developmental delays or mental retardation. The authors were able to identify functions for 62% of cases of self-injury and for 87% of all problem behaviors. Oliver, Murphy and Hall's studies used functional assessment data collected by direct observation in natural settings over periods of up to many months. These studies sometimes also demonstrated the emergence of functions over time within an individual child, illustrating the possibility of functions being learned during the course of development. Thus, the more recently developed methods of functional analysis are beginning to influence research into early intervention. For example, Kurtz et al (2003) went on to develop behavioral interventions for all 30 children in their series and achieved very large reductions in self-injury and combined behavior problems for almost all of their children.

Staff training and dissemination

The earlier section in the chapter indicated that some work has been done on teaching and disseminating skills related to functional analysis. Certification of behavior analysts, post-licensure professional training, the availability of better books and practice manuals for practitioners, better clinical tools to use to conduct a functional analysis will all continue to assist in the dissemination of better, more accurate functional analyses. Nevertheless, there are a large numbers of teachers, classroom assistants, psychologists, behavior analysts, counselors and family members who need support to participate in, conduct and use a functional analysis. At this time we do not have a good empirical basis for determining the training needs of these different audiences. It seems likely that different audiences need training in different skill clusters. Some may only need to accurately report what they have seen. Others may need to accurately complete an assigned procedure, such as a reinforcer assessment. However, professional staff and consultants may need a more complex set of skills.

References

Aikman, G., Garbutt, V. & Furness, F. (2003). Brief probes a method for analyzing the function of disruptive behaviour in the natural environment. *Behavioural and Cognitive Psychotherapy, 31*, 215-220.

Applegate, H., Matson, J. L., & Cherry, K. E. (1999). An evaluation of functional variables affecting severe problem behaviors in adults with mental retardation by using the Questions about Behavioral Function Scale (QABF). *Research in Developmental Disabilities, 20*, 229-237.

Baer, D. M., Wolf, M. M., & Risley, T. R. (1968). Some current dimensions of applied behavior analysis. *Journal of Applied Behavior Analysis, 1*, 91-97.

Berkson, G. (2002). Early development of stereotyped and self-injurious behaviors: II. Age trends. *American Journal on Mental Retardation, 107*, 468-477.

Berkson, G., Tupa, M., & Sherman, L. (2001). Early development of stereotyped and self-injurious behaviors: I. Incidence. *American Journal on Mental Retardation, 106*, 539-547.

Bicard, D. F., & Neef, N. A. (2002). Effects of strategic versus tactical instructions on adaptation to changing contingencies in children with ADHD. *Journal of Applied Behavior Analysis, 35*, 375-389.

Bijou, S. W. (1976). *Child development: The basic stage of early childhood.* Englewood Cliffs, NJ: Prentice-Hall.

Bijou, S. W. & Baer, D. M. (1961). *Child development: A systematic and empirical theory. Volume I,* New York: Appleton-Century-Crofts.

Bijou, S. W. & Baer, D. M. (1965). *Child development: Universal state of infancy. Volume II.* New York: Appleton-Century-Crofts.

Bijou, S. W. & Baer, D. M. (Eds.). (1967). *Child development: Readings in experimental analysis.* New York: Appleton-Century-Crofts.

Buchanan, J. A., & Fisher, J. E. (2002). Functional assessment and noncontingent reinforcement in the treatment of disruptive vocalization in elderly dementia patients. *Journal of Applied Behavior Analysis, 35,* 99-103.

Carr, E. G. (1977). The motivation of self-injurious behavior: A review of some ypotheses. *Psychological Bulletin, 84,* 800-816.

Carr, E. G., Magito, McLaughlin, D., Giacobbe-Grieco, T., & Smith, C. E. (2003). Using mood ratings and mood induction in assessment and intervention for severe problem behavior. *American Journal on Mental Retardation, 108,* 32-55.

Carr, E. G., Newsom, C. D., & Binkoff, J. A. (1980). Escape as a factor in the aggressive behavior of two retarded children. *Journal of Applied Behavior Analysis, 13,* 101-117.

Carr, E. G. , Smith, C. E., Giacin, T. A., Whelan, B. M., & Pancari, J. (2003). Menstrual discomfort as a biological setting event for severe problem behavior: Assessment and intervention. *American Journal on Mental Retardation, 108,* 117-133.

Carr, E. G., Yarbrough, S. C. & Langdon, N. A. (1997). Effects of idiosyncratic stimulus variables on functional analysis outcomes. *Journal of Applied Behavior Analysis, 30,* 673-686.

Chiesa, M. (1994). *Radical behaviorism: The philosophy and the science.* Boston, MA: Authors Cooperative Inc. Publishers.

Cunningham, E., & O'Neill, R. E. (2000). A comparison of results of functional assessment and analysis procedures with young children with autism. *Education and Training in Mental Retardation and Developmental Disabilities, 35,* 406-414.

Dawson, J. E., Matson, J. L., & Cherry, K. E. (1998). An analysis of maladaptive behaviors in persons with autism, PDD-NOS, and mental retardation. *Research in Developmental Disabilities, 19,* 439-448.

DeLeon, I. G., Arnold, K. L., Rodriguez-Catter, V., & Uy, M. L. (2003). Covariation between bizarre and nonbizarre speech as a function of the content of verbal attention. *Journal of Applied Behavior Analysis, 36,* 101-104.

Derby, K. M., Wacker, D. P., Sasso, G., Steege, M., Northup, J., Cigrand, K., et al. (1992). Brief functional assessments techniques to evaluate aberrant behavior in an outpatient setting: A summary of 79 cases. *Journal of Applied Behavior Analysis, 25,* 713-721.

Desrochers, M. N., Hile, M. G., & Williams-Mosely, T. L. (1997). Survey of functional assessment procedures used with individuals who display mental retardation and severe problem behaviors. *American Journal on Mental Retardation, 101,* 535-546.

Dura, J. R. (1991). Controlling extremely dangerous aggressive outbursts when functional analysis fails. *Psychological Reports, 69,* 451-459.

Durand, V. M. & Crimmins, D. B. (1988). Identifying the variables maintaining self-injurious behavior. *Journal of Autism and Developmental Disabilities, 18,* 99-117.

Emerson, E., Reeves, D., Thompson, S., Henderson, D., Robertson, J. & Howard, D. (1996). Time-based lag sequential analysis of the functional assessment of challenging behaviour. *Journal of Intellectual disabilities, 409,* 260-274.

Ferguson, D. L., & Rosales-Ruiz, J. (2001). Loading the problem loader: The effects of target training and shaping on trailer-loading behavior of horses. *Journal of Applied Behavior Analysis, 34,* 409-424.

Fields L., Reeve, K. F., Matneja, P., Varelas, A., Belanich, J., Fitzer, A., et al. (2002). The formation of a generalized categorization repertoire: effect of training with multiple domains, samples, and comparisons. *Journal of the Experimental Analysis of Behavior, 78,* 291-313.

Fisher, W., Piazza, C. C., Bowman, L. G., Hagopian, L. P., Owens, J. C., & Slevin, I. (1992). A comparison of two approaches for identifying reinforcers for persons with severe and profound disabilities. *Journal of Applied Behavior Analysis, 25,_491-498.

Groden, G. & Lantz, S. (2001). The reliability of the Detailed Behavior Report (DBR) in documenting functional assessment observations. *Behavioral Interventions, 16,* 15-25.

Hall, S., Oliver, C., & Murphy, G. (2001a). Early development of self-injurious behavior: an empirical study. *American Journal on Mental Retardation, 106,* 189-199.

Hall, S., Oliver, C., & Murphy, G. (2001b). Self-injurious behaviour in young children with Lesch-Nyhan syndrome. *Developmental Medicine and Childhood Neurology, 43,* 745-749.

Hanley, G. P., Iwata, B. A., & McCord, B. E. (2003). Functional analysis of problem behavior: A review. *Journal of Applied Behavior Analysis, 36,* 147-185.

Haynes, S. N. (1988). Current models and the assessment-treatment relationship in behavior therapy. *Journal of Psychopathology and Behavior Assessment, 10,* 171-183.

Haynes, S. N. & O'Brien, W. H. (1990). Functional analysis in behavior therapy. *Clinical Psychology Review, 10,* 649-668.

Heard, K., & Watson, T. S. (1999). Reducing wandering by persons with dementia using differential reinforcement. *Journal of Applied Behavior Analysis, 32,* 381-384.

Horner, R. H., Day, H. M., & Day, J. R. (1997). Using neutralizing routines to reduce problem behaviors. *Journal of Applied Behavior Analysis, 30,* 601-614.

Individuals With Disabilities Education Act, Amended (1997). Washington, DC: US Department of Education.

Iwata, B. A., Dorsey, M. F., Slifer, K. J., Bauman, K., & Richman, G. S. (1982/ 1994.) Toward a functional analysis of self-injury. *Journal of Applied Behavior Analysis, 27,* 197-209. (Reprinted from *Analysis in Developmental Disabilities, 2,* 3-20, 1982).

Iwata, B. A., Smith, R. G., & Michael, J. L. (2000). Current research on the influence of establishing operations on behavior in applied settings. *Journal of Applied Behavior Analysis, 33,* 411-418.

Iwata, B. A., Wallace, M. D., Kahng, S., Lindberg, J. S., roscoe, E. M., Conners, J., et al. (2000). Skill acquisition in the implantation of functional analysis methodology. *Journal of Applied Behavior Analysis, 33,* 181-194.

Iwata, B. A., Wong, S. E., Riordan, M. M. & Lau, M. M. (1982). Assessment andtraining of clinician interviewing skills: Analogue analysis and field replication. *Journal of Applied Behavior Analysis, 15,* 191-203.

Kahng, S. W., Iwata, B. A., Fisher, S. M., Page, T. J., Treadwell, K. R., Williams, D. E., et al. (1998). Temporal distribution of problem behaviors based on scatter plot analysis. *Journal of Applied Behavior Analysis, 31,* 593-603.

Kroeker, R., Unis, A .S., & Sackett, G. P. (2002). Characteristics of early rhythmic behaviors in children at risk for developmental disorders. *Journal of the American Academy of Child and Adolescent Psychiatry, 41,* 67-74.

Kurtz, P. F., Chin, M. D., Huete, J. M., Tarbox, R. S. F., O'Conner, J. T., Paclawskyj, T. R., et al. (2003). Functional analysis and treatment of self-injurious behavior in young children: A summary of 30 cases. *Journal of Applied Behavior Analysis, 36,* 205-219.

Lavie, T., & Sturmey, P. (2002). Training staff to conduct a paired-stimulus preference assessment. *Journal of Applied Behavior Analysis, 35,* 209-211.

March, R. E. & Horner, R. H. (2002). Feasibility and contributions of functional behavior assessment in schools. *Journal of Emotional and Behavioral Disorders, 10,* 158-170.

Matson, J. L., Bamburg, J. W., Cherry, K. E., & Paclawskyj, T. (1999). A validity study on the Questions About Behavioral Function (QABF) Scale: Predicting treatment success for self-injury, aggression, and stereotypies. *Research in Developmental Disabilities, 20,* 163-1175.

Matson, J. L., Mayville, E. A., & Lott, J. D. (2002). The relationship between behavior motivation and social functioning in persons with intellectual impairment. *British Journal of Clinical Psychology, 41,* 175-1184.

Matson, J. L. & Vollmer, T. (1995). *Questions About Behavioral Function.* Baton Rouge, LA: Disability Consultants, LLC.

McCord, B. E., Thomson, R. J., & Iwata, B. A. (2001). Functional analysis and treatment of self- injury associated with transitions. *Journal of Applied Behavior Analysis, 34,* 195-210.

McGill, P. (1999). Establishing operations: Implications for the assessment, treatment, and prevention of problem behavior. *Journal of Applied Behavior Analysis, 32,* 393-418.

McGill, P., Teer, K., Rye, L., & Hughes, D. (2003). Staff reports of settings events associated with challenging behavior. *Behavior Modification, 27,* 265-282.

McNeill, S. L., Watson, T. S., Henington, C., & Meeks, C. (2002). The effects of training parents in functional behavior assessment on problem identification, problem analysis, and intervention design. *Behavior Modification, 26,* 499-515.

Michael, J. (1982). Distinguishing between discriminative and motivational functions of stimuli. *Journal of the Experimental Analysis of Behavior, 37,* 149-155.

Miltenberger, R. G. & Fuqua, R. W. (1985). Evaluation of a training manual for the acquisition of behavior assessment interviewing skills. *Journal of Applied Behavioral Analysis, 18,* 323-328.

Miltenberger, R. G. & Veltum, L. G. (1988). Evaluation of an instructions and modeling procedure for training behavioral assessment interviewing skills. *Journal of Behavior Therapy and Experimental Psychiatry, 19,* 31-41.

Moore, J. W., Edwards, R. P., Sterling-Turner, H. E., Riley, J., DuBard, M., & McGeorge, A. (2002). Teacher acquisition of functional analysis methodology. *Journal of Applied Behavior Analysis, 35,* 3-7.

Murphy, G., Hall, S., Oliver, C., & Kissi-Debra, R. (1999). Identification of early self-injurious behaviour in young children with intellectual disability. *Journal of Intellectual Disabilities Research, 43,* 149-163.

New York Department of Health (1999a). *Clinical practice guidelines: report of the recommendations. Autism / Pervasive Developmental Disorders. Assessment and intervention for young children (age 0–3 year).* Publication number 4215. Albany: New York Department of Health.

New York Department of Health (1999b). *Clinical practice guidelines: quick reference guide. Autism/Pervasive Developmental Disorders. Assessment and intervention for young children (age 0–3 year).* Publication number 4216. Albany: New York Department of Health

New York Department of Health (1999c). *Clinical practice guidelines: The guideline technical report. Autism / Pervasive Developmental Disorders. Assessment and intervention for young children (age 0–3 year).* Publication number 4217. Albany: New York Department of Health.

Northup, J., Jones, K., Broussard, C., DiGiovanni, G., Herring, M., Fusilier, I., et al. (1997). A preliminary analysis of interactive effects between common classroom contingencies and methylphenidate. *Journal of Applied Behavior Analysis, 30,* 121-125.

Oliver, C., Oxener, G., Hearn, M., & Hall, S. (2001). Effects of social proximity on multiple aggressive behaviors. *Journal of Applied Behavior Analysis, 34,* 85-88.

O'Neil. R., Horner, R. H., Albin, R. W. , Storey, K. & Sprague. (1999*). Functional assessment and program development for problem behavior: A practical handbook (2ⁿᵈ ed.).* Pacific Grove, CA: Brooks/Cole.

O'Reilly, M. F. (1995). Functional analysis and treatment of escape-maintained aggression correlated with sleep deprivation. *Journal of Applied Behavior Analysis, 28,* 225-226.

O'Reilly, M. F. (1996). Assessment and treatment of episodic self-injury: A case study. *Research in Developmental Disabilities, 17,* 349-361.

O'Reilly M. F. (1997). Functional analysis of episodic self-injury correlated with recurrent otitis media. *Journal of Applied Behavior Analysis, 30,* 165-167.

O'Reilly, M. F., Lancioni, G. E, & Emerson, E. (1999). A systematic analysis of the influence of prior social context on aggression and self-injury within analogue analysis assessments. *Behavior Modification, 23,* 578-596.

Paclawskyj, T. R., Matson, J. L., Rush, K. S., Smalls, Y., & Vollmer, T. R. (2000). Questions About Behavioral Function (QABF): A behavioral checklist for functional assessment of aberrant behaviors. *Research in Developmental Disabilities, 21,* 223-229.

Paclawskyj, T. R., Matson, J. L., Rush, K. S., Smalls, Y., & Vollmer, T. R. (2001). Assessment of the convergent validity of the Questions About Behavioral Function scale with analogue functional analysis and the Motivation Assessment Scale. *Journal of Intellectual Disabilities Research, 45,* 484-494.

Piazza, C. C., Bowman, L. G., Contrucci, S. A., Delia, M. D., Adelinis, J. D., & Goh, H. (1999). An evaluation of the properties of attention as reinforcement for destructive and appropriate behavior. *Journal of Applied Behavior Analysis, 32,* 437-449.

Poulson, C. L., Kyparissos, N., Andreatos, M., Kymissis, E., & Parnes, M. (2002). Generalized imitation within three response classes in typically developing infants. *Journal of Experimental Child Psycholology, 81,* 341-357.

Pyles, D. A., Riordan, M. M., & Bailey, J. S. (1997). The stereotypy analysis: An instrument for examining environmental variables associated with differential rates of stereotypic behavior. *Research in Developmental Disabilities, 18,* 11-38.

Reed, H., Thomas, E., Sprague, J. R., & Horner, R. H. (1997). The student guided functional assessment Interview: An analysis of student and teacher agreement. *Journal of Behavioral Education, 7,* 33-49.

Reid, D. H., Rotholz, D., Parsons, M., Morris, Braswell, et al. (2002). Training Human Service Supervisors in Aspects of Positive Behavior Support: Evaluation of a State-Wide, Performance-Based Program. *Journal of Positive Behavioral Interventions.*

Richman, D. M., & Hagopian, L. P. (1999). On the effects of "quality" of attention in the functional analysis of destructive behavior. *Research in Developmental Disabilities, 20,* 51-62.

Rincover, A., Newsom, C. D., & Carr, E. G. (1979). Using sensory extinction procedures in the treatment of compulsive-like behavior of developmentally disabled children. *Journal of Consulting and Clinical Psychology, 47,* 695-701.

Sasso, G. M., Reimers, T. M., Cooper, L. J., Wacker, D., Berg, W., Steege, M., et al. (1992). Use of descriptive and experimental analyses to identify the functional properties of aberrant behavior in school settings. *Journal of Applied Behavior Analysis, 25,* 809-821.

Sawka, K. D., McCurdy, B. L., & Mannella, M. C. (2002). Strengthening emotional support services: An empirically based model for training teachers of students with behavior disorder. *Journal of Emotional and Behavioral Disorders, 10,* 223-

Shore, B. A., Iwata, B. A., Vollmer, T. R., Lerman, D. C., & Zarcone, J. R. (1995). Pyramidal staff training in the extension of treatment for severe behavior disorders. *Journal of Applied Behavior Analysis, 28,* 323-332.

Sigafoos, J., Kerr, M., & Roberts D. (1994). Interrater reliability of the Motivation Assessment Scale: Failure to replicate with aggressive behavior. *Research in Developmental Disabilities, 15,* 333-342.

Sigafoos, J. & Saggers, E. (1995). A discrete trial approach to the functional analysis of aggressive behavior in two boys with autism. *Australia and New Zealand Journal of Developmental Disabilities, 20,* 287-297.

Skinner, B. F. (1953). *Science and Human Behavior.* New York: MacMillan Free Press.

Skinner, B. F. (1969). *Preface of Contingencies of Reinforcement* (1969). New York: Appleton-Century-Crofts.

Smith, E. A. & Van Houten, R. (1996). A comparison of the characteristics of self-stimulatory behaviors in "normal" children and children with developmental delays. *Research in Developmental Disabilities, 17,* 253-268.

Smith, R. G., Iwata, B. A., Goh, H., & Shore, B. A. (1995). Analysis of establishing operations for self-injury maintained by escape. *Journal of Applied Behavior Analysis, 28,* 515-535.

Sturmey, P. (1994a). Assessing the functions of aberrant behaviors: A review of psychometric instruments. *Journal of Autism and Developmental Disorders, 24,* 293-304.

Sturmey, P. (1994b). Assessing the functions of self-injurious behavior: A case of assessment failure. *Journal of Behavior Therapy and Experimental Psychiatry, 25,* 331-336.

Sturmey P. (1995). Analog baselines: A critical review of the methodology. *Research in Developmental Disabilities, 16,* 269-284.

Sturmey, P. (1996). *Functional Analysis In Clinical Psychology.* New York: Wiley.

Sturmey, P. (2001). The reliability of the functional analysis checklist. *Journal of Applied Research in Intellectual Disabilities, 14,* 141 – 146.

Sturmey, P. (2003). Aging-Related Behavioral Interventions. In P. W. Davidson, V. & M. P. Janicki (Eds.) *Mental Health, Intellectual Disabilities, and the Aging Process.* London: Blackwell.

Sturmey, P., Lee, R., Reyer, H., & Robek, A. (2003). Assessing preferences for staff: Some pilot data. *Behavioural and Cognitive Psychotherapy, 31,* 109-112.

Sturmey, P., Reyer, H., Lee, R., & Robek, A. (in press). Applied behavior analysis and dual diagnosis. In: N. Cain & P. Davidson (Eds.), *Training Handbook for Mental Health in Mental Retardation.* Baltimore, MD: Brookes Publishing Co.

Tarrier, N., Wells, A., & Haddock, G. (Eds., 2000). *Treating complex cases: The Cognitive Behavioral Therapy approach.* New York: Wiley. Thelen, E. (1979). Rhythmical stereotypies in normal human infants. *Animal Behaviour, 27,* 699-715.

Thelen, E. (1981). Kicking, rocking, and waving: Contextual analysis of rhythmical stereotypies in normal human infants. *Animal Behaviour, 29,* 3-11.

Touchette, P. E., MacDonald, R. F., & Langer S. N. (1985) A scatter plot for identifying stimulus control of problem behavior. *Journal of Applied Behavior Analysis, 18,* 343-351.

Van Houten, R., Rolider, A., & Ikowitz, J. (1989). *The Functional Analysis Checklist. Unpublished manuscript.* Reprinted in Sturmey, P. (2001). The reliability of the functional analysis checklist. *Journal of Applied Research in Intellectual Disabilities, 14,* 141 – 146.

Vollmer, T. R. (1994). The concept of automatic reinforcement: Implications for behavioral research in developmental disabilities. *Research in Developmental Disabilities, 15,* 187-207.

Vollmer, T. R., Northup, J., Ringdahl, J. E., LeBlanc, L. A., & Chauvin, T. M. (1996). Functional analysis of severe tantrums displayed by children with language delays. *Behavior Modification, 20,* 97-115.

Vollmer, T. R. & Smith, R. G. (1996). Some current themes in functional analysis research. *Research in Developmental Disabilities, 17,* 229-249.

Wacker, D. P., Berg, W. K., Cooper, L. J., Derby, K. M., Steege, M. W., Northup, J., et al. (1994). The impact of functional analysis methodology on outpatient clinic services. *Journal of Applied Behavior Analysis, 27,* 405-407.

Yarborough, S. C. & Carr, E. G. (2000). Some relationships between informant assessment and functional analysis of problem behavior. *American Journal on Mental Retardation, 105,* 130-151.

6

DATA COLLECTION AND OBSERVATION SYSTEMS

Erik A. Mayville
Pathways Strategic Teaching Center
Stephen B. Mayville
Louisiana State University

Introduction

Observation of behavior and collection of data are perhaps the most distinguishing characteristics of the science of behavior modification and applied behavior analysis. Identified as core components of the behavioral assessment approach, these processes facilitate formulation and evaluation of hypotheses regarding a variety of human behavior, and have fueled the evolution of behavioral technology that has occurred during the past 60 years. Interest in behavioral assessment continues to grow; in the past five years alone, at least 10 texts devoted to issues and methods in behavioral assessment have been published (e.g., Bellack & Hersen, 1998; Hawkins, Mathews, & Hamdan, 1999; Haynes & O'Brien, 2000; Lattal, & Perone, 1998; Ramsay, Reynolds, & Kamphaus, 2002; Sharpe & Koperwas, 2003). One peer-reviewed journal is devoted to applications of behavioral assessment (Journal of Psychopathology and Behavioral Assessment), and numerous others routinely feature research based on behavioral assessment procedures (e.g., Journal of Applied Behavior Analysis, Research in Developmental Disabilities, Journal of Behavior Therapy and Experimental Psychiatry, Behavior Modification). Thorough literature bases now exist in the behavioral assessment of mood disorders, anxiety disorders, marital dysfunction, sexual dysfunction and deviation, social skills, health-related disorders, child behavior problems, and appetitive disorders, to name a few (Bellack & Hersen, 1998). Additionally, behavioral assessment was taught in about one-half of all American Psychological

Association approved doctoral training programs in clinical psychology in the early 1990's (Piotrowski & Zalewski, 1993). Given the continued growth and trajectory of behavioral assessment technology, this number has likely increased in the past 10 years.

Researchers in the field of developmental disabilities have applied a variety of innovative data collection and observation procedures to many realms of caregiver and consumer behavior (see Sackett, 1978, and Thompson, Felce, & Symons, 2000, for reviews). Along with these developments has come widespread use of behavioral assessment procedures in both public and private service domains. Behavioral assessment is now a common component of "best practice" treatment approaches for persons with developmental disabilities (Ager & O'May, 2001). Within the broader context of behavior analytic services, behavioral assessment has been recommended by several state service delivery regulators as an indicated methodology for treatment of children with Autism Spectrum Disorders (e.g., California Department of Education, 1997; New York State Department of Health, 1999; Maine Administrators of Services for Children with Disabilities, 2000). Additionally, a number of state courts have rendered decisions favoring plaintiffs seeking applied behavior analytic services for children with Autism Spectrum Disorders in public schools (see Jacobson, 2000, for a review). Thus, behavioral assessment procedures are becoming an increasingly central component of education and treatment for persons with developmental disabilities.

This chapter provides an overview of basic data collection and observation systems as applied to persons with developmental disabilities of all severities. The distinction between direct and indirect methods of assessment is discussed first, followed by an overview of systematic applications of both methods. A review of direct and indirect methods of behavioral observation and data collection follows, and constitutes the bulk of this chapter. Also included is a brief discussion of functional assessment methodologies, as this assessment approach is now often the cornerstone of a comprehensive behavioral assessment system. Absent from this review is a description of technological advancements in behavioral assessment methodologies. Advances in technology during the last decade have yielded dramatic developments in computer-based applications of behavioral assessment procedures. We refer the reader to Thompson and colleagues (2000) for a more thorough survey of technological applications.

Data Collection and Observation Systems

Direct and indirect assessment

Data collection and observation systems are used primarily for assessment. *Direct assessment* refers to the actual observation of the behavior of interest, whereas indirect assessment involves information collection through less objective means, such as self-report from the individual of interest or verbal report through a third party observer. The development and growth of behavior analysis as applied to persons with developmental disabilities has been facilitated by hundreds of studies using direct assessment methods (see Iwata, Bailey, Neef, Wacker, Repp, & Shook, 1997). Data from direct observation of behavior in naturalistic or analogue settings is often used in identifying behavior associated with one or more classification systems (e.g., psychiatric disturbance, social skill, adaptive behavior). Direct observation can also provide an information base from which conclusions can be drawn regarding environment-behavior relations, particularly when target behavior is independently substantiated by two trained observers.

While the methods by which behavior is directly observed and reported are the focus of this chapter, the importance of indirect measures in comprehensive assessment processes should not be underestimated. Researchers in the field of developmental disabilities have recognized the importance of drawing upon information provided by caregivers, family members, and familiar others who have observed the behavior of interest on numerous occasions. Some of the most widely used assessment protocols in the domains of adaptive behavior and psychiatric disturbance are based on indirectly obtained information (e.g., Matson, Gardner, Coe, & Sovner, 1991; Sparrow, Balla, & Cicchetti, 1984; Reiss, 1988). Indirect observation and measurement tools that have been subjected to rigorous psychometric analysis may in some cases provide information that converges with information produced from direct assessment (Paclawskyj, Matson, Rush, Smalls, & Vollmer, 2001). Such measures may compliment direct behavior assessment procedures, or may be used in their stead when resources needed to conduct a comprehensive behavioral assessment are limited (Matson, Mayville, & Laud, 2003). In settings where a large number of individuals receive residential and/or habilitative services, there is often a need for information across many domains (e.g., problem behavior function, adaptive and problem behavior topography, psychiatric disturbance, therapeutic and side effects of psychotropic medications). A number of indirect assessments have been designed to measure these domains of behavior, and may significantly improve identification, classification, and understanding of the behaviors of interest (Kalachnick, 1999; Reiss, 1993; Singh, Sood, Sonenklar, & Ellis, 1991). For both economic and clinical reasons, a system of individual treatment and program evaluation may necessitate the use of indirect assessment procedures.

Systems of data collection and behavioral observation.

In efforts to organize various observational and data recording methods, classification systems have been developed that categorize such methods according to the degree to which they are direct. Cone (1978) detailed such a continuum for the classification of assessment methods typically used within the natural environment. Singh and colleagues (1991) adapted this system to classify observation methods frequently used to assess dual diagnosis among individuals with developmental disabilities. This system is organized along a continuum ranging from the most to least direct methods of behavioral observation. Methods of assessment that form this continuum are listed in Table 1.

Behavioral assessment systems

Over the last two decades, several behavioral assessment systems relevant to individuals with developmental disabilities have been described. Such systems may be employed within the context of a decision-making model that can involve the use of both direct and indirect behavioral observation strategies.

Behavior diagnostics model

Bailey and Pyles (1989) discussed a diagnostic system for challenging behavior in persons with developmental disabilities in which a number of variables (e.g., medical, physical, functional) are systematically examined through assessments that can involve both direct and indirect assessment approaches. Pyles, Muniz, Cade, and Silva (1997) subsequently extended this model to include psychiatric illness and treatment as primary variables to be considered in investigations of problem behavior. The revised system, termed the Howe Developmental Center Paradigm (HDC), is characterized by the use of different flowcharts for each major discipline contributing to an interdisciplinary treatment team (IDT). Flowcharts in the HDC paradigm help guide a process of assessment and hypothesis testing to determine whether problematic behavior is maintained by medical/physical, psychiatric, and/or environmental determinants of behavior. Assessment typically begins with a medical evaluation of the problem to rule out medical/physical discomfort issues before con-

Table 1
Continuum of behavioral assessment methods ranging from direct to indirect

Methods	*Measures*	*References*
Experimental analysis	Experimental manipulation of controlling variables in the natural environment	Iwata, Vollmer, & Zarcone (1990)
Direct behavioral observation in natural settings	A-B-C	Bijou, Peterson, & Ault (1968)
	Scatter plot	Touchette et al. (1985)
	Ecobehavioral assessment	Vyse, Mulick, & Thayer (1984)
Direct behavioral observation in analog settings	Role plays	Senatore, Matson, & Kazdin (1982)
Rating scales and checklists: Client	Zung Self-Rating Depression Scale	Zung (1965)
	PIMRA	Matson (1988)
	Beck Depression Inventory	Beck et al. (1961)
	Fear Survey Schedule	Duff et al. (1981)
	Prout-Strohmer Personality Inventory	Prout & Strohmer (1989)
	Self-Report Depression Questionnaire	Reynolds (1989)
	MMPI-168 (L)	McDaniel (1997)
Self-monitoring	Self-monitoring checklists	Shapiro (1984)
Interviews: Client	Hamilton Rating Scale	Hamilton (1960)
	Clinical Interview Schedule	Ballinger et al (1975)
Rating scales and checklists: Informant	Aberrant Behavior Checklist	Aman & Singh (1986)
	Adolescent Behavior Checklist	Demb et al. (1994)
	Assessment for Dual Diagnosis	Matson (1997)
	Behavior Problems Inventory	Rojahn et al. (2001)
	Diagnostic Assessment for the Severely Handicapped Scale	Matson, Gardner, Coe, & Sovner (1991)
	MESSIER	Matson (1995)
	Motivation Assessment Scale	Durand & Crimmins (1988)
	PAS-ADD	Moss et al. (1993)
	Reiss Screen for Maladaptive Behavior	Reiss (1988)
	Vineland Adaptive Behavior Scale	Sparrow, Balla, & Cicchetti (1984)
Interviews: Informant	Functional Analysis Interview	O'Neil et al. (1990)
	DICA	Herjanic & Reich (1982)
	DISC-P	Costello et al. (1984)
	DIS	Robins et al. (1981)

ducting a functional assessment for environmental determinants of problem behavior. Medical and functional/ecological variables are typically ruled out before an individual is assessed for psychiatric illness. If an individual is assessed for psychiatric illness, diagnostic criteria from the Diagnostic and Statistical Manual of Mental Disorders 4th Edition (APA, 1994) are operationally defined. Pyles and colleagues refer to these target behaviors as operationalized behavioral criteria (OBC's).

Given that problematic behaviors are frequently maintained by multiple functions, feedback loops are included in the flowcharts that allow for a more thorough assessment of such behaviors. This is one of the features that differentiates the HDC paradigm from similar systems of assessment (i.e., Sturmey, 1995). Although the HDC system is a highly structured approach to assessment, it still allows for the use of clinical judgement in prioritizing and implementing interventions. However, in any case, intervention is integrally linked to the results of assessment in the HDC paradigm.

An indirect system of assessment

Systems of observation involving one primary method of assessment across a number of behavioral domains have also been described. A comprehensive assessment system involving indirect observation has been offered by Matson and colleagues (2003). Given the limited resources often available to staff operating in developmental centers, a method of assessment that takes time constraints into account is necessary for the efficient delivery of services. Within the system of assessment described by Matson and colleagues, variables often relevant to comprehensive treatment planning for persons with developmental disabilities are considered. Included in the system are measures for the assessment of psychiatric disturbance, adaptive and maladaptive behavior, feeding disorders, social skill, function of problem behavior, and medication side effects. Given that symptom presentation frequently varies according to level of intellectual disability, domains such as psychopathology and social skills are assessed with different measures according to diagnostic classification of MR. Information gathered from these measures is assimilated and utilized in a manner similar to that of formal decision-making systems such as the HDC paradigm.

Direct assessment: Observation and data collection procedures

Central to systems of behavioral observation are the methods through which behavior is directly observed and recorded. These methods can be used in isolation or in combination to gather and interpret information directly observed in the environment.

Event recording

Event recording has been described simply as "a tally or count of behaviors as they occur" (Cooper, Heron, & Heward, 1987, p. 62). This method of recording has been widely employed with persons with developmental disabilities, and has included a wide range of desired and undesired behavior (Kelly, 1977; Tawney & Gast, 1984). This finding is not surprising given that the goal of many behavioral programs for persons with developmental disabilities is to decrease or increase the number of times a particular behavior occurs. The event recording approach is appropriate for behavior with a discrete beginning and end, and for behavior that lasts for a relatively constant period of time each time it occurs. It is particularly useful for events occurring at a low to moderate frequency; behaviors occurring at high rates may become difficult to accurately record. Pencil and paper measures are commonly used to record events, though a variety of low-tech (e.g., hand-held or wrist counters, tokens, tally boards) and high-tech (e.g., desk-top, lap-top, hand-held computers) methods (see Farrell, 1991, and Kahng & Iwata, 1998 for reviews). Data for event recording is typically collected during a particular interval of time, and then reported either as frequency, rate, or percentage of responding to response opportunities.

Reporting frequency of responding is indicated when there are consistent opportunities and lengths of time available for responding; rate of responding should be used for variation along these dimensions. Frequency is a widely used method of reporting in the assessment and treatment of problem behavior in persons with developmental disabilities (see Whitaker, 1996). Rate of responding is considered the most basic data of behavior analysis (Michael, 1985; Skinner, 1966), appropriate for measurement of behavior that is not controlled by opportunities to respond (Baer & Fowler, 1984). Calculating rate of response is achieved by dividing the total number of responses by the amount of time elapsed in responding. This reporting method is commonly used in assessing proficiency in task performance, particularly academic tasks. Precision teaching, an instructional evaluation system, relies on rate of responding as a primary datum and is becoming an increasingly popular teaching approach for children with autism (Greer, 1997; Kubina, Morrison, & Lee, 2002). Rate of responding is also commonly used in assessment of problem behavior function and treatment outcome assessment (e.g., Fisher, Kuhn, & Thompson, 1998; Vaughn & Horner, 1997). Percentage of responding is used when response opportunities vary and when the observer is not interested in proficiency of responding.

Typically, the number of correct or incorrect responses is divided by the total number of opportunities, and the quotient is multiplied by 100.

Duration recording

Behavior that is continuous, occurs at a frequency too high to accurately count, or occurs for extended periods of time is best measured along the dimension of duration of occurrence. Duration recording involves timing the duration of each episode of a target behavior from beginning to end, and transferring the observed duration value to a data sheet. Measures of duration can be implemented by either recording the total duration of a behavioral episode during an observation period, or through recording the duration per occurrence of multiple episodes during the observation period. The most accurate and commonly used method for duration recording is a stopwatch, though less accurate means such as a clock or wristwatch are also commonly used. Computer programs now exist that will record duration of behavior, and can report data in terms of total events observed, total duration of events, and average duration of observed events (Saunders & Saunders, 2000).

For persons with developmental disabilities, duration recording may be useful for a variety of purposes, including assessment of problem behavior (e.g., Kennedy & Souza, 1995), and in identifying preferred items or activities to be used in a variety of programming activities (Cotter & Toombs, 1966; DeLeon, Iwata, Conners, & Wallace, 1999; Gast, Jacobs, Logan, Murray, Holloway, & Long, 2000; Worsdell, Iwata, & Wallace, 2002). In duration-based preference assessments, the length of time of engagement with items and/or activities is recorded and a preference hierarchy is determined by comparing the duration of engagement for each item or activity presented. For example, Gast and colleagues (2000) used measures of duration of smiling and laughing to evaluate the effectiveness of brief pre-session stimulus preference assessments in predicting the levels of responding of four students with profound multiple disabilities. The duration of laughing and smiling in the presence of particular items presented in the pre-session assessment reliably predicted items that would evoke the same behaviors in social interactions. DeLeon and colleagues (1999) also used duration of engagement with stimuli to help differentiate preference for items for which a clear preference was not established in a traditional, multiple stimulus preference assessment. A duration-based measure improved conclusions about preference of stimuli and regarding predictions of the reinforcing value of the stimuli.

Interval Recording

Interval recording is a procedure wherein the occurrence of a target behavior is noted if the behavior occurs during a predetermined interval of time. Usually a clock or stopwatch is utilized to ensure that intervals are recorded reliably, and occurrence of the target behavior is typically represented in the percentage of intervals within which the target behavior occurred (i.e., number of intervals where the target behavior occurred / total number of intervals x 100).

Interval recording is classified as either partial interval recording or whole interval recording. Partial interval recording occurs when an observer records whether or not a target behavior occurs somewhere within the circumscribed interval. Partial interval recording does not take into account the number of times the behavior occurred, or the duration of the behavior within an interval. Whole interval recording, on the other hand, occurs when a behavior is noted only if it occurs for the entire duration of the interval, thus taking in to account the duration of a target behavior as a criterion for recording. Typically, partial interval procedures are used for behaviors that will be targeted for reduction, while whole interval procedures are typically used for monitoring behaviors that will be targeted for increase (e.g., attention span). When selecting between whole and partial interval techniques, one should keep in mind that whole interval procedures may underestimate the occurrence of behavior whereas partial interval recording may overestimate the occurrence of behavior (Cooper, 1987).

Partial interval recording may be conducted in either a continuous or end-on mode. In a continuous mode, recording intervals are consecutive (see Figure 1). This means that the observer must record the presence of a behavior within an interval where observation is taking place. With end-on partial interval recording, intervals are not consecutive. With the end-on approach, the observer may record the presence or absence target behaviors within an interval where observation does not take place. Thus, in a situation where the observer is observing multiple target behaviors, the likelihood the observer may miss a behavior within an interval of observation may be reduced.

Partial interval recording is one of the more frequent data recording procedures encountered in behavior analytic research·and there are numerous examples of recent well-designed studies that have utilized such procedures (e.g., Hanley, Iwata, Thompson, & Lindberg, 2000; Kennedy, Meyer, Knowles, & Shukla, 2000; Tincani, Castogiavanni, & Axelrod, 1999).

Figure 1.
Partial Interval Data Sheet (10 second)

Individual _____

Primary Observer _____

Reliability Observer _____

A= _____

B= _____

C= _____

Time | Condition _____ Date____

Reliability C — Tot Agr/Agr+Dis ___/___ = ___% | Occ Agr/Occ Agr + Dis ___/___ = ___% | Non Agr/NonAgr + Dis ___/___

Minute 1	A	10	20	30	40	50	60
	B	10	20	30	40	50	60
	C	10	20	30	40	50	60
Minute 2	A	10	20	30	40	50	60
	B	10	20	30	40	50	60
	C	10	20	30	40	50	60
Minute 3	A	10	20	30	40	50	60
	B	10	20	30	40	50	60
	C	10	20	30	40	50	60

Reliability B — Tot Agr/Agr+Dis ___/___ = ___% | Occ Agr/Occ Agr + Dis ___/___ = ___% | Non Agr/NonAgr + Dis ___/___

Minute 4	A	10	20	30	40	50	60
	B	10	20	30	40	50	60
	C	10	20	30	40	50	60
Minute 5	A	10	20	30	40	50	60
	B	10	20	30	40	50	60
	C	10	20	30	40	50	60
Minute 6	A	10	20	30	40	50	60
	B	10	20	30	40	50	60
	C	10	20	30	40	50	60

Reliability A — Tot Agr/Agr+Dis ___/___ = ___% | Occ Agr/Occ Agr + Dis ___/___ = ___% | Non Agr/NonAgr + Dis ___/___

Minute 7	A	10	20	30	40	50	60
	B	10	20	30	40	50	60
	C	10	20	30	40	50	60
Minute 8	A	10	20	30	40	50	60
	B	10	20	30	40	50	60
	C	10	20	30	40	50	60
Minute 9	A	10	20	30	40	50	60
	B	10	20	30	40	50	60
	C	10	20	30	40	50	60
Minute 10	A	10	20	30	40	50	60
	B	10	20	30	40	50	60
	C	10	20	30	40	50	60

A= ___/___ = ___%   B= ___/___ = ___%   RATES

Time | Condition _____ Date____

Reliability C — Tot Agr/Agr+Dis ___/___ = ___% | Occ Agr/Occ Agr + Dis ___/___ = ___% | Non Agr/NonAgr + Dis ___/___

Minute 1	A	10	20	30	40	50	60
	B	10	20	30	40	50	60
	C	10	20	30	40	50	60
Minute 2	A	10	20	30	40	50	60
	B	10	20	30	40	50	60
	C	10	20	30	40	50	60
Minute 3	A	10	20	30	40	50	60
	B	10	20	30	40	50	60
	C	10	20	30	40	50	60

Reliability B — Tot Agr/Agr+Dis ___/___ = ___% | Occ Agr/Occ Agr + Dis ___/___ = ___% | Non Agr/NonAgr + Dis ___/___

Minute 4	A	10	20	30	40	50	60
	B	10	20	30	40	50	60
	C	10	20	30	40	50	60
Minute 5	A	10	20	30	40	50	60
	B	10	20	30	40	50	60
	C	10	20	30	40	50	60
Minute 6	A	10	20	30	40	50	60
	B	10	20	30	40	50	60
	C	10	20	30	40	50	60

Reliability A — Tot Agr/Agr+Dis ___/___ = ___% | Occ Agr/Occ Agr + Dis ___/___ = ___% | Non Agr/NonAgr + Dis ___/___

Minute 7	A	10	20	30	40	50	60
	B	10	20	30	40	50	60
	C	10	20	30	40	50	60
Minute 8	A	10	20	30	40	50	60
	B	10	20	30	40	50	60
	C	10	20	30	40	50	60
Minute 9	A	10	20	30	40	50	60
	B	10	20	30	40	50	60
	C	10	20	30	40	50	60
Minute 10	A	10	20	30	40	50	60
	B	10	20	30	40	50	60
	C	10	20	30	40	50	60

A= ___/___ = ___%   B= ___/___ = ___%   RATES

Momentary time sampling

Momentary time sampling is a procedure that may be indicated when a target behavior is discrete, yet occurs in a protracted manner across time. It is a technique similar to interval recording in that an estimate of behavior frequency is derived. However, unlike interval recording where the occurrence of behavior during an interval is recorded, time sampling is a form of recording where the occurrence of a target

Figure 2
Sample momentary time sample data sheet

Momentary Time Sample Data Sheet

Client: _____

Observer: _____ **Dates:** _____

Target Behavior and Definition: _____

Instructions: For each time listed below, circle "Y" if the client engages in the behavior during that time. If the client does not engage in the behavior, circle "N." At the end of the day, add the number of "Y"'s and divide by the number of observations for the day.

	Sunday	Monday	Tuesday	Wednesday	Thursday	Friday	Saturday
Date							
Time							
	Y N	Y N	Y N	Y N	Y N	Y N	Y N
	Y N	Y N	Y N	Y N	Y N	Y N	Y N
	Y N	Y N	Y N	Y N	Y N	Y N	Y N
	Y N	Y N	Y N	Y N	Y N	Y N	Y N
	Y N	Y N	Y N	Y N	Y N	Y N	Y N
	Y N	Y N	Y N	Y N	Y N	Y N	Y N
	Y N	Y N	Y N	Y N	Y N	Y N	Y N
	Y N	Y N	Y N	Y N	Y N	Y N	Y N
	Y N	Y N	Y N	Y N	Y N	Y N	Y N
	Y N	Y N	Y N	Y N	Y N	Y N	Y N
# YES							
Total							
Percentage							

behavior is observed and noted immediately after the circumscribed time interval. Like interval recording, time sampling may be quantified as a percentage by dividing the number of intervals in which the target behavior was observed by the total number of intervals multiplied by 100 (see Figure 2).

Handmouthing is an example of aberrant behavior that may be particularly well suited to momentary time sampling procedures. For instance, if one were to tally the number of instances that an individual engages in handmouthing across a 30 minute interval period of time, it is likely that only one instance of handmouthing would be recorded even though the behavior may have occurred for the majority of the interval. On the other hand, if an observer were to record whether or not the individual engaged in handmouthing at the end of a one minute interval, a more accurate estimate of the continuous nature of the individuals handmouthing would be highlighted.

Momentary time sampling vs. partial interval recording

There are several considerations that should be made when choosing the between partial interval recording and momentary time sampling techniques. Both techniques have advantages and disadvantages; the appropriateness of the technique varies according to characteristics of the behavior and the measurement goals of the observer (e.g., accuracy of behavior duration, frequency, etc.). In a review of partial interval recording and momentary time sampling, Harrop, Daniels, and Foulkes (1990), concluded that on average, momentary time sampling provides a more accurate estimation of the total duration of the behavior compared with partial interval recording. They also concluded that the accuracy of momentary time sampling increases when the intervals between recording are shortened, when the occurrence of the behavior is of a high frequency, and when the duration of each instance of behavior increases. When momentary time sampling and partial interval recording techniques have been compared, there is evidence to suggest that momentary time sampling results in less observer error than partial interval recording (Murphy & Harrop, 1994). Furthermore, momentary time sampling may be preferred by observers as a data collection procedure when compared to partial interval recording (Murphy & Harrop, 1994).

Although Harrop et al. (1990), suggested that the partial interval recording procedure is not a good estimate of duration or frequency, it appears to be more sensitive than momentary time sampling for detecting short duration, low frequency behaviors. Furthermore, they conclude that partial interval recording may be more sensitive to changes in the duration or frequency of behavior than momentary time sampling.

Permanent products

Permanent products are tangible changes in the environment that may be quantified to assess the occurrence of behavior. Common examples of permanent products include video recordings of behavior and pencil and paper tests. In behavioral observation, permanent products may be used to assess the frequency of behavior, but are not as frequently employed as other data recording procedures. Ayllon (1963) provided a classic example of assessment with permanent products before and during an intervention designed to reduce towel hoarding. The progress of a satiation procedure designed to reduce the towel hoarding of an institutionalized individual was monitored by counting the number of towels in the individual's bedroom.

Cooper (1987) detailed two rules to consider when deciding whether to utilize measurement of permanent products. First, the occurrence of behavior should result in the production of the same permanent product. Secondly, the permanent product should only be produced by the target behavior. Both of these rules may be violated when attempting to record skin damage as an index of self-injury. The presence of cuts or bruises may be the result of an accident or assault by another, and there is not necessarily a direct correspondence to the occurrence of the behavior and the presence of skin damage (Cooper, 1987).

Permanent products that reflect quantifiable changes in the environment and are reliably produced by the target behavior may provide a useful means of assessment.

Latency recording

Latency recording involves measuring the length of time occurring between a stimulus onset and behavior occurrence. Thus, the measurement dimension of interest, as with duration recording, is time elapsed, and a stopwatch is the most frequently used and most accurate recording method. Latency recording is particularly useful in measuring compliance with requests. Mace and colleagues (1988) investigated the effect of "behavioral momentum"; the persistence of behavior following a change in environmental conditions, on compliance using latency recording with two adults with moderate mental retardation. The participants were observed to initiate cleaning tasks following relatively long periods of time following the request. In one of five total experiments, latency for task initiation measured in seconds was recorded following either only the request to complete the tasks (low-probability task sequence) or following several more preferred tasks such as shaking hands with or hugging staff members (high-probability task sequence). Significantly shorter latency periods were noted during the high-probability sequences compared to the low-probability sequences and an attention control condition (provision of positive statements only prior to the low-probability sequence).

Self-monitoring

Self-monitoring refers to procedures in which participants in behavior change interventions attend to and record their own target behavior. This approach has been widely employed within behavior therapy contexts as a primary method of data collection. Common target behaviors that participants independently monitor include number of cigarettes smoked (Brown, Burgess, Sales, Whiteley, Evans, & Miller, 1998; Foxx & Brown, 1979), amount of food intake (Latner & Wilson, 2002), amount of exercise (Wyshogrod, 1985), and frequency of undesired habitual behaviors (Febbaro & Clum, 1998). Self-monitoring is frequently employed as an intervention in and of itself, as merely recording behavior of interest may result in behavior change in the desired direction (Browder & Shapiro, 1985; Korotitsch & Nelson-Gray, 1999; Mace & Kratochwill, 1985). This phenomenon, commonly referred to as *reactivity*, can compromise the accuracy of baseline and treatment data when self-monitoring is the primary method of assessment. As such, independent trained observers are frequently used to collect data on both self-monitoring behavior and the related target behavior.

A common objective for self-monitoring interventions for persons with developmental disabilities is to increase on-task behavior. A number of studies have demonstrated that on-task behavior, typically relevant in educational and vocational settings, can be increased when individuals are taught to record their own on-task behavior (See Gardner & Cole, 1988; Hughes, Korinek, & Gorman, 1991; and Martin & Hrydowy, 1989, for reviews). Hughes and Boyle (1991) used self-monitoring to increase on-task behavior and task productivity for three children classified within the moderate range of developmental disability. The participants were taught to monitor whether or not they had been working on the average of every 45 seconds, with an audible tone cueing the students to place checks in one of two columns on a worksheet. The columns represented "yes" or "no" answers to the question, "Was I working?" A multiple baseline design across pre-vocational tasks revealed clear, significant increases in on-task behavior for each task. Task productivity also increased for all participants, though productivity improvements were less dramatic.

While self-monitoring is commonly used for increasing behavior in persons with developmental disabilities, often it is only one of several procedures used in a multi-component treatment package. Relatively few published reports have evaluated the efficacy of self-monitoring interventions independent of other intervention components (Hughes et al., 1991; Martin & Hrydowy, 1989), though some evidence does exist demonstrating the efficacy of self-monitoring when used as the exclusive intervention (Blick & Test, 1987; Hughes et al., 1991; Sugai & Rowe, 1984). An additional criticism involves the practicality of maintaining self-monitoring interventions in applied settings; these interventions may be intrusive and/or cumbersome in actual workplace settings (Martin & Hrydowy, 1989). Nonetheless, the substantial body of literature on self-monitoring indicates that this procedure can be an important component in creating lasting behavior change in a variety of relevant settings, and can help individuals with developmental disabilities learn to independently record and manage their own behavior.

Direct assessment: Analogue and natural observation

Direct assessment consists of both analogue assessment and natural observation.

Natural observation, as the name implies, consists of the observation of behavior in the environment as it naturally occurs. With natural observation, an individual may be observed unobtrusively across a wide range of settings to examine the topographical and temporal nature of target behaviors. Analogue assessment, on the other hand, is frequently conducted outside of the flow of an individual's life as it normally occurs. Analogue assessment typically consists of a series of contrived environmental conditions that are controlled by the experimenter and designed to evoke target behavior. Analogue assessment is frequently used to assess aberrant behavior among individuals with developmental disabilities, though various forms of analogue assessment have been used with the population at large for a wide array of behavior problems, including anxiety disorders, substance-use disorders, mood disorders, and family discord (Mash & Foster, 2001).

There are advantages and disadvantages to both natural observation and analogue assessment. For natural observation, the greatest advantage consists of the observation of the behavior as it naturally occurs in the environment. Observations occur directly in the individual's natural environment, so there is little question about the generalizability of observation so long as it is conducted across relevant settings. With analogue assessment, behavior is observed in a setting contrived by the observer that may not replicate the same stimulus conditions that occur in the natural environment. Some more notable limitations of natural observation include: 1) its time consuming nature; 2) some behaviors cannot be observed in the natural environment for ethical reasons (e.g., sexual or aggressive behavior); and, 3) the observation might not be valid representation of the target behavior as it normally occurs (Sloan & Mizes, 1999).

The strength of analogue assessment is control over antecedent conditions (Iwata, Kahng, Wallace, & Lindberg , 2000). Analogue assessment frequently occurs in settings where the observer has a high degree of control over environmental contingencies that may initiate or maintain target behavior. With analogue assessment, an observer may be able to "turn on" and "turn off" behavior by varying stimulus conditions rather than waiting for the conditions to naturally occur. In this vein, analogue assessment may be more cost effective than natural observation (Mash & Foster, 2001). Researchers have found that for individuals with MR, analogue methodology may be particularly helpful for identifying antecedent conditions that are related to the occurrence of problem, thus aiding in the design of intervention (Iwata, et al., 2000; Kahng, Iwata, & Lewin, 2002; Mace, Lalli, & Pinter-Lalli, 1991).

Reliability of natural and analogue assessment

Analogue assessment typically affords more control over contingencies related to the occurrence of behavior when compared with natural observation. In analogue assessment, the observer may set the stage for target behaviors to occur by creating environmental conditions thought to be related to the onset and/or maintenance of problem behavior. With natural observation, it may be difficult to establish the reliability of behavior occurrence since the observer has no control over the individual and/or the contingencies that typically elicit or maintain target behaviors.

Although analogue assessment appears to be the most reliable direct assessment method, its reliability may still be questionable. Sturmey (1996) cited three potential problems for the reliability of analogue assessment of problem behavior in persons with developmental diasabilities. First, the behavioral function of a target behavior may not be identified until after numerous analogue sessions have been conducted. Second, graphical data analysis (the method of choice for analogue assessment) may produce unreliable interpretation if the variance in the data is high or the data are not stable. Lastly, it is unclear how the observer's behavior may effect the data. For example, the choice of different experimental designs may affect the reliability of the data.

More recently, Martin, Gaffan, and Williams (1999) reported estimates of convergent validity for three methods of data interpretation for analogue assessments along with estimates of test-retest reliability. Across 27 separate analogue assessments, the agreement between three forms of data interpretation was low. Similarly, estimates of test-retest reliability across intervals of two weeks, one month, and 3 months were disappointing. Further research is needed to assess the utility of various methods of data interpretation for analogue assessment, and factors that may have effected the low estimates of test-retest reliability found by Martin and colleagues.

Indirect Assessment

Indirect assessment refers to a host of data collection methods that involve either self-report or informant-report to assess various dimensions of behavior. Typically, indirect methods of assessment are conducted through interview or checklist format, and are administered to caregivers that are familiar with the target behavior in question. Less frequent are self-report measures designed for individuals with mild developmental disabilities. The content of indirect assessment covers a wide array of behavior (problematic and adaptive), and wide-ranging systems of assessment have been based primarily on indirect methods (Matson, Mayville, & Laud, 2003).

There are numerous benefits to indirect assessment. The primary benefit of indirect assessment is time efficiency. Resources for individuals with developmental disabilities are frequently spread thin, and indirect methods of assessment are usually less labor-intensive than more direct means of assessment. Thus, the incremental validity and cost-effectiveness of more direct measures (i.e., analogue assessment) may depend in part on the unavailability of valid, less direct means of assessment (Haynes, 2001).

Numerous indirect assessment measures with favorable psychometric properties have been described in the research literature (Matson, Mayville, & Laud, 2003; Singh et al., 1991). Although self-report rating scales and interviews have been designed, limitations such as acquiescent response patterns may lessen the utility of self-report versions of such measures (Sigelman, Budd, Spanhel, & Schoenrock, 1981). Far more prevalent are informant-based interviews and rating scales. Such measures have been found reliable and valid for the assessment of adaptive behavior (e.g., the Vineland Adaptive Behavior Scales; Sparrow, et al., 1984), maladaptive behavior (e.g., the Aberrant Behavior Checklist; Aman, Singh, Stewart, & Field, 1985), behavior function (e.g., Questions About Behavioral Function; Paclawskyj, et al., 2000), social skills (e.g., Matson Evaluation of Social Skills for Individuals with Severe Retardation; Matson, 1995), psychiatric disorders (e.g., The Diagnostic Assessment for the Severely Handicapped; Matson, 1994), and medication side-effects (e.g., the Matson Evaluation of Drug Side Effects; Matson, Mayville, Bielecki, Barnes, Bamburg, & Baglio 1998).

While indirect assessment measures have yielded data demonstrating reliability and validity, there are conditions in which the reliability and validity of indirect assessment methods may be attenuated. In a description of the limitations of indirect assessment of functional relations, Repp and Horner (2000) detailed several variables that may lessen the utility of indirect measures of assessment. This includes response biases, limitations of the informant to accurately describe behavior, and lack of familiarity with the client. Furthermore, if the results of numerous methods of indirect assessment fail to provide a clear diagnostic picture, the use of more direct, labor-intensive methods such as analogue assessment may be indicated.

Functional Assessment

Methods that involve the assessment of environment-behavior relations are collectively referred to as methods of functional assessment. While determining the exact nature of environment-behavior relations can only be achieved through an experimental analysis (Cooper et al., 1987), observational methods can yield valuable information that can assist in developing an effective function-based treatment. Such methods are frequently the focus of behavioral observation systems for problem behavior displayed by persons with developmental disabilities. The chapter on functional assessment in this book provides a thorough review of functional assessment methodologies; only introductory concepts are discussed here.

Antecedent-behavior-consequence (ABC) assessment

Assessment within the ABC format involves recording a description of events that happen directly before, during, and after the occurrence of target behavior (Bijou, Peterson, & Ault, 1968). From this data, graphical representations may indicate that the target behavior is most closely associated with specific antecedents and consequences. Although data collected in this format typically results in the development of inferences that are correlational in nature, a clear picture of the functional nature of target behavior may emerge utilizing the ABC method (see Figure 3).

Figure 3.
Maladaptive Behavior Record

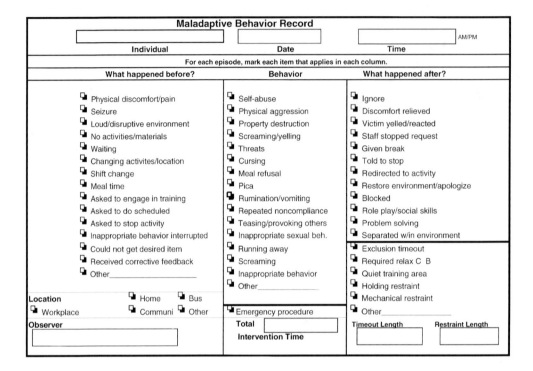

Scatter plot analysis

A scatter plot is a specific behavioral recording method described in detail by Touchette, MacDonald, and Langer (1985). The scatter plot typically consists of a grid designed for the recording of problem behavior across time. Time is typically recorded along the abscissa, while the frequency of behavior is scaled on the ordinate. Intervals for scatterplots typically consist of 30 minute blocks of time that are prevalent enough to allow for observation of behavior both within and across days. Through graphing behavior with a scatterplot, stimulus control problems may be identified by differential rates in the frequency of problem behavior across time. Scatter plots have also be developed to assess the occurrence of problem behaviors across staff members, particular settings, etc.

Given that the original data presented by Touchette, et al., (1985) was limited by the small number of subjects reported in their study, Kahng, et al., (1998) attempted to replicate the findings of Touchete, et al., (1985) with a larger sample of participants. Through conducting continuous observations across 20 individuals, Kahng, et al.,

(1998) failed to replicate the findings of Touchette, et al., (1985). None of the scatterplots yielded clear temporal relationships discernable through visual inspection. Although statistical procedures utilized in the study may have indicated that temporal relationships existed, the apparent insensitivity of visual inspection to identify temporal relationships may call in to question the way scatter plots are frequently used and analyzed.

Indirect functional assessment

Methods for indirectly assessing functions of behavior have emerged during past 15 years, and include semi-structured interviews of informants (e.g., O'Neil, Horner, Albin, Storey, & Sprague, 1990), as well as informant-completed checklists (e.g., Durand, 1990; Paclawskyj, Matson, Rush, Smalls, & Vollmer, 2000). Checklists such as the Motivation Assessment Scale (MAS; Durand, 1990) and the Questions About Behavior Function (QABF; Paclawskyj, Matson, Rush, Smalls, & Vollmer, 2000) may be useful for the determination of behavior function in settings where time constraints are a concern (Matson, Bamburg, Cherry, & Paclawskyj, 1999; Paclawskyj, Matson, Rush, Smalls, & Vollmer, 2001).

Conclusions

The use of behavioral observation and data collection systems has become standard in best practice models of behavioral, educational, and habilitative programming for individuals with developmental disabilities. Behavioral assessment methodologies allow professionals to collect and compile information that is integral in facilitating person-centered goal development, as well as for evaluation of treatment outcome and effectiveness. Both direct and indirect assessment strategies are often necessary in identifying relevant objectives and evaluating treatment outcomes, particularly in settings where relatively large numbers of individuals are served.

Research in behavioral assessment methodology and systems for persons with developmental disabilities has been generated at a rapid and steady pace for almost 30 years, and no signs of abatement are evident. Direct observation methods have been the most widespread in both research and clinical practice, a result of the proliferation of applied behavior analytic technology to the field of developmental disabilities. While direct observation can be labor intensive and cumbersome to implement in a system-based approach, technological advancements will likely help minimize these obstacles. Advances in palmtop and voice-activated technology are likely to significantly influence the methods in which behavioral data is collected, organized, and analyzed; such options are already routinely used in a number of academic-affiliated and private organizations.

Indirect assessment approaches, informant-completed checklists in particular, have become more widespread during the past 15 years. Researchers have acknowledged the importance of differentiating indirect measures according to level of individual impairment, and several measures accounting for this variable have emerged. Additionally, to establish that such measures are rooted in science, several experimenters have gone to great lengths to investigate the psychometric properties of indirect assessment measures. A significant addition to the informant-based rating scale literature would be information regarding the influence of individual rater characteristics on the integrity of ratings. Currently, little is known about how variables such as education, training, length of time working with the client, relationship to the client, and cultural background may influence informant responding to rating scale questions. This point may be particularly relevant for rating psychiatric symptomotology, as such behavior can often be difficult to recognize and interpret, particularly for persons with severe and profound impairments.

Given the advantages that indirect and direct assessment approaches present for researchers and clinicians working with persons with developmental disabilities, structured data collection and observation systems based on both are sensible. Such approaches are commonly used in clinical practice, particularly within the context of a functional assessment of challenging behavior. Research on how each methodology can compliment the other within a structured protocol would be useful, particularly for clinicians responsible for coordinating assessment systems for large groups of individuals. Several assessment paradigms exist that encourage the use of data from both direct and indirect sources, (e.g., Pyles et al., 1997) but research regarding how the combination of each methodology influences assessment and treatment outcome integrity is needed. Conversely, direct comparisons of each methodology to determine which might provide more reliable and valid information across a variety of domains, as well as cost-benefit analyses of each when used in isolation are also needed.

For a number of populations for whom behavioral assessment technology is applied, systems for conducting behavioral observation and collecting data continue to evolve. Given the continued interest in and development of behavioral assessment methodologies for persons with developmental disabilities, further significant advances in data collection and observation systems for this population are likely.

References

Ager, A. & O'May, F. (2001). Issues in the definition and implementation of "best practice" for staff delivery of interventions for challenging behaviour. *Journal of Intellectual and Developmental Disability, 26,* 243-256.

Aman, M.G., & Singh, N.N. (1986). *Aberrant Behavior Checklist: Manual.* East Aurora, NY: Slosson Educational Publications.

Aman, M.G., Singh, N.N., Stewart, W., & Field, C.J. (1985). Psychometric characteristics of the Aberrant Behavior Checklist. *American Journal of Mental Deficiency, 89,* 492-502.

American Psychiatric Association (1994). *Diagnostic and Statistical Manual of Mental Disorders (4th ed., rev.).* Washington DC: Author.

Ayllon, T. (1963). Intensive treatment of psychotic behaviour by stimulus satiation and food reinforcement. *Behaviour Research and Therapy, 1,* 53-61.

Baer, D.M., & Fowler, S.A. (1984). How should we measure the potential of self-control procedures for generalized education outcomes? In W.L. Heward, T.E. Heron, D.S. Hill, & J. Trap-Porter (Eds.), *Focus on behavior analysis in education* (pp. 145-161). Columbus, OH: Charles E. Merrill.

Bailey, J.S., & Pyles, D.A.M. (1989). Behavioral diagnostics. In E. Cipani (Ed), *The treatment of severe behavior disorders: Behavior analysis approaches. Monographs of the American Association on Mental Retardation, No. 12* (pp. 85-107). Washington, DC: American Association on Mental Retardation.

Ballinger, B.R., Armstrong, J., Presely, A.J., & Reid, A.H. (1975). Use of a standardized psychiatric interview in mentally handicapped patients. *British Journal of Psychiatry, 127,* 540-544.

Beck, A.T., Ward, C.H., Mendelson, M., Mock, J., & Erbaugh, J. (1961). An inventory for measuring depression. *Archives of General Psychiatry, 4,* 561-571.

Bellack, A.S. & Hersen, M. (1998). *Behavioral assessment: A practical handbook (4th ed).* Needham Heights, MA., Allyn & Bacon.

Bijou, S.W., Peterson, R.F., & Ault, M.H. (1968). A method to integrate descriptive and experimental field studies at the level of data and empirical concepts. *Journal of Applied Behavior Analysis, 1,* 175-191.

Blick, D. W., & Test, D. W. (1987). Effects of self-recording on high-school students' on-task behavior. *Learning Disability Quarterly, 10,* 203-213.

Brown, R.A., Burgess, E.S., Sales, S.D., Whiteley, J.A., Evans, D.M., & Miller, I.W. (1998). Reliability and validity of a smoking timeline follow-back interview. *Psychology of Addictive Behaviors, 12,* 101-112.

Browder, D.M., & Shapiro, E.S. (1985). Applications of self-management to individuals with severe handicaps: A review. *Journal of the Association for Persons with Severe Handicaps, 12,* 125-130.

California Department of Education (1997). *Best practices for designing and delivering effective programs for individuals with autistic spectrum disorders.* Sacramento, California: Resources in Special Education, California Department of Education.

Cone, J.D. (1978). The behavioral assessment grid (BAG): A conceptual framework and a taxonomy. *Behavior Therapy, 2,* 882-888.

Cooper, J.O. (1987). Measuring and recording behavior. In Cooper, J.O., Heron, T.E., & Heward, W.L. (Eds.). *Applied Behavior Analysis.* Merril-Prentice Hall: Upper Saddle River: New Jersey

Cooper, J.O., Heron, T.E., & Heward, W.L. (1987). *Applied Behavior Analysis.* Columbus, OH.: Merrill Publishing.

Costello, A.J., Edelbrock, C., Dulcan, M.K., Kalas, R., & Klaric, S. (1984). *Report on the NIMH Diagnostic Interview Schedule for Children (DISC).* Washington, DC: National Institute of Mental Health.

Cotter, V.W. & Toombs, S. (1966). A procedure for determining the music preferences of mental retardates. *Journal of Music Therapy, 3,* 57-64.

DeLeon, I.G., Iwata, B.A., Conners, J., & Wallace, M.D. (1999). Examination of ambiguous stimulus preferences with duration-based measures. *Journal of Applied Behavior Analysis, 32,* 111-114.

Demb, H.B., Brier, N., Huron, R., & Tomor, E. (1994). The Adolescent Behavior Checklist: Normative data and sensitivity and specificity of a screening tool for diagnosable psychiatric disorders in adolescents with mental retardation and other developmental disabilities. *Research in Developmental Disabilities 15,* 151-165.

Duff, R., LaRocca, J., Lizzet, A., Martin, P., Pearce, L., Williams, M., & Peck, C. (1981). A comparison of the fears of mildly retarded adults with children of their mental age and chronological age matched controls. *Journal of Behavior Therapy and Experimental Psychiatry, 12,* 121-124.

Durand, V.M. (1990). *Severe behavior problems: A functional communication approach.* New York, N.Y.: Guilford Press.

Durand, V.M., & Crimmins, D.B. (1988). Identifying the variables maintaining self-injurious behavior. *Journal of Autism and Developmental Disorders, 18,* 99-117.

Farrell, A.D. (1991). Computers and behavioral assessment: Current applications, future possibilities, and obstacles to routine use. *Behavioral Assessment, 13,* 159-179.

Febbaro, G.A.R., & Clum, G.A. (1998). Meta-analytic investigation of the effectiveness of self-regulatory components in the treatment of adult problem behaviors. *Clinical Psychology Review, 18,* 143-161.

Fisher, W.W., Kuhn, D.E., & Thompson, R.H. (1998). Establishing discriminative control of responding using functional and alternative reinforcers during functional communication training. *Journal of Applied Behavior Analysis, 31,* 543-560.

Foxx, R.M., & Brown, R.A. (1979). Nicotine fading and self-monitoring for cigarette abstinence or controlled smoking. *Journal of Applied Behavior Analysis, 12,* 111-125.

Gardner, W. I., & Cole, C. L. (1988). Self-monitoring procedures. In E. S. Shapiro & T. R. Kratochwill (Eds.), *Behavioral assessment in schools* (pp. 206-246). New York: Guilford Press.

Gast, D.L., Jacobs, H.A., Logan, K.R., Murray, A.S., Holloway, A., & Long, L. (2000). Pre-session assessment of preferences for students with profound multiple disabilities. *Education and Training in Mental Retardation and Developmental Disabilities, 35,* 393-405.

Greer, R.D. (1997). The Comprehensive Application of Behavior Analysis to Schooling (CABAS(R)). *Behavior and Social Issues, 7,* 59-63.

Hamilton, M. (1960). A rating scale for depression. *Journal of Neurology, Neurosurgey, and Psychiatry, 23,* 56-62.

Hanley, G.P., Iwata, B.A., Thompson, R.H., & Lindberg, J.S. (2000). A component analysis of "stereotypy as reinforcement" for alternative behavior. *Journal of Applied Behavior Analysis, 33,* 285-297.

Harrop, A., Daniels, M., & Foulkes, C. (1990). The use of momentary time sampling and partial interval recording in behavioral research. *Behavioral Psychotherapy, 18,* 121-127.

Hawkins, R.P, Mathews, J.R., & Hamdan, L. (1999). *Measuring behavioral health outcomes: A practical guide.* Dordrecht, Netherlands: Kluwer Academic Publishers.

Haynes, S.N. (2001). Clinical applications of analogue behavioral observation: Dimensions of psychometric evaluation. *Psychological Assessment, 13,* 73-85.

Haynes, S.N., & O'Brien, W.H. (2000). *Principles and practice of behavioral assessment.* Dordrecht, Netherlands: Kluwer.

Herjanic, B. & Reich, W. (1982). Development of a structured psychiatric interview for children: Agreement between child and parent on individual symptoms. *Journal of Abnormal Child Psychology, 10,* 307-324.

Hughes, C.A., & Boyle, J.R. (1991). Effects of self-monitoring for on-task behavior and task productivity on elementary students with moderate mental retardation. *Education and Treatment of Children, 14,* 96-111.

Hughes, C. A., Korinek, L., & Gorman, J. (1991). Self-management with student with mental retardation in school settings: A research review. *Education and Training in Mental Retardation, 26,* 271-291.

Iwata, B.A., Bailey, J.S., Neef, N.A., Wacker, D.P., Repp, A.C., & Shook, G.L. (Eds.) (1997). *Behavior analysis in developmental disabilities* (third edition). Lawrence, Kansas: Society for the Experimental Analysis of Behavior.

Iwata, B.A., Kahng, S.W., Wallace, M.D., & Lindberg, J.S. (2000). The functional analysis model of behavioral assessment. In Austin, J., & Carr, J.E. (Eds.). *Handbook of Applied Behavior Analysis.* Reno NV.: Context Press.

Iwata, B.A., Vollmer, T.R., & Zarcone, J.R. (1990). The experimental (functional) analysis of behavior disorders: Methodology, applications, and limitations. In Repp, A.C., & Singh, N.N. (Eds.). *Perspectives on the use of nonaversive and aversive interventions for persons with developmental disabilities.* Sycamore, IL.: Sycamore Publishing Company.

Jacobson, J.W. (2000). Early intensive behavioral intervention: Emergence of a consumer-driven service model. *The Behavior Analyst, 23,* 149-171.

Kahng, S., & Iwata, B.A. (1998). Computerized systems for recording real-time observational data. *Journal of Applied Behavior Analysis, 31,* 253-261.

Kanhg, S.W., Iwata, B.A., Fischer, S.M., Page, T.J., Treadwell, K.R.H., Williams, D.E., & Smith, R.G. (1998). Temporal distributions of problem behavior based on scatter plot analysis. *Journal of Applied Behavior Analysis, 31,* 593-604.

Kahng, S.W., Iwata, B.A., & Lewin, A.B. (2002). The impact of functional assessment on the treatment of self-injurious behavior. In Schroeder, S.R., Oster-Granite, M.L., & Thompson, T (Eds.). *Self-Injurious Behavior: gene-brain-behavior relationships.* Washington, D.C.: American Psychological Association.

Kalachnik, J.E. (1999). Measuring side effects of psychopharmacologic medication in individuals with mental retardation and developmental disabilities. *Mental Retardation and Developmental Disabilities Research Reviews, 5,* 348-359.

Kelly, M. B. (1977). A review of the observational data-collection and reliability procedures reported in the Journal of Applied Behavior Analysis. *Journal of Applied Behavior Analysis, 10,* 97-101.

Kennedy, C.H., Meyer, K.A., Knowles, T., & Shulka, S. (2000). Analyzing the multiple functions of stereotypical behavior for students with autism: Implications for assessment and treatment. *Journal of Applied Behavior Analysis, 33,* 559-571.

Kennedy, C.H., & Souza, G. (1995). Functional analysis and treatment of eye poking. *Journal of Applied Behavior Analysis, 28,* 27-37.

Korotitsch, W.J., & Nelson-Gray, R.O. (1999). An overview of self-monitoring research in assessment and treatment. *Psychological Assessment, 11,* 415-425.

Kubina, R.M. JR, Morrison, R., Lee, D.L. (2002). Benefits of adding precision teaching to behavioral interventions for students with autism. *Behavioral Interventions, 17,* 233-246.

Lattal, K.A., & Perone, M. (Eds.). (1998). Handbook of research methods in human operant behavior. New York: Plenum Press.

Latner, J.D, & Wilson, G.T. (2002). Self-monitoring and the assessment of binge eating. *Behavior Therapy, 33,* 465-477.

Mace, F.C., Hock, M.L., Lalli, J.S., West, B.J., Belfiore, P., Pinter, E., & Brown, D.K. (1988). Behavioral momentum in the treatment of noncompliance. *Journal of Applied Behavior Analysis, 21,* 123-141.

Mace, F.C., & Kratochwill, T.R. (1985). Theories of reactivity in self-monitoring: A comparison of cognitive-behavioral and operant models. *Behavior Modification, 9,* 323-343.

Mace, R.C., Lalli, J.S., & Pinter-Lalli, E. (1991). Functional analysis and treatment of aberrant behavior. *Research in Developmental Disabilities, 12,* 155-180.

Maine Administrators of Services for Children with Disabilities (2000). *Report of the MADSEC task force.* Manchester, Maine: Maine Administrators of Services for Children with Disabilities.

Martin, G.L., & Hrydowy, E. R. (1989). Self-monitoring and self-managed reinforcement procedures for improving work productivity of developmentally disabled workers: A review. *Behavior Modification, 13,* 322-339.

Martin, N.T., Gaffan, E.A., & Williams, T. (1999). Experimental functional analyses for challenging behavior: A study of validity and reliability. *Research in Developmental Disabilities, 20,* 125-146.

Mash, E.J. & Foster, S.L. (2001). Exporting analogue behavioral observation from research to clinical practice: Useful or Cost-Defective? *Psychological Assessment, 13,* 86-98.

Matson, J.L. (1988). *The PIMRA manual.* Orland Park, IL:International Diagnostic Systems.

Matson, J.L. (1994). *The Diagnostic Assessment for the Severely Handicapped II (DASH-II). User's guide.* Baton Rouge, LA: Scientific Publishers, Inc.

Matson, J.L. (1995). *Manual for the Matson Evaluation of Social Skills for Individuals with Severe Retardation.* Baton Rouge, LA: Scientific Publishers Inc.

Matson, J.L. (1997). *The Assessment for Dual Diagnosis: Manual.* Baton Rouge, LA: Disability Consultants.

Matson, J.L., Bamburg, J.W., Cherry, K.E., & Paclawskyj, T.R. (1999). A validity study on the Questions About Behavioral Function (QABF) Scale: Predicting treatment success for self-injury, aggression, and stereotypies. *Research in Developmental Disabilities, 20,* 142-160.

Matson, J. L., Gardner, W. I., Coe, D. A., & Sovner, R. (1991). A scale for evaluating emotional disorders in severely and profoundly mentally retarded persons: Development of the Diagnostic Assessment for the Severely Handicapped. *British Journal of Psychiatry, 159,* 404-409.

Matson, J.L., Mayville, E.A., Bielecki, J., Barnes, W.H., Bamburg, J.W., & Baglio, C.S. (1998). Reliability of the Matson Evaluation of Drug Side-Effects Scale (MEDS). *Research in Developmental Disabilities, 19,* 501-506.

Matson, J.L., Mayville, S.B., & Laud, R.B. (2003). A system of assessment for adaptive behavior, social skills, behavioral function, medication side-effects, and psychiatric disorders. *Research in Developmental Disabilities, 24,* 75-81.

McDaniel, W.F. (1997). Criterion-related diagnostic validity and test-retest reliability of the MMPI-168(L) in mentally retarded adolescents and adults. *Journal of Clinical Psychology, 53,* 485-489.

Michael, J. L. (1985). Behavioral analysis: A radical perspective. In B.L. Hammonds (Ed). *Psychology and learning* (pp. 99-121). Washington, DC: American Psychological Association.

Moss, S., Patel, P., Prosser, H., Goldberg, D., Simpson, N., Rowe, S., & Lucchino, R. (1993). Psychiatric morbidity in older people with moderate and severe learning disability: I. Development and reliability of the patient interview (PAS-ADD). *British Journal of Psychiatry, 163,* 471-480.

Murphy, M.J. & Harrop, A. (1994). Observer error in the use of momentary time sampling and partial interval recording. *British Journal of Psychology, 85,* 169-179.

New York State Department of Health (1999). *Clinical practice guideline: The guideline technical report – Autism/pervasive developmental disorders, assessment and intervention.* Albany, New York: Early Intervention Program, New York State Department of Health.

O'Neil, R.E., Horner, R.H., Albin, R.W., Storey, K., & Sprague, J.R. (1990). *Functional analysis of problem behavior: A practical assessment guide.* Sycamore, IL: Sycamore Publishing Company.

Paclawskyj, T.R., Matson, J.L., Rush, K.S., Smalls, Y., & Vollmer, T.R. (2000). Questions About Behavioral Function (QABF): A behavioral checklist for functional assessment of aberrant behavior. *Research in Developmental Disabilities, 21,* 223-229.

Paclawskyj, T. R, Matson, J. L., Rush, K. S., Smalls, Y, & Vollmer, T. R. (2001). Assessment of the convergent validity of the Questions About Behavioral Function scale with analogue functional analysis and the Motivation Assessment Scale. *Journal of Intellectual Disability Research, 45,* 484-494.

Piotrowski, C., & Zalewski, C. (1993). Training in psychodiagnostic testing in APA approved PsyD. and Ph.D. clinical psychology programs. *Journal of Personality Assessment, 61,* 394-405.

Prout, H.T., & Strohmer, D.C. (1989). *Prout-Strohmer Personality Inventory manual.* Schenectady, NY: Genium.

Pyles, D.A.M., Muniz, K., Cade, A., Silva, R. (1997). A behavioral diagnostic paradigm for integrating behavior-analytic and psychopharmacological interventions for people with a dual diagnosis. *Research in Developmental Disabilities, 18,* 185-214.

Ramsay, M.C., Reynolds, C.R., & Kamphaus, R.W. (2002). Essentials of behavioral assessment. New York: John Wiley and Sons, Inc.

Reiss, S. (1988). *The Reiss Screen for Maladaptive Behavior test manual.* Orland Park, IL: International Diagnostic Systems.

Reiss, S. (1993). Assessment of psychopathology in persons with mental retardation. In J.L. Matson & R.P. Barrett (Eds.), *Psychopathology in the mentally retarded (2nd ed.),* pp. 17-40. Needham Heights, MA: Allyn and Bacon.

Repp, A.C. & Horner, R.H. (2000). *Functional analysis of problem behavior: From effective assessment to effective support.* Belmont, CA.: Wadsworth Publishing.

Reynolds, W.M. (1989). *Self-Report Depression Questionnaire: Administration booklet.* Odessa, FL: Psychological Assessment Resources.

Robins, L.N., Helzer, J.E., Crougan, J., & Ratcliff, K.S. (1981). National Institute of Mental Heath: Diagnostic Interview Schedule. *Archives of General Psychiatry, 38,* 381-389.

Rojahn, J., Matson, J.L., Lott, D., Esbensen, A.J., & Smalls, Y. (2001). The Behavior Problems Inventory: An instrument for the assessment of self-injury, stereotyped behavior, and aggression/destruction in individuals with developmental disabilities. *Journal of Autism and Developmental Disorders, 31,* 577-588.

Sackett, G. P. (Ed.), (1978). *Observing behavior: Proceedings of the conference "Application of Obsrevational/Ethological Methods to the Study of Mental Retardation"* (2 vols.) [NICHD mental retardation research centers series]. Baltimore: University Park Press.

Saunders, R.R. & Saunders, J.L. (2000). Monitoring staff and consumer behavior in residential settings. In T. Thompson, D. Felce, & F.J. Symons, *Behavioral observation: Technology and applications in developmental disabilities* (pp. 115-142). Baltimore: Brookes Publishing Co.

Shapiro, E.S. (1984). Self-monitoring. In T.H. Ollendick & M. Hersen (Eds.), *Child behavior assessment: Principles and procedures* (pp. 148-165). New York: Pergamon.

Senatore, V., Matson, J.L., & Kazdin, A.E. (1982). A comparison of behavioral methods to train social skills to mentally retarded adults. *Behavior Therapy, 13,* 313-324.

Sharpe, T., & Koperwas, J. (2003). *Behavior and sequential analyses: Principles and practice.* Thousand Oaks, CA, US: Sage Publications, Inc.

Sigelmann, C., Budd, E.C., Spanhel, C.L., & Schoenrock, C.J. (1981). When in doubt, say yes: Acquiescence in interviews with mentally retarded persons. *Mental Retardation, 19,* 53-58.

Singh, N.N., Sood, A., Sonenklar, N., & Ellis, C. (1991). Assessment and diagnosis of mental illness in persons with mental retardation. *Behavior Modification, 15,* 419-443.

Skinner, B.F. (1966). Operant behavior. In W.K. Honing (Ed.), *Operant behavior: Areas of research and application* (pp. 12-32). New York: Appleton Century Crofts.

Sloan, D.M. & Mizes, J.S. (1999). Foundations of behavior therapy in the contemporary healthcare context. *Clinical Psychology Review, 19,* 255-274.

Sparrow, S. S., Balla, D. A., & Cicchetti, D. V. (1984). *Vineland Adaptive Behavior Scales.* Circle Pines, MN: American Guidance Service.

Sturmey, P. (1995). Diagnostic-based pharmacological treatment of behavior disorders in persons with developmental disabilities: A review and decision-making typology. *Research in Developmental Disabilities, 16,* 235-252.

Sturmey, P. (1996). <u>Functional Analysis in Clinical Psychology</u>. West Sussex: John Wiley & Sons.

Sugai, G., & Rowe, P. (1984). The effect of self-recording on out-of-seat behavior of an EMR student. <u>Education and Training of the Mentally Retarded, 19,</u> 23-28.

Tawney, J. W., & Gast, D. L. (1984). <u>Single subject research in special education</u>. Upper Saddle River, NJ: Merril.

Thompson, T., Felce, D., & Symons, F. J. (2000). <u>Behavioral observation: Technology and applications in developmental disabilities</u>. Baltimore: Brookes Publishing Co.

Tincani, M.J., Castrogiavanni, A., & Axelrod, S. (1999). A comparison of the effectiveness of brief versus traditional functional analysis. <u>Research in Developmental Disabilities, 20,</u> 327-338.

Touchette, P.E., MacDonald, R.R., & Langer, S.N. (1985). A scatter plot for identifying stimulus control of problem behavior. <u>Journal of Applied Behavior Analysis, 18,</u> 343-351.

Vaughn, B.J., & Horner, R.H. (1997). Identifying instructional tasks that occasion problem behaviors and assessing the effects of student versus teacher choice among these tasks. <u>Journal of Applied Behavior Analysis, 30,</u> 299-312.

Vyse, S., Mulick, J.A., & Thayer, B.M. (1984). An ecobehavioral assessment of a special education classroom. <u>Applied Research in Mental Retardation, 5,</u> 395-408.

Whitaker, S. (1996). A review of DRO: The influence of the degree of intellectual disability and the frequency of the target behaviour. <u>Journal of Applied Research in Intellectual Disabilities, 9,</u> 61-79.

Worsdell, A.S, Iwata, B.A., &Wallace, M.D. (2002). Duration-based measures of preference for vocational tasks. <u>Journal of Applied Behavior Analysis, 35,</u> 287-290.

Wyshogrod, D. (1985). Current treatment of obesity exemplified in a case study. <u>Journal of Behavior Therapy and Experimental Psychiatry, 16,</u> 151-157.

Zung, W.W.K. (1965). A self-rating depression scale. <u>Archives of General Psychiatry, 12,</u> 63-70.

7

Rating Instruments

Luc Lecavalier, Ph.D. & Michael G. Aman, Ph.D.
Nisonger Center, The Ohio State University

Introduction

The field of mental retardation has progressed significantly over the past 30 years. At the heart of this is an increased ability to recognize certain disorders. The advances in the areas of dual diagnosis, genetic disorders, and autism spectrum disorders represent this point well. Valid and reliable measurement of behavioral and emotional functioning is central to diagnosis, classification, and intervention. Most professionals in the field of developmental disabilities use and rely on rating instruments in their research and clinical activities. This chapter focuses on rating instruments. First, generic issues related to this method of measurement will be covered. Then, selected instruments will be described briefly and reviewed. Instruments were chosen because of their solid empirical foundations, widespread use, unique applications, and/or recent development. This section is not meant to be an exhaustive review of the literature on rating instruments. Interested readers are encouraged to consult the sources directly.

Definition of Rating Instrument

For the purposes of this discussion, rating instruments are defined as standardized tools, usually comprising multiple items, with a built-in system for quantifying behaviors and emotional states. By *standardized*, we mean that the content of the scale does not change with use. The method for quantifying behaviors is usually a metric relating to severity or frequency.

An example of a very simple informant-based scale is the *Clinical Global Impression* (CGI) Scale, which has two main subscales of one item each (NIMH, 1976). The Severity of Illness subscale asks the clinician to rate the subject's condition on a seven-point Likert scale from one (not at all ill) through seven (among the most severely ill). The Global Improvement subscale asks the researcher to rate any change on a scale that extends from seven (very much worse) through four (no change) to one (very much improved). The CGI is almost ubiquitous in drug research, and it is respected because it provides the "bottom line" (i.e., the clinician's best appraisal of the drug effect for each participant). The *Minnesota Multiphasic Personality Inventory* (MMPI) is characteristic of the other extreme (see Goldman et al., 2000). The MMPI is a self-report scale comprising up to 567 items, which are scored onto eight syndrome scales (e.g., Depression, Hysteria) and several other supplementary subscales.

Strengths and Weaknesses of Rating Scales

Rating instruments have a variety of strengths and weaknesses (Aman & White, 1986). Among the strengths of rating scales are the following. First, compared to other assessment modalities such as behavioral observations and interviews, they are quick. Second, they are usually inexpensive, as they can typically be completed by a wide range of informants (parent, staff member, or the person him/herself). Third, they can be very flexible, enabling the rater to consider behavior over a broad time period and/or across a range of settings. Fourth, they are usually consumer-friendly in that they often focus on behaviors that caregivers consider important to the client. Fifth, normative data are available for many rating scales. This approach makes it possible to (a) identify clients who are extreme on a given dimension, (b) know with certainty the direction in which behavior should be changed, and (c) judge when a behavior has been "normalized." Finally, the standardized content facilitates communication between researchers and clinicians.

Among the disadvantages of rating scales are the following. First, many rating scales invite the raters to make judgments about another person's behavior or to infer emotional states. To the extent that this is the case, such instruments can be subjective. Second, some raters are prone to "halo errors," which are described as a general tendency of the rater to assess the person as consistently high or low on various subscales intended to identify different facets of behavior. Thus, it is possible for the overall appraisal of the individual to water down important subscale differences. Third, when individuals with extreme behavior are identified, there is a likelihood that subsequent ratings of problematic behavior will spontaneously decline. This factor is a reflection of the statistical phenomenon known as regression towards the mean. If workers are not aware of this tendency of scores to decline between first and second ratings, they may misconstrue such change as reflecting true improvement.

Development of Rating Scales and Basic Psychometric Concepts

Rating instruments, broadband or specific, can be developed from an a priori theoretical model or established psychiatric taxonomy (such as the DSM or ICD) or by empirical studies. Instruments based on a priori models or psychiatric classifications are driven by the criteria of their taxonomy. For instance, the *Assessment for Dual Diagnosis* (ADD; Matson, 1997) was developed to be consistent with DSM-IV disorders (American Psychiatric Association, 1994).

Empirically driven scales are usually developed with factor analytic techniques and rely on the covariation of behavioral descriptors. An example of an empirically-driven scale is the *Aberrant Behavior Checklist* (ABC; Aman, Singh, Stewart, & Field, 1985a).

Other instruments such as the *Reiss Screen for Maladaptive Behavior* (RSMB; Reiss, 1988) or the *Strohmer-Prout Behavior Rating Scale* (SPBRS; Strohmer & Prout, 1989) represent combinations of these two approaches in that both psychometric methodology and established psychiatric taxonomies were used in the selection and retention of items.

Regardless of the method underlying their development, rating instruments need to be evaluated in terms of their reliability and validity. Reliability refers to the consistency of ratings and has three major components: internal consistency, temporal stability, and interrater agreement. Two sources of error can decrease the reliability of a rating scale: factors related to the rater and factors related to the instrument. Different levels of training, experience, and motivation to complete the instrument are examples of rater-related sources of error. Studies have consistently shown that different raters, especially those playing different roles in the lives of the individual they are rating (e.g., teacher and parent), often do not perfectly agree on adaptive or problem behaviors (e.g., Tassé & Lecavalier, 2000).

Population variables are an example of instrument-related error. For instance, Havercamp (1996) examined the impact of the level of intellectual functioning on the internal and interrater reliability of the RSMB and *Psychopathology Instrument for Mentally Retarded Adults* (PIMRA; Matson, Kazdin, & Senatore, 1984) in a sample of 277 adolescents and adults with mental retardation. She found that both types of reliability decreased substantially for individuals functioning in the profound range of intellectual deficits.

Validity refers to the extent to which the instrument measures what it claims to measure (Anastasi & Urbina, 1997). Validation is an ongoing process and has the objective of addressing two fundamental questions: (a) What does the instrument measure? and (b) How precise is the measurement? The three general types of validity are: content, construct, and criterion validity. Content validity refers to the extent to which items represent the universe of behaviors of interest. Criterion validity refers to the relationship between a predictor (e.g., the score on the instrument) and an independent external criterion (e.g., a diagnosis). Concurrent and predictive validity are two types of criterion validity. With concurrent validity, the predictor and criterion are obtained at the same moment in time, whereas with predictive validity the predictor is obtained before the criterion. Construct validity is the extent to which an instrument measures the theoretical construct it claims to measure. Construct validity encompasses other forms of validity and can be established by several methods such as factor analysis, measures of internal consistency, and correlations with other measures of the same construct.

Considerations for Enhancing Quality of Behavior Ratings

Most of the following considerations are common sense, but it is worth reviewing these simple procedures to avoid some common mistakes in administering rating scales. Here are some simple rules of thumb. 1. Always read the manual and/or supporting documentation before administering any scale. 2. Instruments with existing psychometric data should be preferred over others that lack this basic information. In the same vein, all else being equal, scales with better psychometric characteristics are to be preferred over other instruments. 3. The rater should always be properly introduced to the rating instrument. The clinician should orient the rater to the time period to be considered, the settings covered, the metric (scale) to be used, and the standards to be applied when judging behavior (e.g., who constitutes the comparison group?). 4. The clinician should be prepared to assist raters if they experience difficulties reading items. Not all raters with reading difficulties will divulge it, and offering to read the items and record responses should be considered in certain circumstances. 5. Especially when dealing with internalizing disorders (e.g., generalized anxiety disorder, major depressive disorder) the clinician should consider having the client rate him- or herself. Naturally, this will not be possible in the case of people with severe or profound intellectual deficits. But in the case of clients with mild mental retardation, the client may be the best informant as to his or her internal state. 6. Be suspicious of ratings in which all items are scored as uniformly high or low. In such cases, it may be worth enlisting a second informant. 7. Be wary of "advocates." By this, we are referring to informants who have some social agenda when conducting ratings and whose ratings may not reflect the behaviors that they are observing. To avoid this, the clinician has to keep both feet planted squarely on the ground and be appropriately alert to apparent discrepancies. 8. As there is a tendency for extreme scores to regress to the mean between first and second rating, it is wise to delay introduction of any new treatment until the second rating has been obtained. Naturally, this is not always possible, but it is desirable when it can be done. 9. When there is a change of raters in the course of a client's treatment, it is only natural to expect different levels of stringency as a function of the different raters. In the past, we have developed a solution to this problem but this can only work in the short term. We have photocopied the last rating by the previous rater and instructed the new rater (who also has known the client) to judge behavior relative to the last rating: lack of change is reflected by circling the *same* score whereas improvements or worsening are signified by circling *higher* or *lower* scores, as appropriate, relative to the previous ratings.

Screening and Diagnostic Tools

Reiss Screen for Maladaptive Behavior (RSMB)

The RSMB (Reiss, 1988) was designed to assess the likelihood that adolescents or adults with mental retardation may have a mental health problem. The instrument has 38 items that are scored on a scale ranging from 0 (No problem) through 2 (Major problem). Based on factor analysis of 306 individuals (most with dual diagnoses), 26 items were found to load onto the following seven clinical subscales: (1) Aggressive Behavior, (2) Psychosis, (3) Paranoia, (4) Depression (Behavior Signs), (5) Depression (Physical Signs), (6) Dependent Personality Disorder, and (7) Avoidant Disorder. Each subscale has 5 contributing items; some items score onto more than one subscale. An eighth scale, Autism, was added later. There are also six special maladaptive behavior items (e.g., suicidal tendencies or self injurious behavior) that do not load on any factor, but represent serious mental health or behavioral problems. In order to increase the validity of findings in clinical settings, Reiss (1988) recommended using the average score of two or more informants. The manual provides cut-off scores for each subscale (4.0, 5.0, or 6.0, depending on the subscale) and for the total score (9.0).

Aman (1991) reviewed the RSMB and concluded that its psychometric characteristics were significantly better than average. Internal consistency was generally adequate, although Depression (Physical Signs) had an alpha coefficient below .70. Interrater reliability for items was good, but it was not reported for subscales. Construct validity for the scale is based on its factor analytic origins. Using differences between dually diagnosed clients and a standardization group, Reiss developed a set of cutoff scores for clinical and research use.

The RSMB has been translated into several languages (e.g., Gustafsson & Sonnander, 2002; Lecavalier & Tassé, 2001; Van Minnen, Savelsberg, & Hoogduin, 1995). Van Minnen et al (1995) assessed a Dutch translation of the RSMB in 48 residents with dual diagnoses and 41 residents without a psychiatric diagnosis. Coefficient alpha ranged from .46 (Autism subscale) to .87 (Aggressive behavior) with a median value of .72. Interrater reliability ranged from .50 (Avoidant behavior) to .84 (Depression - Physical signs), with a median r of .69. The diagnosis group was rated significantly higher on all subscales and on the total score than the no-diagnosis group. In fact the total score for the diagnosis group was nearly four times that of the no-diagnosis group. Although, this study provided mixed evidence for internal consistency, interrater reliability and validity data were very good.

The RSMB is relatively brief and easy to use and has been used in many studies. It can be helpful for screening individuals who need a more intensive work-up and for epidemiological research.

Reiss Scales for Children's Dual Diagnosis (Reiss Scales)

The Reiss Scales is a downward extension of the RSMB. It was developed to screen children and adolescents aged 4 to 21 years, for presence of dual diagnoses. The instrument comprises 60 items. There are 10 subscales with five items each and 10 additional items that flag significant behavior difficulties. Items are rated on a three-point scale ranging from 0 (No problem) through 2 (Major problem). The first nine subscales were derived by factor analysis of ratings on 313 young people being seen at 15 community-based agencies serving individuals with developmental disabilities (Reiss & Valenti-Hein, 1990, 1994). The subscales were labeled as follows: (1) Anger/Self-Control, (2) Anxiety Disorder, (3) Attention Deficit, (4) Autism, (5) Conduct Disorder, (6) Depression, (7) Poor Self-Esteem, (8) Psychosis, (9) Somatoform Disorder, and (10) Withdrawn/Isolated. Because no "Depression" subscale emerged in the factor analysis, the developers constructed this subscale on an a priori basis using content from DSM and clinical reference works. As only two items loaded onto the Somatoform Behavior factor in the factor analyses, the authors added three new items to round out the subscale to five items (Reiss & Valenti-Hein, 1994). The manual provides cut-off scores for each subscale (5.0 or 6.0, depending on the subscale) and for the total score (29.0).

Psychometric data for the Reiss Scales are generally positive. Coefficient alpha ranged from .57 to .86 across subscales (median = .81). Interrater reliability data at the item level for 50 pairs of raters ranged from .26 to .74 (average $r = .46$). Construct validity was provided for most subscales through the factor analysis, although Depression, Somatoform Behavior, Autism, and Poor Self Esteem could benefit from further analysis. Evidence for criterion group validity was presented by demonstrating that young people with dual diagnoses differed from non-diagnosed subjects on all subscales except Attention Deficit. Further criterion group validity data were presented for groups of young people who had diagnoses of autistic disorder, psychosis, conduct disorder, and affective disorder. In each case, the diagnosed subgroup scored significantly higher than non-diagnosed subjects on subscales congruent with the diagnoses (Reiss & Valenti-Hein, 1994).

To conclude, the psychometric data of the Reiss Scales are generally favorable, although further construct validity data on the Depression and Somatoform Behavior subscales would be helpful. The cut-off rule calls for children to be screened if they surpass the cut-off on *two* subscales. Thus, it is possible that some children with a single psychiatric disorder may be missed. Depending upon the purposes for which the Reiss Scales are being used, some professionals may choose to scrutinize children who meet the cut-off score on one subscale only.

Assessment of Dual Diagnosis (ADD)

The ADD (Matson, 1997) is the successor of the well-known PIMRA and was developed to screen adults with mild and moderate mental retardation for psychopathology. It contains 79 items distributed on 13 subscales based on DSM-IV symptoms. Each item of the ADD is scored on a three-point Likert scale for the last month in terms of its frequency (0 = not at all, through 2 = more than 10 times), duration (0 = less than 1 month, through 2 = over 12 months), and severity (0 = no disruptions or damage, through 2 = caused property damage or injury). The subscales are: (1) Mania, (2) Depression, (3) Anxiety, (4) Post Traumatic Stress Disorder, (5)

Substance Abuse, (6) Somatoform Disorder, (7) Dementia, (8) Conduct Disorder, (9) Pervasive Developmental Disorder, (10) Schizophrenia, (11) Personality Disorders, (12) Eating Disorders, and (13) Sexual Disorders. The ADD was standardized and validated by having trained interviewers score the responses of direct care staff.

Few studies have been published on the ADD at the time of this writing, but preliminary data indicate good reliability. Matson and Bamburg (1998) examined the ratings obtained on a sample of 101 adults living in residential facilities and group homes. Internal consistency for the 13 subscales ranged from .77 to .95; Interrater reliability for the 13 subscales, based on Spearman ranked correlations, ranged between .82 and 1.00, and test-retest reliability for the 13 subscales, based on Pearson's product-moment coefficient for a two-week interval, ranged from .82 to 1.00.

Few diagnostic instruments are available for adults with mild and moderate mental retardation. The ADD measures a broad range of behaviors and is the only one based solely on DSM-IV taxonomy. The initial reliability data are encouraging, although it is difficult to know the effects of having interviewers complete the scale (e.g., it could add a source of error or decrease the generalizability of the data). In all likelihood, the instrument will be used as a rating scale and future studies need to examine its reliability and validity with this format.

Minnesota Multiphasic Personality Inventory (MMPI)

In a series of studies, McDaniel and his colleagues (Johns & McDaniel, 1998; McDaniel, 1997; McDaniel, & Harris, 1999) examined the psychometric properties of the MMPI – 168 in adults with mild and moderate mental retardation. The MMPI – 168 (Overall & Gomez-Mont, 1974) is a short version of the MMPI with good psychometric properties in individuals with average intellectual functioning. The scale was administered orally to participants who responded *yes* or *no*. In addition, the authors reported using simplified items when participants failed to understand. McDaniel (1997) reported good test-retest reliability for nine of the 13 MMPI subscales and good criterion validity based on previous diagnosis in participants' charts. Modest correlation coefficients between five of the MMPI-168 subscales and four of the RSMB subscales were also reported (Johns & McDaniel, 1998).

Although the authors contended that the MMPI-168 could be used with adaptations as a screening instrument, more research needs to be done to overcome methodological shortcomings (e.g., standardization of administration and criterion contamination). Methodological problems with self-report measures in general will be discussed later.

Multidimensional Informant-Based Adult Rating Scales

Aberrant Behavior Checklist (ABC)

The *Aberrant Behavior Checklist* (ABC) was primarily developed as an outcome measure in treatment studies. The ABC was derived by factor analysis and then cross validated in a second factor analysis (Aman, Singh, Stewart, & Field, 1985a). It has five factors comprising 58 items, as follows: I. Irritability, Agitation, Crying (15 items); II. Lethargy, Social Withdrawal (16 items); III. Stereotypic Behavior (7 items); IV. Hyperactivity/Noncompliance (16 items); and V. Inappropriate Speech (4 items). The developmental sample on which the ABC was derived was primarily made up of adults and adolescents, which has caused some workers to view it as an adult-only instrument. However, the ABC has also been used with children and adolescents and has essentially been found to have a consistent factor structure over the age span (Brown, Aman, & Havercamp, 2002; Marshburn & Aman, 1992; Rojahn & Helsel, 1991). Norms are available for both young people (Brown, et al., 2002; Marshburn & Aman, 1992) and for adults (Aman & Singh, 1994; Aman et al., 1985a). However, for reasons of brevity, we have assigned the ABC to the Adult Scales section.

The original reports on the ABC provided substantial psychometric data (Aman, Singh, Stewart, & Field, 1985b). Internal consistency as determined by coefficient alpha was high. Interrater reliability varied across raters and subscales but on average was quite satisfactory (mean $r = .63$). Validity was addressed in a variety of ways, including (a) comparison of groups that should differ in problem behavior (criterion group validity), (b) relation of ABC subscale scores with maladaptive scores on the *AAMD Adaptive Behavior Scale* (congruent validity), and (c) comparison of direct observation scores with ABC rating scores. In each case, the data supported the ABC's validity, although the evidence was best for the first four subscales; the last, Inappropriate Speech, was dubbed as "experimental" at the time (Aman et al., 1985b).

About 150 studies using the ABC have been published (Aman, 2003). These include (a) psychometric studies; (b) behavioral phenotype investigations; (c) drug trials; and (d) miscellaneous studies. The psychometric reports have consistently been positive and supportive of the original factor structure and reliability/validity estimate. The ABC has also consistently been sensitive to meaningful pharmacological and subject comparisons (Aman, 2003). This scale is one of the most researched and proven instruments in the developmental disabilities literature.

Diagnostic Assessment of the Severely Handicapped – II (DASH–II)

The DASH-II (Matson, 1995; Matson, Gardner, Coe, & Sovner, 1991) is for persons with severe and profound mental retardation, and along with the ADD replaces and expands on the PIMRA. The scale is a revision of a previous version and contains 84 items representing 13 diagnostic categories based on the DSM-III-R. It is intended for adults with severe and profound mental retardation and was developed with the ratings of trained interviewers who scored the responses of direct care staff persons who knew well the person being evaluated. The disorders are not exhaustive of DSM conditions but cover conditions commonly seen in adolescents and adults with mental retardation (e.g., PDD, Stereotypic and Elimination Disorders) as well as conditions commonly seen in the general population (e.g., Mood and Sleep Disorders). Each item of the DASH is scored on three dimensions for the previous two weeks: (a) Frequency (0 = not at all, through 2 = more than 10 times); (b) Duration (0 = less than 1 month, through 2 = over 12 months); and (c) Severity [0 = no disruptions or damage, through 2 = property damage or injury to person(s)]. The subscales are: (1) Anxiety, (2) Depression, (3) Mania, (4) Autism and other PDDs, (5) Schizophrenia, (6) Stereotypies, (7) Self-Injurious Behavior, (8) Elimination Disorders, (9) Eating Disorders, (10) Sleep Disorders, (11) Sexual Disorders, (12) Organic Syndromes, and (13) Impulse Control and Other Miscellaneous Behaviors. The items have been factor analyzed into six factors, namely (a) Emotional Lability, (b) Antisocial, (c) Language Disorder, (d) Social Withdrawal, (e) Eating Disorder, and (f) Sleeping Disorder.

Individuals who obtain scores of one standard deviation above the mean on certain subscales (e.g., Anxiety or Mania) or scores of one or two on the severity domain for items on other subscales (Self-Injurious Behaviors or Sleep Disorder) are considered to be at high risk for psychopathology. These cut-off scores were established arbitrarily but follow DSM considerations and have been found to be associated with psychopathology (Matson, 1995).

The manual reported standardization data from 658 persons with severe and profound mental retardation. Internal consistency was reported to be variable with values ranging from .39 to .83 for subscales and factor scores. Test-retest and interrater reliability was also reported to vary significantly by subscale and dimension rated.

In a series of studies, the validity of the Mania, Anxiety, PDD/Autism, Depression, Stereotypies, and Self-Injury subscales of the DASH-II were evaluated (Matson, et al., 1996; Matson et al., 1997; Matson et al., 1999; Matson & Smiroldo, 1997; Matson, Smiroldo, Hamilton, & Baglio, 1997). Packlowskyj, Matson, Bamburg, and Baglio (1997) obtained a correlation of 0.75 between the DASH-II total score and the overall ABC score as well as significant subscale correlations. There has been a significant amount of empirical work on the DASH-II and despite the fact that certain subscale scores have low reliability, it is one of the most widely-used scales for adolescents and adults with severe and profound mental retardation.

Strohmer-Prout Behavior Rating Scale (SPBRS)

The SPBRS (Strohmer & Prout, 1989) is a 135-item instrument for rating adolescents and adults with mild mental retardation or borderline intellectual functioning. Its 12 subscales were designated as follows: (1) Thought/Behavior Disorder (15 items), (2) Verbal Aggression (8 items), (3) Physical Aggression (10 items), (4) Sexual Maladjustment (8 items), (5) Noncompliance (15 items), (6) Hyperactivity (10 items), (7) Distractibility (10 items), (8) Anxiety (11 items), (9) Somatic Concerns (12 items), (10) Withdrawal (10 items), (11) Depression (11 items), and (12) Low Self-Esteem (15 items). In addition, broadband Externalizing and Internalizing factors are also derived from combinations of the subscale scores. The authors of the SPBRS reported that it was derived by a "rational clinical" method, which we presume means that it was derived from the DSM that was current at the time and by the authors' clinical experiences with the population.

A modicum of reliability and validity data were provided in the original manual (Strohmer & Prout, 1989; Aman, 1991). In general, there were good standardization data, interrater reliability was good, and test-retest data were not reported. Validity data were generally supportive, but the confirmatory factor analysis was not described in sufficient detail to judge the results. There are no norms for ratings by family member informants. We have not seen a great deal of work on the SPBRS since its appearance in 1989. It is possible that, at 135 items, it is too long for many research or clinical applications. Likewise, the fact that it was designed only for people with mild retardation and borderline IQ may have limited its use. Nevertheless, it appears to be a soundly-developed tool which may be helpful for certain applications.

AAMR Adaptive Behavior Scales–Residential and Community (ABS–RC:2) (Part II)

The most widely-used adaptive behavior scales, such as the *Vineland Adaptive Behavior Scales* (Sparrow, Balla, & Cichetti, 1984) and the *Scales of Independent Behavior–Revised* (Bruininks, Woodcock, Weatherman, & Hill, 1996), contain problem behavior sections. Because of space limitations and because they are usually administered by interview format, adaptive behavior scales will not be discussed in this section. However, we describe the ABS-PC briefly because it has a lengthy history and substantial research data have accumulated.

The ABS-RC:2 is the revision of the 1969 and 1974 *AAMD Adaptive Behavior Scales* (Nihira, Leland, & Lambert, 1993). The ABS-RC: 2 is primarily designed to analyze criterion-referenced adaptive behaviors. As with its predecessors, the ABS-PC is well standardized, with normative data on more than 4,000 individuals. As with its predecessors, Part II contains an inventory of problem behaviors. Also, like its predecessors, Part II is broken down into several domains as follows: (1) Social Behavior, (2) Conformity, (3) Trustworthiness, (4) Stereotyped and Hyperactive Behavior, (5) Sexual Behavior, (6) Self Abusive Behavior, (7) Social Engagement, and (8) Disturbing Interpersonal Behavior. In addition, elements of the Part II domains can be scored onto two empirically derived factors, designated as Social Adjustment and Personal Adjustment.

The biggest weakness of Part II the ABS-PC is consistent with that of its predecessors, namely a lack of construct validity for the domains. The items were originally taken from "critical incident reports" completed by direct care providers. These behaviors were later classified by judges into domains and sub-domains. However, this allocation of domains is not consistent with the DSM or ICD taxonomies (although there are points of similarity), and previous factor analysis at the item level did not consistently assign items to their respective domains (see Aman, 1991). Although the two overarching factors for Part II were empirically derived and do have a degree of construct validity, they are likely to be much too global to be very helpful clinically. Perhaps the greatest utility may be to "flag" individuals with problematic behavior. Given certain advances in assessment instruments in the field, it would be difficult to argue that this should be a core part of most assessment systems. However, given the history of the ABS, it may be fruitful to continue tracking clients who were assessed earlier with it.

Multidimensional Informant-Based Child Rating Scales

Developmental Behaviour Checklist (DBC)

Einfeld and Tonge (1992) modeled the scoring of the DBC after the well-known *Child Behavior Checklist* (Achenbach, 1991). Items for the DBC were extracted from case records in a clinic that cared for children with developmental disabilities. Raters are asked to assess the young person on a three-point scale that ranges from 0 (not true) to 2 (very true or often true). There are a total of 96 items on the parent version and 93 items on the teacher version of the DBC (items covering sleep disturbances were removed from the teacher version), 10 of which are not scored onto subscales. Some 1,093 children and adolescents were then rated on these items by parents, teachers, and residential workers. Principal components factor analysis produced six factors, which became the subscales for the first DBC. The first manual described a number of reliability comparisons and provided a variety of validity data (see Einfeld & Tonge, 1992).

Einfeld and Tonge (2002) have since revised the DBC. The factor structure was reanalyzed with improved statistical methods, a large international sample, and more children with mild mental retardation (Dekker, Nunn, Einfeld, Tonge, & Koot, 2002). Items and anchor points of the rating scale have remained unchanged. The second edition of the DBC has five subscales derived from factor analysis (n = 1536 parents and 1155 teachers), which include (a) Disruptive and Antisocial Behavior (27 items), (b) Self-Absorbed (31items), (c), Communication Disturbance (13 items), (d) Anxiety (9 items), and (e) Social Relating Disturbance (10 items). A larger proportion of the variance was explained in the revised version of the scale (44% compared to 33% with the original version). The Self Absorbed subscale contains a number of items (pica, self injury, making non-speech sounds) that appear to be related to lower functional level. Examination of the manual in fact shows that scores on this domain are higher for individuals with severe retardation compared to those with mild mental retardation. A total behavior problem score is tabulated by summing up all 96-items. A score of 46 or greater has been shown to be the clinical cut-off point.

Over the years, Einfeld and Tonge (2002) and others (e.g., Hastings, Brown, Mount, & Cormack, 2001) have provided a significant amount of psychometric analysis and supportive data on the DBC. The internal consistency for the Disruptive/Antisocial and Self-Absorbed subscales for both parent and teacher versions are at or above 0.89, but the other subscales have internal consistencies varying between .62 and .73. Test-retest and interrater reliability are all within acceptable ranges and data support the validity of the total and subscale scores (see Einfeld & Tonge, 2002). The instrument has been used in a number of studies, including a longitudinal study (Tonge & Einfeld, in press) and for exploring the profiles of several clinical and genetic disorders (see Einfeld & Tonge, 2002). Clark, Tongue, Einfeld, and Mackinnon (2003) reported the correspondence between change in total score as reported by the parent and an expert clinician to be $r = 0.86$ and concluded that this supports the scale's use in measurement of outcome in treatment studies. Brereton, Tonge, Mackinnon, and Einfeld (2002) reported that the DBC could be helpful in screening children with autism. The DBC-Autism Scoring Algorithm (DBC-ASA) consists of 29 items that have proven to differentiate autistic from nonautistic children with mental retardation matched for age, sex, and IQ level. The DBC-ASA had a sensitivity of 0.86 and a specificity of 0.69 in a total sample of 360 children.

This tool from Australia is one of the more conscientiously derived instruments in the field. It was carefully assembled and has sound psychometric characteristics. Its developers have pursued a programmatic line of research that has resulted in progressive refinement of the DBC. There is at least one potential weakness with the scale. The DBC has no ADHD or hyperactivity dimension which may be problematic, because ADHD is so common in young people with mental retardation.Nisonger Child Behavior Rating Form (NCBRF) The NCBRF was begun as an adaptation of the *Child Behavior Rating Form* (CBRF; Edelbrock, 1985), which in turn was used to rate typically-developing inpatient children and adolescents with psychiatric disorders. Aman, Tassé, Rojahn, and Hammer (1996) revised the CBRF by adding items (such as examples of stereotyped behavior and self injury) relevant to mental retardation and disabilities and modified others to make them more concrete. There were 10 pro-social items and 71 problem behavior items on the revised scale. Then, 369 outpatients at a university affiliated program for MR/DD were rated on the new instrument (326 by their parents and 260 by their teachers). These data were factor analyzed, and items with substantial loadings on the resulting factors were retained on the final scale (Aman et al., 1996). The subscale composition of the parent NCBRF is as follows: *A. Prosocial Section:* (1) Compliant/Calm and (2) Adaptive/ Social; *B. Problem Behavior Section*: (1) Conduct Problem, (2) Insecure/Anxious, (3) Hyperactive, (4) Self-Injury/Stereotypic, (5) Self-Isolated/Ritualistic, and (6) Overly Sensitive. Factor analysis of the teacher ratings produced essentially the same subscales except for the last from the *Problem Behavior* section, which was labeled *Irritable* instead of *Overly Sensitive*. Comparison of NCBRF scores with *Aberrant Behavior Checklist* scores indicated a high level of congruent validity (Aman et al.,

1996). Tassé, Aman, Hammer, and Rojahn (1996) analyzed the data as a function of age and gender. Gender was found not to affect scores, whereas age did for certain subscales. Tassé et al. (1996) also provided normative tables for these subjects.

Several other studies have been conducted to evaluate the NCBRF. Tassé, Morin, and Girouard (2000) examined the factor structure of a French translation of the NCBRF in French-Canadian children with mild to severe retardation. Factor structures of both the parent and teacher French-language versions were remarkably similar to the original NCBRF versions (congruence coefficients of .93 and .91, respectively). Girouard, Morin, and Tassé (1998) assessed one-month test-retest reliability and found it to range from .69 to .93 across subscales. Interrater reliability between parents and teachers ranged from .51 to .86, which is considered high. Tassé and Lecavalier (2000) had parents and teachers rate 109 children on the French-Canadian translation. Interrater reliability ranged from .42 to .63 across the subscales, which is high for raters having different roles. Lecavalier, Aman, Hammer, Stoica, and Matthews (in press) had parents and teachers of 330 children with autism spectrum disorders rate them on the NCBRF. Results of the factor analyses suggested that the original factor structure for the NCBRF held fundamentally true for these children. Finally, the NCBRF has been used as the primary outcome measure in large clinical trials of risperidone in children with disruptive behavior disorders, and the Conduct Problems subscale in particular was remarkably sensitive to the effects of treatment (Aman et al., 2002; Snyder et al., 2002). There is a growing and largely supportive data base on the NCBRF. The instrument has the advantage of parallel parent and teacher versions, it has both Prosocial and Problem Behavior sections, and it is in the public domain. These features should make it attractive for many research and clinical applications.

Specific Purpose Rating Scales

Affective and Anxiety Disorders

In addition to the multi-purpose instruments described above, several instruments have been specifically developed to measure affective and anxiety disorders. The *Anxiety, Depression and Mood Scale* (ADAMS; Esbensen, Rojahn, Aman, & Ruedrich, in press) is an empirically driven informant-based measure containing 28-items distributed on five subscales. Two factor analyses on a total sample of 533 adults with mild through profound mental retardation resulted in a five-factor solution. Factors were labeled: (1) Manic/Hyperactive Behavior (5 items), (2) Depressed Mood

(7 items), (3) Social Avoidance (7 items), (4) General Anxiety (7 items), and (5) Compulsive Behavior (3 items). One item loaded on two subscales. Items are rated on a four-point Likert scale ranging from "not a problem" to "severe problem," indicating the frequency and severity with which a particular behavior or symptom is present. Internal consistency for the five subscales ranged from .75 to .83, test-retest reliability from .72 to .83, and interrater reliability from .37 to .62. Data on a clinical sample of 129 individuals having a variety of psychiatric diagnosis provided support for the validity of the subscales. The ADAMS appears to be a psychometrically sound instrument for screening anxiety, depression, and mood disorders among individuals with mental retardation.

The *Emotional Disorder Rating Scale for Developmental Disabilities* (EDRS-DD; Feinstein, Kaminer, Barrett, & Tylenda, 1988) is a 59-item rating scale developed for children and adolescents with mild and moderate mental retardation. Items are rated on four-point Likert scales for severity and frequency. The instrument has eight subscales, six of which were based on DSM-III categories. The subscales are: (1) Anxiety (6 items), (2) Hostility/Anger (7 items), (3) Psychomotor Retardation (9 items), (4) Depressive Mood (14 items), (5) Somatic/Vegetative (3 items), (6) Sleep Disturbance (5 items), (7) Irritability (6 items), and (8) Elated/Manic Mood (9 items).

Although psychometric characteristics have been reported for a sample of typically developing children (Kaminer, Feinstein, Seifer, & Stevens, 1990), there are relatively few psychometric data available on the instrument for children with mental retardation. The available data suggest that the internal consistency and stability of the instrument are low and that interrater reliability is satisfactory (Aman, 1991; Feinstein et al., 1988).

A number of self-report instruments for measuring mood and anxiety have also been used in published studies. Some of these instruments were developed specifically for people with mental retardation, while others were developed for typically-developing people and adapted for individuals with mental retardation. For instance, Reynolds and Baker (1988) developed the *Self-Report Depression Scale* (SRDQ), a 32-item instrument designed specifically for adolescents and adults with mild to severe mental retardation. The SRDQ was based on DSM-III-R symptoms of major depression and its authors reported good psychometric properties in a sample of 89 individuals. Internal consistency was .90, test-retest reliability was .63, and a correlation of .67 was obtained with the *Hamilton Depression Rating Scale*.

Unlike the SRDQ, the *Beck Depression Inventory* (BDI; Beck & Steer, 1993) and the *Zung Self-Rating Depression Scale* (ZDS; Zung, 1965) were developed for individuals without mental retardation but have been used frequently with adults with mental retardation (e.g. Helsel & Matson, 1988; Prout & Schaefer, 1985; Kazdin, Matson, & Senatore, 1983; Powell, 2003). The BDI contains 21 items rated on a four-point scale ranging from 0 to 3 while the ZDS contains 20 items scored on a five-point scale ranging from 0 to 4. Kazdin et al. (1983) used a 13-item BDI and a simplified version of the ZDS as well as other measures of depression (SRDQ, MMPI-Depression scale, TAT, PIMRA, *Hamilton Rating Scale for Depression*) and reported significant associations between measures in a sample of 110 adults. In a sample of 120 adults functioning predominantly in the range of mild and moderate mental retardation, Powell (2003) reported alpha coefficients of .86 and .58 for the BDI and the ZDS, respectively. The correlation between instruments was not reported.

The *Zung Self-Rating Anxiety Scale* (ZAS; Zung, 1971) and the *Fear Survey Schedule for Children-Revised* (FSSC-R; Ollendick, 1983) are two instruments measuring symptoms of anxiety that have been adapted to be used as self-report measures in individuals with mental retardation. The *Fear Survey for Children With and Without Mental Retardation* (FSCMR; Ramirez & Kratochwill, 1990) is an adaptation of the FFSC-R for use in children with and without mental retardation between the ages of 6 and 13. It contains 60 items assessing fear stimuli. The authors reported good psychometric characteristics in a sample of 271 children. Lindsay and Mitchie (1988) attempted to modify the ZAS by rewording certain items to facilitate comprehension for use in adults with mild and moderate mental retardation. In a sample of 29 adults, they reported that a response format using presence or absence of anxiety symptoms was the most reliable.

In many studies using self-report measures, the content of the scale and administration procedures were modified by reading the questions to participants, simplifying the content of questions and rating system, or by using visual aids to facilitate judgments. These strategies are intended to increase reliability and *could* prove fruitful, but their efficacy has yet to be demonstrated. Such strategies could decrease reliability and the ability to generalize findings. For instance, reading questions in a face-to-face interview can lead to better comprehension but may also lead to the under-reporting or over-reporting of certain behaviors. Adding visual aids to anchor points of rating scales could help people remember available options without increasing the reliability of their judgments. In many studies, it is not clear which participants benefited from adaptations and what these adaptations consisted of. It is worth remembering that rating scale are no longer standardized if clinicians make their own adaptations when and as they see fit. Unfortunately, this is a common problem and is to be avoided. These issues do not only pertain to the scales mentioned in this chapter, but to all self-report scales used in the field of mental retardation. For a good review on methodological issues related to self-report instruments in individuals with mental retardation, readers are encouraged to consult Finaly and Lyons (2001).

Repetitive Behaviors

The *Behavior Problems Inventory* (BPI) is presented in this section because two of its three subscales measure repetitive behaviors. The BPI was derived from a direct observation system for evaluating self-injury. It was subsequently used to conduct a nation-wide survey of self-injurious behavior in West Germany (Rojahn, 1986). The instrument has undergone a series of changes through the years. The last major change occurred when the independently developed *Stereotyped Behavior Scale* (SBS; Rojahn, Matlock, & Tassé, 2000; Rojahn, Tassé, & Sturmey, 1997) replaced the original five stereotyped behavior items. Rojahn et al. (2000) reported good reliability and criterion related validity and presented norms based on 550 adults with mild to profound mental retardation for the SBS. One shortcoming of the SBS is the small amount of explained variance.

The current version of the BPI (designated as *BPI-01*) is a 49-item rating scale for assessing adults and young people with mental retardation (Rojahn, Matson, Lott, Esbensen, & Smalls, 2001). The subscales are (a) Self-Injurious Behavior (14 items), (b) Stereotyped Behavior (24 items), and (c) Aggressive/Destructive Behavior (11 items). Each of the three sections has a broad definition describing the range of behaviors to be rated in the past two months. Each item is rated on a frequency (0 = never, through 4 = hourly) and a severity scale (0 = no problem, 3 = severe problem). Rojahn et al. (2001) reported an $r = .90$ between the frequency and severity scales, so if time and resources are an issue users may opt for the scaling method that seems more appropriate.

Although the BPI items were originally arbitrarily assigned to its three subscales, its structure has been confirmed by factor analysis (Rojahn et al., 2001). Reliability and validity data are reasonably strong (Rojahn et al., 2001; Sturmey, Sevin, & Williams, 1995). The BPI was recently used in two trials of risperidone, and the Aggressive subscale was sensitive to treatment in both instances (Aman et al., 2002; Snyder et al., 2002). Self-injury, stereotypy, and aggression are all fairly common in individuals with mental retardation. When these behaviors are the main targets of investigation, the BPI can be recommended as a very sound tool.

Bodfish, Symons, Parker, and Lewis (2000) recently developed the *Repetitive Behavior Scale-Revised* (RBS-R). The RBS-R is an empirically-derived scale containing 43 items measuring six dimensions of repetitive behavior: stereotyped behavior, self-injurious behavior, compulsive behavior, ritualistic behavior, sameness behavior, and restricted behavior. The scale was developed by compiling items from existing behavior rating scales measuring repetitive behaviors and from clinical experience. Items are evaluated on a four-point Likert scale ranging from (0) "behavior does not occur" to (3) "behavior occurs and is a severe problem." The scale has been used to measure repetitive behavior in people with mental retardation and autism spectrum disorders. Preliminary data suggest good psychometric properties.

Autism Spectrum Disorders (ASDs)

The heterogeneity of ASDs, the changing nature of the diagnostic criteria, and the advances made in the field have led to the development of a number of rating scales over the past 40 years. Most of these instruments are diagnostic in nature. Instruments such as the *Autism Diagnostic Interview-Revised* (ADI-R; Lord, Rutter, & LeCouteur, 1994), the *Autism Diagnostic Observation Schedule* (ADOS; Lord et al., 2000) and the *Childhood Autism Rating Scale* (CARS; Schopler, Richter, DeVellis, & Daly, 1980) are the most widely used and respected instruments in the field, but will not be covered because they are not rating scales in the usual sense. Having said that, the CARS has been used successfully as a rating scale completed by parents in at least four studies (see Tobin & Glenwick, 2002) and the *Autism Screening Questionnaire* (ASQ) is a 40-item rating scale based on the ADI-R that recently became commercially available. Berument, Rutter, Lord, Pickles, and Bailey (1999) reported good discriminant validity for the ASQ in a sample of 200 children with and without ASDs. The scoring algorithm varies depending on the presence or absence of language and age of the individual being rated.

The *Autism Behavior Checklist* (Krug, Arick, & Almond, 1980a) is one of five components of the *Autism Screening Instrument for Educational Planning* (ASIEP; Krug, Arick, & Almond, 1980b). It was developed for individuals with more severe forms of mental retardation and contains 57 dichotomously-scored (yes/no) items grouped into five subscales: Sensory, Relating, Body and Object Use, Language, and Social and Self-Help Skills. Items were assigned to subscales based on face validity and were assigned a weight from 1 to 4, based on their ability to differentiate between children with and without autism. The *Autism Behavior Checklist* provides profile charts for different age groups ranging from 18 months to 35 years and recommends cutoff scores. Although Krug et al. (1980a) reported good validity and reliability, the ABC has been the object of many psychometric studies and results have varied widely (e.g., see Miranda-Linne & Lennart, 2002; Volkmar, Cichetti, Dyukens, Sparrow, Leckman, & Cohen, 1988; Wadden et al., 1991).

The *Gilliam Autism Rating Scale* (GARS; Gilliam, 1995) is intended for use with individuals aged 3 to 22 years. It contains 56 items divided into four subscales: Social Interaction, Communication, Stereotyped Behaviors, and Developmental Disturbance. The Developmental Disturbance addresses behaviors and milestones in the first 36-months of life, while the other three subscales focus on current behaviors. Items on the three behavioral domains are rated on a four-point Likert scale ranging from "Never Observed" (0) to "Frequently Observed" (3), while items on the Developmental Disturbance subscale are rated dichotomously as "yes" or "no." The sum of subscales yields a total autism score called the "autism quotient." Gilliam (1995) provided normative information for a sample of 1,092 individuals with a diagnosis of autism from across the United States, Puerto Rico, and Canada.

The GARS is gaining in popularity. Some studies have used it to measure severity of symptoms or to confirm a diagnosis of autism (e.g., Schreck & Mulick, 2000). Despite its increasing popularity, the scale has not been the object of many studies and certain questions need to be addressed empirically. For instance, norms are not broken by age and gender, diagnosis of the standardization group was not confirmed by independent clinicians, and reliability data are provided for small sample sizes. At the time of this writing, two independent studies were located on the validity of the instrument. South et al. (2002) reported that the GARS consistently underestimated the likelihood that autistic children would be classified as having autism compared to the ADI-R and ADOS-G, with a sensitivity of .48. Lecavalier (in press) reported an overemphasis of items measuring repetitive and stereotyped behaviors, poor to good reliability coefficients, and low sensitivity.

The *Gilliam Asperger's Disorder Scale* (Gilliam, 2001) was based on DSM-IV and normed on 371 individuals between the ages of 3 and 22 years who had been previously diagnosed with Asperger's Disorder. Items are rated on a four point rating scale and the Asperger's Quotient is tabulated by summing up the items of four behavioral subscales: Social Interaction, Restricted Patterns of Behavior, Cognitive Patterns, and Pragmatic Skills. The development and standardization, scoring system, and limitations of the GADS are all similar to those of the GARS.

The *Autism Spectrum Screening Questionnaire* (ASSQ; Ehlers, Gillberg, & Wing, 1999) is a 27-item screening instrument rated on a three-point Likert scale. This instrument was initially developed for a prevalence study of Asperger's Disorder in Sweden (Elhers & Gillberg, 1993) and subsequently translated to English. The authors generated a pool of items judged to reflect best the behavioral characteristics of children with Asperger's Disorder between the ages of 7 and 16 years. Eleven items tap social interactions, six communication, five restrictive and repetitive behavior, and five associated symptoms (e.g., clumsiness, tics). The data obtained from the epidemiological sample indicated high interrater reliability and stability over an eight-month period (n = 139; r = .90). Most children in the sample did not have Asperger's Disorder, which made it difficult to estimate reliability due to a restriction in the range of scores. Authors followed up by examining test-retest and interrater reliability as well as divergent and concurrent validity in a clinical sample of children with ASDs, behavior problems, and learning disabilities. Good reliability and validity were noted and suggested that the ASSQ is a useful screening device for the identification of high-functioning ASDs in clinical settings.

The *Pervasive Developmental Disorder - Behavior Inventory* (PDD-BI; Cohen, 2003; Cohen, Schmidt-Lackner, Romanczyk, & Sudhalter, 2003) is an instrument designed to measure response to treatment and contains both adaptive and problem behavior sections. There is a parent and teacher version, and items are rated on a four-point rating scale ranging from "Does not show the behavior" (0) to "Often/Typically shows the behavior" (3). There are two other rating options for items, "Don't know" and "Used to show the behavior." These options provide clinical information and are not scored. There are 176 items distributed onto ten subscales on the parent version and 144 items distributed onto eight subscales on the teacher version. The subscales were defined on an a priori basis and were further divided into subcategories containing four items each. Problem behavior subscales include: (1) Sensory/Perceptual Approach Behaviors (complex rituals and stereotyped behaviors), (2) Specific Fears, (3) Arousal Problems, (4) Aggressiveness, (5) Social Pragmatic Problems, and (6) Semantic Pragmatic Problems. Adaptive subscales include: (1) Social Approach Behaviors, (2) Learning, Memory, and Receptive Language, (3) Phonological Skills, and (4) Semantic/Pragmatic Ability. An overall severity of autism score can be obtained by tabulating scores from certain subscales that bear a strong relation to DSM-IV criteria.

The authors reported good internal consistency and interrater reliability. A series of factor analyses lent support to the validity of most subscales and of the two general dimensions of maladaptive-adaptive and approach-withdrawal behaviours. These analyses also indicated a need to refine further certain areas of the adaptive subscales. Correlations between subscales of the PDD-BI and measures of problem behavior, adaptive behavior, and autistic symptomatology were supportive of their validity. The PDD-BI seems to be a well-constructed instrument. The subscales can be administered separately, and the presence of adaptive and problem behavior might also make it appealing for certain applications. Another advantage of the instrument is that its scores can be adjusted for expected developmental change.

Conclusions

In the field of developmental disabilities, researchers and clinicians alike rely significantly on rating scales. Rating instruments are imperfect but have many advantages and play an important role in assessment. They are also an important part of many successful initiatives to understand the causes of behavioral and emotional problems through research or to take proper administrative actions.

In the last several decades, a variety of instruments have been developed to measure behavioral and emotional functioning of individuals with developmental disabilities. The selection of an instrument hinges on the objectives of the assessment and scale characteristics. Some instruments, such as the ABC, are "universal" in the sense that they assess generic behaviors likely to be found in any samples of individuals with developmental disabilities. When a particular behavioral disorder is the focus of measurement, specific purpose instruments may be preferred, especially from a measurement reliability standpoint. An instrument's sensitivity (number of people accurately identified as having a disorder) and specificity (number of people accurately identified as not having the disorder) should also be given serious consideration, especially when used in the context of diagnostic or screening.

Close attention should be paid to psychometric characteristics and features of the population needing assessment. Threats to reliability are important because reliability determines the maximum amount of validity (Anastasi & Urbina, 1997). People with mental retardation and autism spectrum disorders are a heterogeneous group and we should not assume that any single measure is useful for the entire population. Readers are encouraged to consult Floyd and Widaman (1995) for issues germane to factor analysis and Cichetti (1994) for matters relevant to the reliability and validity of standardized rating scales.

Rating scales cannot be expected to perform well if used improperly. Simple procedures to avoid common mistakes when using rating scales were presented. Instruments cannot be ahead of the field and problems related to the taxonomy and identification of psychopathology remain important obstacles for successful instrumentation development and refinement. More research is needed to better understand the nature of the relationship between mental retardation and psychopathology and to develop a reliable and valid taxonomy of psychopathology for all individuals with developmental disabilities. Despite the significant progress made in the last decades, additional research is needed on both informant-based and self-report measures in the field of developmental disabilities.

References

Achenbach, T. M. (1991). *Integrative guide for the 1991 CBCL/4-18, YSR, and TRF profiles.* Burlington, VT: University of Vermont, Department of Psychiatry.

Aman, M. G. (1991). Assessing psychopathology and behavior problems in persons with mental retardation: A review of available instruments. [DHHS Publication No. (ADM) 01-1712] Rockville, MD: U.S. Department of Health and Human Services.

Aman, M. G. (2003). *Annotated Bibliography on the Aberrant Behavior Checklist (June 2003 update).* Columbus, OH: Ohio State University.

Aman, M. G., DeSmedt, G., Derivan, A., Lyons, B., Findling, R. L., and the Risperidone Disruptive Behavior Study Group. (2002). Double–blind, placebo-controlled study of Risperidone for the treatment of Disruptive Behaviors in Children with Sub average Intelligence. *American Journal of Psychiatry, 159,* 1337-1346.

Aman, M. G. & Singh, N. N. (1994). *Aberrant Behavior Checklist - Community. Supplementary Manual.* East Aurora, NY: Slosson Educational Publications.

Aman, M. G., Singh, N. N., Stewart, A. W., & Field, C. J. (1985a). The Aberrant Behavior Checklist: A behavior rating scale for the assessment of treatment effects. *American Journal of Mental Deficiency, 89,* 485-491.

Aman, M. G., Singh, N. N., Stewart, A. W., & Field, C. J. (1985b). Psychometric characteristics of the Aberrant Behavior Checklist. *American Journal of Mental Deficiency, 89,* 492-502.

Aman, M. G., Tassé, M. J., Rojahn, J., & Hammer, D. (1996). The Nisonger CBRF: A child behavior rating form for children with developmental disabilities. *Research in Developmental Disabilities, 17,* 41-57.

Aman, M. G., & White, A. J. (1986). Measures of drug change in mental retardation. In K. D. Gadow & C. T. Greenwich (Eds.), *Advances in learning and behavioural difficulties, 5,* 157-202.

American Psychiatric Association (1994). *Diagnostic and statistical manual of mental disorders* (4th ed.). Washington, DC: Author.

Anastasi, A., & Urbina, S. (1997). *Psychological testing (7th Ed.).* Upper Saddle River, NJ: Prentice Hall.

Beck, A. T., & Steer, R. A. (1993). *Beck Depression Inventory.* San Antonio: Psychological Corporation.

Berument, S. B., Rutter, M., Lord, C., Pickles, A., & Bailey, A. (1999) Autism Screening Questionnaire: Diagnostic validity. *British Journal of Psychiatry, 175,* 444-451.

Bodfish, J. W., Symons, F. J., Parker, D. E., & Lewis, M. H. (2000). Varieties of Repetitive Behavior in Autism: Comparisons to Mental Retardation. *Journal of Autism and Developmental Disorders, 30,* 237-243.

Brereton, A. V., Tonge, B. J., Mackinnon, A. J., & Einfeld, S. L. (2002). Screening young people for autism with the Development Behavior Checklist. *Journal of the American Academy of Child and Adolescent Psychiatry, 41,* 1369-1375.

Brown, E. C., Aman, M. G., & Havercamp, S. M. (2002). Factor analysis and norms for parent ratings on the Aberrant Behavior Checklist-Community for young people in special education. *Research in Developmental Disabilities, 23,* 45-60.

Bruininks, R. H., Woodcock, R. W., Weatherman, R. F., & Hill, B. K. (1996). *Scales of Independent Behavior - Revised: Manual.* Boston: The Riverside Publishing Co.

Cichetti, D. V. (1994). Guidelines, criteria, and rule of thumb for evaluating normed and standardized assessment instruments in psychology. *Psychological Assessment, 6,* 284-290.

Clark, A. R., Tonge, B. J., Einfeld, S. L., & Mackinnon, A. (2003). Assessment of change with the Developmental Behaviour Checklist. *Journal of Intellectual Disability Research, 47,* 210-212.

Cohen, I. L. (2003). Criterion-related validity of the PDD Behavior Inventory. *Journal of Autism and Developmental Disorders, 33,* 47-53.

Cohen, I. L., Schmidt-Lackner, S., Romanczyk, R., & Sudhalter, V. (2003). The PDD Behavior Inventory: A rating scale for assessing response to intervention in children with pervasive developmental disorder. *Journal of Autism and Developmental Disorders, 33,* 31-45.

Dekker, M.C., Nunn, R. J., Einfeld, S. E., Tonge, B. J., & Koot, H. M. (2002). Assessing emotional and behavioral problems in children with intellectual disability: Revisiting the factor structure of the Developmental Behavior Checklist. *Journal of Autism and Developmental Disorders, 32*, 601-610.

Edelbrock, C. S. (1985). Child Behavior Rating Form. *Psychopharmacology Bulletin, 21*, 835-837.

Ehlers, S., & Gillberg, C. (1993). The epidemiology of Asperger syndrome: A total population study. *Journal of Child Psychology and Psychiatry and Allied Disciplines, 34*, 1327-1350.

Ehlers, S., Gillberg, C., & Wing, L. (1999). A screening questionnaire for Asperger syndrome and other high functioning autism spectrum disorders in school age children. *Journal of Autism and Developmental Disorders, 29*, 129-141.

Einfeld, S. L., & Tonge, B. J. (1992). *Manual for the Developmental Behaviour Checklist.* Clayton, Malbourne, and Aydney: Monash University Center for Developmental Psychiatry and School of Psychiatry, University of New South Wales.

Einfeld, S. L., & Tonge, B. J. (2002). *Manual for the Developmental Behaviour Checklist (2nd ed.).* Clayton, Malbourne, and Sydney: Monash University Center for Developmental Psychiatry and School of Psychiatry, University of New South Wales.

Esbensen, A. J., Rojahn, J., Aman, M. G., & Ruedrich, S. (in press). The reliability and validity of an assessment instrument for anxiety, depression and mood among individuals with mental retardation. *Journal of Autism and Developmental Disorders.*

Feinstein, C., Kaminer, Y., Barrett, R. P., & Tylenda, B. (1988). The assessment of mood and affect in developmentally disabled children and adolescents: The Emotional Disorders Rating Scale. *Research in Developmental Disabilities, 9*, 109-121.

Finlay, W. M. L., & Lyons, E. (2001). Methodological issues in interviewing and using self-report questionnaires with people with mental retardation. *Psychological Assessment, 13*, 319-335.

Floyd, F., & Widaman, K. F. (1995). Factor analysis in the development and refinement of clinical assessment instruments. *Psychological Assessment, 7*, 286-299.

Gilliam, J. E. (1995). *Gilliam Autism Rating Scale.* ProEd: Austin, Texas.

Gilliam, J. E. (2001). *Gilliam Asperger's Disorder Scale.* ProEd: Austin, Texas.

Girouard, N., Morin, I. N., & Tassé, M. J. (1998). Étude de fidelité test-retest et accord interjuges de la Grille d'évaluation comprtementale pour enfants Nisonger (GÉCEN). [Test-retest and interrater reliability of the French version of the Nisonger Child Behavior Rating From.] *Revue Francophone de la Déficience Intellectuelle, 9,* 127-136.

Goldman, R. S., Robinson, D., Grube, B. S., Hanks, R. A., Putnam, K., Walder, D. J., etr al. (2000). General psychiatric symptoms measures. In A. J. Rush, Jr., H. A. Pincus, M. B. First, D. Blacker, J. Endicott, S. J. Keith, et al. (Eds.), *Handbook of psychiatric measures* (pp. 71-92). Washington, DC: American Psychiatric Association.

Gustafsson, C., & Sonnander, K. (2002) Psychometric evaluation of a Swedish version of the Reiss Screen for Maladaptive Behavior. *Journal of Intellectual Disability Research, 46,* 218-229.

Hastings, R. P., Brown, T., Mount, R. H., & Cormack, K. F. M. (2001). Exploration of the psychometric properties of the Developmental Behaviour Checklist. *Journal of Autism and Developmental Disorders, 31,* 423-431.

Havercamp, S. M. (1996). *Psychiatric symptoms and mental retardation: Reliability of rating scales as a function of IQ.* Unpublished masters thesis, Ohio State University, Columbus, OH.

Helsel, W. J., & Matson, J. L. (1988). The relationship of depression to social skills and intellectual functioning in mentally retarded adults. *Journal of Mental Deficiency Research, 32,* 411-418.

Johns, M. R., & McDaniel, W. F. (1998). Areas of convergence and discordance between the MMPI-168 and the Reiss Screen for Maladaptive Behavior in mentally retarded clients. *Journal of Clinical Psychology, 54,* 529-535.

Kaminer, Y., Feinstein, C., Seifer, R., & Stevens, L. (1990). An observationally based rating scale for affective symptomatology in child psychiatry. *Journal of Nervous and Mental Disease, 178,* 750-754.

Kazdin, A. E., Matson, J. L.., & Senatore, V. (1983). Assessment of depression in mentally retarded adults. *American Journal of Psychiatry, 140,* 1040-1043.

Krug, D. A., Arick, J. R., and Almond, P. J. (1980a). Behavior checklist for identifying severely handicapped individuals with high levels of autistic behavior. *Journal of Child Psychology and Psychiatry, 21,* 221-229.

Krug, D. A., Arick, J. R., & Almond, P. J. (1980b). Autism Screening Instrument for Educational Planning. Portland, OR: ASIEP Educational Co.

Lecavalier, L. (in press). An evaluation of the Gilliam Autism Rating Scale. *Journal of Autism and Developmental Disorders.*

Lecavalier, L., Aman, M. G., Hammer, D., Stoica, W., & Matthews, G. L. (in press). *Factor analysis of Nisonger Child Behavior Rating Form in children with autism spectrum disorders*. Journal of Autism and Developmental Disorders.

Lecavalier, L., & Tassé, M. J. (2001). Traduction et adaptation transculturelle du Reiss Screen for Maladaptive Behavior [Translation and cross-cultural adaptation of the Reiss Screen for Maladaptive Behavior]. *Revue Francophone de la déficience intellectuelle [French Journal on Mental Retardation], 12,* 31-44.

Lindsay, W. R., & Michie, A. M. (1988). Adaptation of the Zung Self-Rating Anxiety Scale for people with a mental handicap. *Journal of Mental Deficiency Research, 32,* 485-490.

Lord, C., Risi, S., Lambrecht, L., Leventhal, B. L., DiLavore, P., Pickles, A., et al. (2000). The Autism Diagnostic Observation Schedule – Generic: A standard measure of social and communication deficits associated with the spectrum of autism. *Journal of Autism and Developmental Disorders, 30,* 205-223.

Lord, C., Rutter, M., & Le Couteur, A. (1994). Autism Diagnostic Interview-Revised: A revised version of a diagnostic interview for caregivers of individuals with possible pervasive developmental disorders. *Journal of Autism and Developmental Disorders, 24,* 659-685.

Marshburn, E. C., & Aman, M. G. (1992). Factor validity and norms for the Aberrant Behavior Checklist in a community sample of children with mental retardation. *Journal of Autism and Developmental Disorders, 22,* 357-373.

Matson, J. L. (1995). *Manual for the Diagnostic Assessment for the Severely Handicapped-II*. Baton Rouge, LA: Louisiana State University.

Matson, J. L. (1997). *Manual for the Assessment of Dual Diagnosis*. Baton Rouge, LA: Louisiana State University.

Matson, J. L., Baglio, C. S., Smiroldo, B. B., Hamilton, M., & Packlowskyj, T. (1996). Characteristics of autism as assessed by the Diagnostic Assessment for the Severely Handicapped – II (DASH-II). *Research in Developmental Disabilities, 17,* 1-9.

Matson, J. L., & Bamburg, J. A. (1998). Reliability of the Assessment of Dual Diagnosis (ADD). *Research in Developmental Disabilities, 19,* 89-95.

Matson, J.L., Gardner, W. I., Coe, D. A., & Sovner, R. (1991). A scale for evaluating emotional disorders in severely and profoundly mentally retarded persons. *British Journal of Psychiatry, 159,* 404-409.

Matson, J. L., Hamilton, M., Duncan, D., Bamburg, J., Smiroldo, B. B., Anderson, S., et al. (1997). Characteristic of stereotypic movement disorder and self-injurious behavior as assessed by the Diagnostic Assessment for the Severely

Handicapped II (DASH-II). *Research in Developmental Disabilities, 18*, 457-469.

Matson, J. L., Kazdin, A. E, & Senatore, V. (1984). Psychometric properties of the Psychopathology Instrument for Mentally Retarded Adults. *Applied Research in Mental Retardation, 5*, 81-89.

Matson, J. L., Rush, K. S., Hamilton, A., Anderson, S. J., Bamburg, J. W., Baglio, C. S., et al. (1999). Characteristics of depression as assessed by the Diagnostic Assessment for the Severely Handicapped-II (DASH-II). *Research in Developmental Disabilities, 20*, 305-313.

Matson, J. L., & Smiroldo, B. B. (1997). Validity of the mania subscale of the Diagnostic Assessment for the Severely Handicapped – II (DASH-II). *Research in Developmental Disabilities, 18*, 1-5.

Matson, J. L., Smiroldo, B. B., Hamilton, M., & Baglio, C. S. (1997). Do anxiety disorders exist in people with severe and profound mental retardation? *Research in Developmental Disabilities, 18*, 39-44.

McDaniel, W.F. (1997). Criterion-Related Diagnostic validity and test-retest reliability ofthe MMPI-168 (L) in mentally retarded adolescents and adults. *Journal of Clinical Psychology, 53*, 485-489.

McDaniel, W. F., & Harris, D. W. (1999). Mental health outcomes in dually diagnosed individuals with mental retardation assessed with the MMPI-168(L): Case Studies. *Journal of Clinical Psychology, 55*, 487-496.

Miranda-Linne, F. M., & Lennart, M. (2002). A factor analytic study of the Autism Behavior Checklist. *Journal of Autism and Developmental Disorders, 32*, 181-188.

National Institute of Mental Health. (1976). Clinical Global Impressions (CGI). In W. Guy (Ed). *ECDEU assessment manual for psychopharmacology revised* (pp.217-222). Rockville, MD: U.S. National Institutes of Health, Psychopharmacology Research Branch.

Nihira, K., Leland, H., & Lambert, N. (1993). Adaptive Behavior Scale–Residential and Community (2nd ed.). Examiners manual. Austin TX: Pro-Ed.

Ollendick, T. H. (1983). Reliability and validity of the Revised Fear Survey Schedule for Children (FSSC-R). *Behaviour Research and Therapy, 21*, 685-692.

Overall, J. E., & Gomez-Mont, F. (1974). The MMPI-168 for psychiatric screening. *Educational and Psychological Measurement, 34*, 315-319

Paclawskyj, T. R., Matson, J. L., Bamburg, J. W., & Baglio, C. (1997). A comparison of the Diagnostic Assessment for the Severely Handicapped – II (DASH-II) and the Aberrant Behavior Checklist (ABC). *Research in Developmental Disabilities, 18*, 189-298.

Powell, R. (2003). Psychometric properties of the Beck Depression Inventory and the Zung Self Rating Depression Scale in adults with mental retardation. *Mental Retardation, 41*, 88-95.

Prout, T. H., & Schaefer, B. M. (1985). Self-reports of depression by community-based mildly mentally retarded adults. *American Journal of Mental Deficiency, 90*, 220-222.

Ramirez, S. Z., & Kratochwill, T. R. (1990). Development of the Fear Survey for Children with and without Mental Retardation. *Behavioral Assessment, 12*, 457-470.

Reiss, S. (1988). *The Reiss Screen for Maladaptive Behavior test manual.* Worthington, OH: IDS Publishing Corporation.

Reiss, S., & Valenti-Hein, D. (1990). *Reiss Scales for Children's Dual Diagnosis: Test Manual (2nd Edition).* Worthington, OH: International Diagnostic Services.

Reiss, S., & Valenti-Hein, D. (1994). Development of a psychopathology rating scale for children with mental retardation. *Journal of Consulting and Clinical Psychology, 61*, 28-33.

Reynolds, W. M., & Baker, J. A. (1988). Assessment of depression in persons with mental retardation. *American Journal on Mental Retardation, 93*, 93-103.

Rojahn, J. (1986). Self-injurious and stereotypic behavior of non-institutionalized mentally retarded people: Prevalence and classification. *American Journal on Mental Deficiency, 91*, 268-276.

Rojahn, J., & Helsel, W. J. (1991). The Aberrant Behavior Checklist in children and adolescents with dual diagnosis. *Journal of Autism and Developmental Disorders, 21*, 17-28.

Rojahn, J., Matlock, S. T., & Tassé, M. J. (2000). The Stereotyped Behavior Scale: Psychometric properties and norms. *Research in Developmental Disabilities, 21*, 437-454.

Rojahn, J., Matson, J. L., Lott, D., Esbensen, A. J., & Smalls, Y. (2001). The Behavior Problems Inventory: An instrument for the assessment of self-injury, stereotyped behavior and aggression/destruction in individuals with developmental disabilities. *Journal of Autism and Developmental Disorders, 31*, 577-588.

Rojahn, J., Tassé, M. J., & Sturmey, P. (1997). The Stereotyped Behavior Scale for adolescents and adults with mental retardation. *American Journal on Mental Retardation, 102*, 137-146.

Schopler, E., Richter, R. J., DeVellis, R. F., & Daly, K. (1980). Toward objective classification of childhood autism: Childhood Autism Rating Scale (CARS). *Journal of Autism and Developmental Disorders, 10*, 91-103.

Schreck, K. A., & Mulick, J. A. (2000). Parental report of sleep problems in children with autism. *Journal of Autism and Developmental Disorders, 30,* 127-135.

South, M., Williams, B. J., McMahon, W. M., Owley, T., Filipek, P.A., Shernoff, E., et al. (2002). Utility of the Gilliam Autism Rating Scale in research and clinical populations. *Journal of Autism and Developmental Disorders, 32,* 593-599.

Sparrow, S., Balla, D., & Cichetti, D. (1984). *The Vineland Adaptive Behavior Scales: Interview Edition, Survey Form.* Circle Pines, MN: American Guidance Service.

Snyder, R., Turgay, A., Aman, M.G., Binder, C., & Fisman, S., & The Risperidone Conduct Study Group (2002). Effects of risperidone on conduct and disruptive disorders in children with subaverage IQ's. *Journal of the American Academy of Child and Adolescent Psychiatry, 41,* 1026-1036.

Strohmer, D. C., & Prout, H. T. (1989). *Strohmer-Prout Behavior Rating Scale.* Schenectady, NY: Genium Publishing.

Sturmey, P., Sevin, J. A., & Williams, D. E. (1995). The Behavior Problem Inventory: A further replication of its factor structure. *Journal of Intellectual Disability Research, 39,* 353-356.

Tassé, M., Aman, M.G., Hammer, D., & Rojahn, J. (1996). The Nisonger Child Behavior Rating Form: Age and gender effects and norms. *Research in Developmental Disorders, 17,* 59-75.

Tassé, M.J., & Lecavalier, L. (2000). Comparing parent and teacher ratings of social competence and problem behavior. *American Journal on Mental Retardation, 105,* 252-259.

Tassé, M. J., Morin, I., N., & Girouard, N. (2000). French Canadian translation and validation of the Nisonger Child Behavior Rating Form. *Canadian Psychology, 41,* 116-123.

Tobin, L. E., & Glenwick, D. S. (2002). Relation of the Childhood Autism Rating Scale-Parent version to diagnosis, stress, and age. *Research in Developmental Disabilities, 23,* 211-223.

Tonge, B., J. & Einfeld, S. L. (in press). Psychopathology and intellectual disability: The Australian child to adult longitudinal study. In L.M. Glidden (Ed), *International Review of Research in Mental Retardation.* San Diego, CA: Academic Press.

Van Minnen, A., Savelsberg, P.M., & Hoogduin, K.A.L. (1995). A Dutch version of the Reiss Screen of Maladaptive Behavior. *Research in Developmental Disabilities, 16,* 43-49.

Volkmar, F. R., Cichetti, D. V., Dykens, E,. M., Sparrow, S. S., Leckman, J. F., & Cohen, D. J. (1988). An evaluation of the Autism Behavior Checklist. *Journal of Autism and Developmental Disorders, 18,* 81-97.

8

Self-Injurious Behavior
in Mental Retardation

Theodore A. Hoch, Kristin E. Long, Megan M. McPeak,
and Johannes Rojahn
George Mason University

Introduction

According to the two latest editions of the manual on the definition and classification of mental retardation published by the American Association on Mental Retardation (1992, 2002) individuals with mental retardation are classified by their varying needs of support. Supports for the enhancement of a dignified and high-quality life are not only needed due to inherent cognitive and behavioral deficits, but also because of the multiple vulnerabilities associated with the condition itself. For instance, neuro-pathologies such as seizure disorders, cerebral palsy, and spina bifida are common, particularly among individuals with exhibiting greater mental retardation, and so are a variety of mental illnesses such as mood disorders, anxiety disorders and schizophrenia. In addition, individuals with mental retardation are at risk for chronic and severe behavior disorders, sometimes referred to as problem behavior, maladaptive behavior, or—somewhat euphemistically—challenging behavior. The most common and troublesome behavior problems are aggressive outbursts against others, destruction of property (see Chapter 10 in this book), and self-injurious behavior.

Self-injurious behavior or SIB refers to an array of heterogeneous behaviors that typically create exasperating problems for the affected individual and for the surrounding human support system including parents and family members, teachers, direct care staff, paraprofessionals and professionals. The primary concern is that SIB poses a threat of lasting and irreversible physical harm. For instance, it has been reported time and again that head banging had led to blindness due to detachment of the retinas. Cases have been reported of broken limbs from banging against walls and dropping to the floor, of life-threatening internal bleeding caused either by physical trauma or by the ingestion of sharp-edged metal objects, and of other self-inflicted damage severe enough to even have caused death. However, almost equally detrimental are the psychosocial effects of SIB. Anyone who has experienced a bout of serious head banging, for instance, will be able to relate to the finding that watching somebody engage in SIB takes its emotional toll on teachers or staff persons (Mossman, Hastings, & Brown, 2002). It is easy to imagine how a vicious spiral of events is set in motion, where SIB upsets caregivers to the point where they avoid contact, except for the most basic functions of care, which is likely to lead to further social isolation denying the individual of the requisite stimulation to maximize cognitive and socio-emotional development and the acquisition of adaptive skills. That in turn decreases the likelihood of a joyful and satisfied life and overall well-being. In addition, SIB often absorbs or exhausts tremendous financial resources and seriously strains the service system.

This chapter was designed to provide an overview of current behavioral management and treatment issues. Our intention was not to present a comprehensive quantitative literature review on behavioral treatment of SIB, such as the one that has recently been published by Kahng, Iwata, and Lewin (2002)[1].

Characteristics of SIB

1. Epidemiology of SIB

SIB prevalence rates among people with mental retardation vary greatly from study to study. This finding comes as no surprise considering the variety of different reference populations, sampling strategies, case ascertainment procedures, case definitions, settings, and assessment tools that were used across studies (Rojahn & Esbensen, 2002). Part of the problem has been that very few of the published studies received the financial grant support necessary to reach the rigorous scientific standards expected from epidemiological research in areas with broader political appeal.

1 Also beyond the scope of this chapter is a discussion of the increasingly important role of psychopharmacology of SIB. For a recent review of the literature on psychopharmacology and SIB see Matson et al. (2000).

Perhaps the most robust and frequently replicated finding is that there is a negative correlation between the prevalence of SIB and the level of mental retardation (McClintock, Hall & Oliver, 2003; Rojahn & Esbensen, 2002). For instance, the largest epidemiological data base analyzed showed that the prevalence of clinically significant SIB among 10 to 45 year olds who received developmental disabilities services in either California or New York was as follows: four percent among individuals with mild mental retardation, 7% for individuals with moderate mental retardation, 16% in severe and 25% in profound mental retardation. The overall prevalence rate of serious SIB was eight percent (Rojahn, Borthwick-Duffy & Jacobson, 1993; Rojahn, Matson, Lott, Esbensen, & Smalls, 1999). Researchers also point to an association between receptive and expressive communication and SIB, suggesting that individuals with communication deficits are more likely to develop SIB than individuals without a communication deficit (McClintock et al., 2003). Since the degrees of mental retardation and communication skills are highly correlated, the extent of their independent contributions as risk factors of SIB is unclear.

Evidence of the relationship between other demographic variables and SIB are less clear. Sex ratio estimates for instance, are inconsistent across studies and may vary with different SIB topographies (McClintock et al., 2003; Rojahn and Esbensen, 2002). Overall, it seems that the prevalence of SIB as a broad behavior category does not differ significantly between sexes. The exception of course, are x-linked conditions strongly associated with SIB. These disorders include the Lesch-Nyhan syndrome (Anderson & Ernst, 1994) or other conditions associated with SIB that occur disproportionately in males (e.g., autism spectrum disorders). Cross-sectional studies suggest that SIB is related to chronological age with larger proportions of middle-aged individuals (teens, adolesents and young adults) affected than young children and elderly people (Jacobson, 1982; Oliver, Murphy, & Corbett, 1987; Rojahn, 1986). However, those data need to be viewed with caution, particularly with regard to the very young because SIB in young children may be under reported. As Murphy, Hall, Oliver, and Kissi-Debra (1999) have shown, SIB at that age may not be as dramatic yet or may not be recognized for what it is. In a very carefully conducted study Berkson, Tupa, and Sherman (2001) followed a group of 39 very young children (three to 40 months of age) with severe disabilities who were referred for being at risk for or manifesting stereotyped behavior or SIB. Risk factors were defined as severe visual impairment, significant developmental disability, and social withdrawal. Of these children, six (15.4%) engaged in repeated, non-transient SIB. Most of these children engaged in only one SIB topography, and all were directed against the head (except biting).

Incidence refers to the ratio of emerging new cases within a specified time period relative to a reference population. Despite the fact that much could be learned about the conditions that contribute to the emergence of SIB and its prevention, longitudinal studies involving infants and young children at risk for SIB are rare. Financial resources necessary to conduct a study involving tracking cohorts of such vulnerable individuals over a long period of time are by and large even greater than in cross-sectional studies. In one of the very few incidence studies of newly emerging SIB, Murphy et al. (1999) interviewed teachers of children with severe mental retardation and autism. Screening more than 600 children 11 years and younger revealed that the incidence of recent onset SIB during a period of one year was 3%.

Researchers have debated whether and to what extent maladaptive behaviors in general and SIB in particular may be an atypical manifestation of psychiatric disorders such as schizophrenia or mood disorders ("psychosocial masking"). The notion that SIB may be associated with psychiatric disorders is rooted in the fact that "self-mutilation", as it is typically referred to in the psychiatric literature, is symptomatic for several psychiatric disorders, including borderline personality disorder, acute psychotic episodes, schizophrenia, depression, obsessive-compulsive disorder, post-traumatic stress disorder, anxiety disorders, and impulse control disorders (Favazza, 1996). Rojahn, Matson, Naglieri, and Mayville (in press) studied a group of 180 individuals with predominantly severe and profound mental retardation and found that SIB tended to be especially correlated with conditions that are conventionally known to be associated with behavior problems, namely impulse control problems and conduct problems. Depression, mania, anxiety, and schizophrenic conditions, on the other hand, were less strongly associated with SIB. However, it was also found that individuals with SIB had substantially higher psychopathology scores across almost all assessed conditions than individuals without behavior problems. The same held true for stereotyped or aggressive/destructive behavior. In other words, and as others have argued (e.g., Thompson and Caruso, 2002; Tsiouris, Mann, Patti & Sturmey, 2003), SIB did not appear to be a population-specific behavioral equivalent of common psychiatric disorders.

Thompson and Caruso (2002) proposed that SIB has common characteristics that distinguish it from self-mutilation associated with the typical psychiatric population. In their view, SIB in mental retardation (a) involves repetitive movements that produce actual or potential damage when repeated frequently, (b) occurs episodically, either in punctuated bouts, or in protracted periods, (c) may be initiated by a particular event, but may continue autonomously once it has begun, and (d) causes injury to particular bodily locations that vary with etiology of the disability and the function of the behavior. Interestingly, the taxonomy of "pathological self mutilation" introduced by Favazza (1996), is consistent with Thompson and Caruso's distinction between SIB in mental retardation and self-mutilation in the general psychiatric population, despite radically different theoretical orientations. Favazza a cultural psychiatrist, proposes three distinct types of self-mutilation, one of which is equivalent with SIB as it is the topic of this chapter: *Stereotypic self-mutilation*, which is repetitive in nature and associated with mental retardation and several disorders (Autistic Disorder, Lesch-Nyhan disease, DeLange syndrome, etc.)[2].

2. Topographies and Targeted Body Areas

One of the characteristics of SIB is that it is relatively invariant. Like stereotyped behavior, individuals engage in their very own, idiosyncratic form of SIB, rarely with any noticeable changes from bout to bout. Since SIB topographies are relatively stagnant, and since the topography of SIB determines the targeted areas of the body as well as the type of damage it caused, neither the targeted areas nor the inflicted damage are random. A consistent finding across different epidemiological studies is that the most common SIB among individuals with mental retardation is self-hitting or banging (i.e., butting, hitting, striking, slapping) that is either directed at the head or face, or at some other body parts. Some individuals prefer to bang themselves with their own body parts (i.e., palms, fists, knees), or they use stable, hard objects against which to bang themselves. The second most common form of SIB is self-biting. Other frequently reported SIBs were scratching, pinching, hair pulling, deliberate vomiting and rumination, and different forms of digging, poking or gouging (Iwata et al., 1994; Rojahn & Esbensen, 2002).

Symons and Thompson (1997) studied the SIB of 29 individuals with mental retardation, and reported that about 80% of the injuries occurred on only 5% of the body surface – forehead, temples, and the hands. The head areas are typically struck with the hands, fist or hard objects, while the hand areas are typically the targets of biting.

2 *The second category is* major self-mutilation, *often associated with psychosis, occurs suddenly, is highly dramatic, and causes serious tissue damage (e.g., enucleated eye, amputated body parts), while the third category is* moderate/superficial self-mutilation, *which includes cutting, carving, burning, hair pulling and others that are alleged to be symptoms of a variety of psychiatric disorders.*

Other topographies cause damage to other areas of the body. For instance, hair pulling is typically restricted to the scalp, while skin picking is typically focused on the arms and thighs. Iwata, Pace, Kissel, Nau, and Farber (1990) developed a useful assessment technique to classify and quantify surface tissue damage of SIB.

Mechanisms Controlling the Emergence and Maintenance of SIB

At first glance SIB seems utterly paradoxical. How can we explain that a person repeatedly engages in seemingly painful and obviously self-damaging behavior? Recent research clearly leads to the conclusion that SIB is the product of a complex interplay of genetic, neurobiological, neurochemical and environmental mechanisms (Schroeder, Oster-Granite & Thompson, 2002).

Carr's (1977) crucial conceptual paper on the motivation of SIB followed a few years later by the methodological contribution of functional analysis by Iwata, Dorsey, Slifer, Bauman, and Richman (1982) on how to ascertain controlling variables, brought into focus that, in most cases and to a significant extent, SIB is subject to basic principles of operant conditioning, biological factors notwithstanding. As such, motivation of SIB and its controlling variables can be conceptualized in a functional-behavioral framework, including predisposing genetic and biological variables. This means that any variable that contributes to the cause, development, maintenance, and change of any parameter of SIB, be it genetic, biological or environmental, be it temporary or lasting; or be it relatively accessible or inaccessible for manipulation, can be conceptualized within a behavior analytic framework as either distal or proximal variables (see Figure 1).

1. Distal Variables

Distal variables are those that predispose a person to a greater likelihood to develop a certain behavior as compared to peers who are similar in most other respects, with the exception of the predisposing attribute. SIB as a behavioral phenotype is a case in point. Several conditions such as Lesch-Nyhan disease, Cornelia de Lange syndrome, Smith-Magenis syndrome, and Prader-Willi syndrome are associated with SIB. For instance, the most common first type of SIB in Lesch-Nyhan cases is biting of lips and/or fingers (e.g., Robey, Reck, Giacomini, Barabas & Eddey, 2003). Other behavior problems included head banging, extension of arms when being wheeled through doorways, tipping of wheelchairs, eye poking, fingers in wheelchair spokes, and rubbing behaviors. Individuals with Cornelia de Lange syndrome are prone to insert fingers into the mouth and to bite their finger tips (Berney, Ireland, & Burn, 1999). Prader-Willi syndrome is associated with in skin picking (Dykens & Smith, 1999; Symons, Butler, Sanders, Feuer, & Thompson, 1999), and Smith-Magenis syndrome is known for the pulling of nails (Dykens & Smith, 1999). Obviously, such predisposing biological variables are currently inaccessible for systematic behavior analytic manipulations at this point in time. However, they signal the presence of biological forces that may require special considerations in behavioral programming. For instance, Anderson and Ernst (1994) observed that SIB among individuals with Lesch-Nyhan disorder was treatment resistant to behavioral intervention.

Figure 1. Distal and proximal variables that determine the emergence and maintenance of SIB (EO = establishing operations).

2. Proximal Variables

Proximal variables are those that control SIB more immediately from one occurrence to the next and are the primary targets of manipulation in a behavior program. Proximal variables can be antecedent events (such as establishing operations, discriminative stimuli and evocative stimuli), or consequent events.

Establishing operations are events that temporarily affect the effectiveness of a reinforcer, and simultaneously change the probability of occurrence of the operant that had produced that reinforcer in the past (Michael, 2000). A host of potential establishing operations for SIB has been reported in the form of physiological conditions including sleep deprivation, menses, anxiety, stress and over or under arousal of the CNS (Romanczyk, Lockshin & O'Conner, 1992; Romanczyk & Matthews, 1998; Symons, Sutton, Walker & Bodfish, 2003). Similarly, psychotropic medication can function as an establishing operation (e.g., the anhedonic effect of neuroleptics may impact the effectiveness of primary reinforcers), as well as the availability of desirable behavioral alternatives or the lack thereof, or reinforcer satiation. Establishing operations have become a particularly fruitful focus of innovative applied behavior analytic research on SIB in recent years (McGill, 1999; Wilder & Carr, 1998).

Functional Assessment and Analysis

Functional analysis and functional assessment are procedures designed to identify both response antecedent and consequent events that control the target behavior in order to select proper intervention strategies. While the terms "functional analysis" and "functional assessment" were introduced in the early 1980s as a consequence of Iwata et al.'s (1982) breakthrough methodological contribution, the role of behavioral assessment in selecting treatments based on the specific controlling variables of the target behavior of a specific individual has been a mainstay of behavior therapy from its beginning (Kanfer & Saslow, 1969). Functional assessment typically encompasses empirical, but non-experimental assessments that do not involve the removal of the individual from the natural environment in which the target behavior occurs. Functional assessment procedures can include casual or structured interviews with staff members, parents, and other people familiar with the individual and the behavior, or observations in the natural environment that can range from simple unstructured observations, to systematic and structured data collection in the form of scatter plots (Touchette, MacDonald & Langer, 1985) or contingency observations and rating scales, such as the *Motivation Assessment Scale* (Durand & Crimmins, 1988, 1992) or the *Questions About Behavioral Functions* (Matson & Vollmer, 1995). Functional analysis, on the other hand, refers to the systematic, experimentally controlled exposure of the individual to stimulus conditions, so called analog conditions, suspected to be maintaining SIB. Introduction of functional analysis methodology by Iwata et al. (1982) had a tremendous impact on the treatment of SIB and other behavior problems (Kahng et al., 2002). Regardless of the method, the purpose is to identify variables that are systemically related the SIB to permit individualized, function-relevant treatments. Functional analysis combined with proper medical evaluations can not only produce effective behavioral treatment programs but is also said to reduce the likelihood of unwarranted and unnecessary psychopharmacological treatment or intrusive punishment procedures (Pelios, Morren, Tesch & Axelrod, 1999). Several excellent books and manuals are available with practical guidelines and useful examples of data collection instruments (e.g., O'Neill, Horner, Albin, Sprague, Storey, & Newton, 1997).

Figure 2. Percentage of various functional properties of SIB from Iwata et al. (1993) and Kurtz et al (2003).

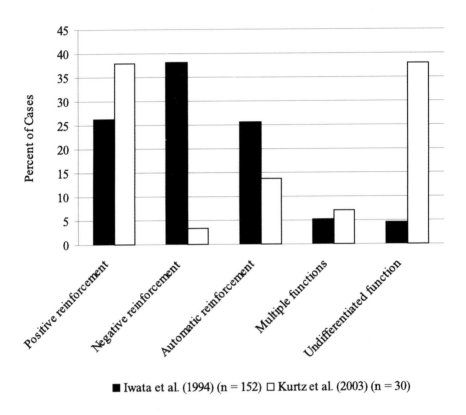

■ Iwata et al. (1994) (n = 152) □ Kurtz et al. (2003) (n = 30)

Figure 2 presents a summary of two studies on the functional properties of SIB. Iwata et al. (1994) studied the functional properties of 152 SIB cases including children and adults that were seen for treatment during an 11-year period. They found that negative reinforcement (social) was the predominant behavioral function in 38.1% of the cases, positive reinforcement (social) in 26.3%, and automatic reinforcement in 25.7%. Multiple controlling functions were identified in only 5.3%, and inconsistent controlling functions in 4.6%. The surprising and encouraging conclusion we can draw is that the great majority of SIB seems to have a single functional purpose, which simplifies the task of fitting a treatment program to it. Moreover, almost 65% are under the control of contingencies that are relatively accessible for experimental manipulation (social-negative reinforcement or escape-motivated behavior and social positive reinforcement for attention or access to food or materials).

A slightly different picture emerged in a study on young children with SIB (Kurtz et al., 2003). Among the 30 children (mean age 2 years 9 months) with SIB, functional properties were undifferentiated in almost 40% of the cases. Most of the children's SIB was controlled by positive reinforcement (37.9%), while SIB was controlled by negative reinforcement in only 3.4% of the cases. Automatic reinforcement was identified in 13.8% and a combination of positive and negative reinforcement in 7.0% of the cases.

In comparing the two studies, the difference in the proportion of cases in which SIB is controlled by negative reinforcement is remarkable. In fact, among the young children in Kurtz et al. (2003), the SIB of only one child was controlled by escape motivation. The second most striking difference between the two data sets is the proportion of cases in which the SIB functions are undifferentiated or unclear. Whether these differences can be accounted for by the age difference in the two samples or other unknown variables remains unclear at this point.

Some researchers have begun to incorporate functional analysis or assessment to evaluate effects of psychoactive medication (e.g., Crosland et al., 2003; Garcia, & Smith, 1999; Mace, Blum, Sierp, Delaney, & Mauk, 2001; Symons, Fox, & Thompson, 1998). While medications directly affect biochemical substrates of SIB, they may thereby also change establishing operations. For instance, the anhedonic effects of neuroleptic drugs may alter the effectiveness of certain reinforcers. In other instances, combining pharmacological and function-relevant environmental manipulations has been effective (Frazier, Doyle, Chiu, & Coyle, 2002; Symons et al., 1998).

Behavioral Interventions

In many instances, multiple controlling variables are functionally related to SIB. Therefore, effective interventions must often be comprised of multiple components (Carr & Smith, 1995; O'Neill et al., 1997). The focus of function-relevant treatment is not so much suppression of SIB, as it is altering contingencies to render the SIB irrelevant, inefficient, and ineffective, and to replace it with behavior that is more beneficial to the focus person and those around her or him as represented in Figure 3

(O'Neill et al., 1997). It is in this vein that intervention for SIB is now discussed. For the reader interested in more detail on specific intervention procedures and their effectives, a selection of representative studies is provided in Table 1.

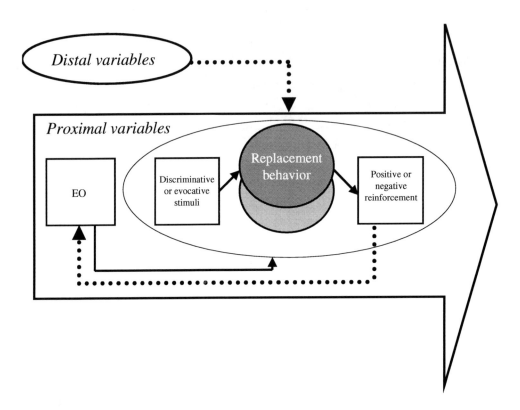

Though biological determinants may increase probability of a particular topography's emergence, or contribute to sustenance, it that does not mean that the behavior is immune to environmental influence. A number of authors have demonstrated functional relations between environmental events and SIB in people with genetic syndromes and with acquired brain injury, and have likewise demonstrated behavioral improvements when the environmental contingencies are altered (Dykens & Smith, 1999; Hall, Oliver, & Murphy, 2001; Persel, Persel, Ashley, & Krych, 1997; Symons et al., 1999; Treadwell & Page, 1996). Clearly, functional analysis and function relevant treatment can be beneficial for people exhibiting behavior problems that are said to have a physiological basis.

Table 1
Selected Studies on Behavioral Interventions for SIB

Intervention Type	References
Manipulating Establishing Operations	Brylewski & Wiggs (1999); Carr et al. (2003); DeLeon et al. (2000); Derby et al. (1995); Fischer et al. (1997); Healy et al. (2001); Horner et al. (1997); Kahng et al. (2001); Lindauer et al. (1999); McCord et al. (2001); O'Reilly (1996); O'Reilly et al. (2001); O'Reilly & Lancioni (2000); O'Reilly et al. (1999); Sigafoos et al. (1996); Van Camp et al. (2002); Vollmer et al. (1998); Wacker et al. (1996); Zarcone et al. (1993)
Manipulating Discriminative Stimuli	Oliver et al. (1998); Saunders et al. (1996); Van Camp et al. (2002)
Response Based Interventions	Bowman et al. (1997); Braithwaite & Richdale (2000); Durand & Merges (2001); Kahng et al. (2001); Kern et al. (1997); Obi (1997); Shore et al. (1997); Sigafoos & Meikle (1996); Van Houten (1993); Zhou et al. (2000)
Manipulating Consequences	Arntzen & Werner (1999); Barton et al. (1985); Bird et al. (199); Grace et al. (1996); Healy et al. (2001); Luiselli (1992); Luiselli & Waldstein (1994) Matson & Keyes (1990); McCord et al. (2001); McKerchar et al. (2001); Patel et al. (2000); Rapp et al. (1999); Roberts et al. (1995); Rush et al. (2001); Sigafoos & Pennell (1995); Thompson et al. (1999); Van Camp et al. (2002); Zarcone et al. (1993)

1. Manipulations of Antecedents

When functional analysis or assessment implicates establishing operations, discriminative stimuli, or combinations of these in maintaining SIB, function-relevant treatment may involve manipulating these types of variables. Additionally, when functional analysis or assessment implicates consequences in maintaining SIB, antecedent manipulation may also be indicated. These types of intervention do not directly contact the behavior, but instead alter the circumstances under which the behavior is most or least likely to occur, thereby indirectly affecting the behavior, and have been called "passive behavior management" (Bailey & Pyles, 1989). Various types of passive behavior management are discussed next.

a) Manipulating Establishing Operations

Establishing operations (EOs) are motivating antecedents that enhance or degrade the relative momentary effectiveness of a reinforcer (Michael, 2000). Brylewski and Wiggs (1999) and O'Reilly and Lancioni (2000) identified sleep deprivation as an establishing operation that increased probability of SIB for some people with developmental disabilities. Physical discomfort related to menstrual periods (Carr, Smith, Ciacin, Whelan, & Pancari, 2003) and otitis (O'Reilly, 1997) have been shown to increase probability of SIB for some, as well. Food-deprivation or satiation may also influence probability of SIB (Wacker et al., 1996). In general, allergies, illnesses, or other medical issues may function as establishing operations that are functionally related to self- injury (Bailey & Pyles, 1989). Establishing regular sleep patterns, medically addressing physical discomfort and illness, ensuring adequate dietary intake, and otherwise addressing physiology relevant establishing operations may substantially reduce or eliminate SIB for some individuals.

Sensorially or materially impoverished environments have been implicated as establishing operations promoting value of various reinforcers by a number of researchers, and remedying these environmental deficits has produced decline or elimination in SIB for some people with developmental disabilities. For example, Lindauer, DeLeon, and Fisher (1999) found an environment enriched with empirically identified preferred stimuli decreased SIB rate for a woman diagnosed with mental retardation and a mood disorder. Often, however, additional procedures are needed to produce clinically significant declines in SIB. When Van Camp, Vollmer, and Daniel (2002) incorporated empirically identified preferences into task routines for a boy with autism, they found greater decline in SIB when this environmental enrichment was combined with other procedures. Similarly, Sigafoos, Pennell, and Verslius (1996) found that non-contingent access to preferred toys combined with mand training reduced head banging for an 11-year-old boy with multiple disabilities. Kahng, Abt, and Wilder (2001) found an environment enriched with empirically identified sensorially relevant stimuli eliminated hand to head SIB, but additional intervention was needed to decelerate head banging.

Transition from one activity or location to another may also be an establishing operation that promotes SIB for some. However, both McCord, Thomson, and Iwata (2001) and Mace, Shapiro, and Mace (1999) report advanced notice of transitions was insufficient to decelerate SIB, and that additional intervention was needed.

A number of researchers examined clinical utility of altering value of reinforcers initially accessed contingent on SIB, by presenting those (or equivalent) reinforcers noncontingently. For example, noncontingent access to social attention (O'Reilly, Lacey, & Lancioni, 2001), and to matched, alternative sensory stimulation (Healy, Ahearn, Graff, & Libby, 2001) produced clinically significant reductions in SIB for all participants involved. However, multiple determination of SIB has sometimes necessitated additional intervention. Rush, Crockett, and Hagopian (2001) found non-contingent social attention reduced other, socially mediated problem behaviors, but that non-socially mediated SIB required additional intervention (e.g., facial screening). Sigafoos and Pennell (1995) found that contingently removing otherwise non-contingently available, sensorially matched alternative stimuli when SIB occurred produced a greater reduction than did non-contingent access to the alternative stimuli alone.

Much of the literature on non-contingent access to reinforcers indicates social attention delivered on a fixed time schedule as a potential partial remedy for socially mediated SIB. Other studies have shown that temporally proximal (O'Reilly, Lancioni, & Emerson, 1999) and more temporally distant social phenomena (O'Reilly, 1996) can exert adverse or idiosyncratic effects on SIB. While these prior social phenomena can be altered and reductions in SIB sometimes subsequently obtained, possibility of idiosyncratic responding to such stimuli suggests that some caution is needed both when interpreting and applying findings from the literature. Individually measured response to treatment must remain among the utmost determinants of treatment efficacy.

Preferred stimulus satiation is also a phenomenon that can promote SIB. Initial within-session reduction was seen in SIB when preferred stimuli were made non-contingently available, but DeLeon, Anders, Rodrigues-Catter, and Neidert (2000) found this effect to attenuate across 20 minute sessions. They subsequently found that varying the sets of empirically identified stimuli used to enrich an environment produced more sustained suppression in SIB.

b) Manipulating Discriminative Stimuli

Contrary to an EO, discriminative stimuli (S^Ds or S^{Δ}s) are not motivative antecedents. S^Ds increase the momentary probability of a behavior by having preceded the response when it was reinforced in the past. S^{A}s decrease momentary probability of a behavior by having been present in the past when the behavior was not reinforced. Discriminative stimuli, then, do not alter momentary potency of consequences, as is done by EOs. Instead, they more directly alter momentary probability of a particular response class by virtue of their presence when prior occurrences of the response class were followed by particular consequence operations. Altering discriminative stimuli can reduce SIB and is often done in conjunction with other contingency manipulations. For instance, Van Camp et al. (2002) reported that by establishing s-delta antecedent control of environmental features present when SIB was occasioned, in addition to other manipulations, frequency was substantially decreased for a 13-year-old boy with autism. Saunders, Saunders, Brewer, and Roach (1996) ensured more timely delivery of task prompts and produced a decrease one subject's SIB, and eliminated another subject's SIB by altering instructions and other discriminative stimuli associated with mealtime. In general, when providing prompts in the treatment of SIB or any other behavioral difficulty to the extent that the prompts are delivered only once, are stated as instructions rather than requests, are meant to engage in a particular behavior rather than to cease the SIB, and to the extent that functional reinforcers or other functional consequences are delivered contingent on compliance or noncompliance with the instructions, the result is the greater the probability that the prompts will acquire discriminative stimulus control over the behaviors prompted (Cooper, Heron, & Heward, 1987).

2. Response Based Interventions

Discussion thus far has focused on conducting passive behavior management to treat SIB. Reinforcement contingencies maintaining SIB can be disrupted by providing the reinforcing stimuli on a fixed time schedule, or by treating medical or other physiological, social, or environmental conditions that establish various stimuli as reinforcers. Altering non-salient discriminative stimuli, or establishing inhibitory discriminative stimulus control for SIB or discriminative control for alternative behaviors can also reduce probability of SIB.

Active behavior management, in contrast, operates directly on the SIB (Bailey & Pyles, 1989). This approach involves altering properties of the response itself, such as effort required to attain reinforcement, or by altering consequence aspects of contingencies. Increased response effort, achieved through use of arm splints or wrist restraints that permit some joint flexion, has been an effective component in treatment packages for hand to head self injury for individuals with Lesch-Nyhan syndrome

(Obi, 1997), and some people with severe or profound mental retardation (Kahng, et al., 2001; Shore, Iwata, DeLeon, Kahng, & Smith, 1997; Zhou, Goff, & Iwata, 2000). Use of these devices did not preclude the hand to head SIB, but instead increased amount of effort needed for the subject to contact his head with his hand. Contingencies requiring less response effort were set in place for alternative behaviors. Increasing the response effort required to satisfy the ongoing schedule of reinforcement, while providing a less effortful contingency for an alternative behavior, enhanced the efficiency of the alternative behavior in each of these cases, producing decreases in SIB and increases in functional alternative responding.

These studies illustrate that one must attend closely to reinforcement parameters of concurrent schedules when altering SIB response effort. In the instances reported above, lesser response effort was required for the alternative responses to attain the same or greater magnitude of reinforcement. Response efficiency and reinforcer magnitude must also be attended to when shaping or accelerating alternative behaviors to temporally or physically displace, or to assume the same function served by, the SIB.

This subject is often done through social skills training, and is often a combination of active and passive behavior management. In general, people with developmental disabilities who display SIB exhibit a more restricted range of social behaviors compared with those who do not exhibit SIB (Duncan, Matson, Bamburg, Cherry, & Buckley, 1999). When SIB is maintained by contingent access to social stimuli or tangibles, or by escape or avoidance of task demands or other environmental variables, the social skill taught is often a mand, and the procedure is often termed "functional communication training." Mand training is appropriate when the SIB is under antecedent control of an establishing operation, and consequence control of a stimulus change that is specific to that establishing operation. For instance, if a food deprived subject (e.g., colloquially, a hunger child) exhibited SIB, and the SIB is maintained by gaining access to food; and if the reinforcing function of access to food is found to vary directly with magnitude of food deprivation, then the SIB may be said to function as a mand. Training manding has been effective in eliminating or reducing SIB when combined with other, consequence based procedures for people diagnosed with a variety of disabilities (Braithwaite & Richdale, 2000; Kern, Carberry, & Haidara, 1997; Obi, 1997), and to be sufficient to eliminate SIB without additional intervention for some (Bowman, Fisher, Thompson, & Piazza, 1997; Durand & Merges, 2001; Sigafoos & Meikle, 1996). These procedures may involve selecting a response modality for the mand that is salient for the individual; prompting the mand response and following it with the reinforcer that previously followed SIB; and blocking reinforcement for SIB, or otherwise altering contingencies such that SIB is less efficient. Mand topographies may include signing, speaking, picture-exchange, and use of an augmentative communication device. The topography that is targeted must require no more (and preferably less) response effort than the self-injurious response it is to replace, and must be reinforced as rapidly as, or more rapidly than the SIB, with reinforcers that at least quantitatively and qualitatively match (and preferably exceed) those available contingent on SIB.

3. Manipulating Consequences

Numerous treatment packages, particularly those involving differential reinforcement, incorporate an extinction schedule for self-injurious responding and a reinforcement schedule for one or more other topographies. Cautions we raised earlier regarding concurrently available schedules also apply to the implementation of differential reinforcement procedures. Practitioners or researchers can exert greater control over various social and tangible consequences than can be directly exerted in many instances of automatic, sensory reinforcement. Current literature advocates taking functional analysis a step beyond identifying contingencies maintaining SIB, to identifying properties of consequences that exert reinforcer function. Healey et al. (2001), McKerchar, Kahng, Casioppo, and Wilson (2001), Patel, Carr, Kim, Robes, and Eastridge (2000), Sigafoos and Pennell (1995), and Van Camp et al. (2002) describe procedures by which therapist controlled stimuli were identified that were substitutable for sensory stimuli produced via automatic reinforcement hypothesized to maintain SIB. Providing sensory experience that successfully competes with that produced by SIB, irrespective of the SIB, can render the SIB inefficient and irrelevant.

Multi-component treatment packages also sometimes involve punishment procedures. Rush et al. (2001) found greatest reduction of automatically reinforced SIB when facial screening was added to a treatment package also involving non-contingent attention and social extinction. Thompson, Iwata, Conners, and Roscoe (1999) report greater SIB suppression when reprimands or brief manual restraint were combined with reinforcement for manipulating leisure materials, than when the punishment procedure was implemented alone. Finally, Sigafoos and Pennel (1995) report removing non-contingently accessed sensory stimuli matched to those hypothesized as automatically reinforcing SIB, contingent on SIB, produced a greater reduction than did non-contingent access to the sensory stimuli alone. Punishment has a long history in behavioral treatment of SIB (Iwata et al., 1982), and with the advent of functional analysis and assessment, and the function relevant treatment thus afforded, exposing those exhibiting SIB to punishment contingencies has been reduced, given attention devoted to other aspects of maintaining contingencies (Mace, 1994; Pelios et al., 1999).

Restraining devices or other forms of protective equipment are sometimes used with people who display SIB to prevent serious tissue damage. Some devices, such as helmets used with people who display head banging or hand to head SIB, do not prevent SIB, but instead provide a protective barrier that can preclude serious damage. Other devices, such as arm splints, may be used to either increase effort expenditure required to emit SIB, or may be used to prevent occurrence of SIB altogether. Using such devices is often regulated by state, agency, or funding source policy. Although a primary concern must be ensuring the client's well being, systematic elimination or minimization of restraining devices must be part of treatment planning whenever they are used.

Oliver, Hall, Hales, Murphy, and Watts (1998) report elimination of hand to head SIB for two participants, and reduction for a third when rigid arm splints were introduced. They then systematically increased arm flexion by reducing rigidity of initially inflexible arm. They coupled this procedure simultaneously with additional alternative behavior training, and reductions in SIB were maintained although the splints eventually permitted greater arm flexion. The authors opine the procedure established inhibitory stimulus control exerted by the terminally flexible splints over the SIB.

Others have used splints that increased SIB response effort, while providing reinforcement for less effortful alternative behavior on a denser schedule. For example, Zhou et al. (2000) used flexible arm sleeves with four middle-aged participants exhibiting self-injurious hand mouthing maintained by automatic reinforcement, such hand mouthing required greater effort. Concurrently, they provided access to empirically identified preferred leisure items. Hand mouthing showed greater decrease, and object engagement greater increase, when both procedures were coupled, than when leisure item access occurred alone. Kahng et al. (2001) report a similar procedure, but found head banging increased when hand to head SIB was made more effortful by flexible splints. Contingent exercise was added, which reduced head banging.

Obi (1997) replaced rigid wrist restraints with a hard helmet to permit shaping and generalizing completion of activities of daily living and work related tasks for a man with Lesch-Nyhan syndrome. Following acquisition of the alternative behaviors, the hard helmet was successfully faded, and reductions in SIB and restraint use, and increases in adaptive and social skills were maintained for at least 26 months' follow-up.

In other instances, devices are used that mask sensory stimulation obtained by SIB. Luiselli and Waldstein (1994) evaluated effects of wearing a glove in a sensory extinction procedure combined with alternative behavior training for a woman with profound mental retardation who exhibited hand to eye SIB. Prior management was preventive, with the woman's left wrist tied to a bedrail. (She had no functional use of her right arm.) Hand to eye SIB was effectively decelerated using the sensory extinction procedure, with zero instances noted in a follow-up session conducted one month later. The device used in this procedure did not prevent the hand to eye behavior, but altered its sensory consequences. Rapp, Miltenberger, Galenski, Ellingson and Long (1999) found similar suppression when a woman diagnosed with severe mental retardation who exhibited Trichotillomania wore gloves.

Contingent personal, or physical restraint has also been reported. Thompson et al. (1999) report efficacy of a reprimand or brief personal restraint in suppressing SIB when combined with reinforcement for leisure material manipulation for four people with mental retardation. More than a decade earlier, Barton, Repp, and Brulle (1985) reported on a similar procedure with similar findings with four children diagnosed with severe or profound mental retardation and multiple physical disabilities.

Although efficacy can be demonstrated for either mechanical or physical restraint procedures in suppressing SIB, this type of procedure often remains controversial, and carries with it risks for iatrogenic injury or exacerbation of behavioral difficulties. Spreat, Lipinski, Hill, and Halpin (1986) reported more than three-times greater likelihood of injury to the restrained party when physical restraint was used, as opposed to mechanical restraint, for their sample of 231 people with mental retardation living in a residential facility. Mechanical restraint can be particularly risky when used with elderly or infirm people, with possible untoward effects of long term use including decrease in muscle mass, muscle strength, and bone density; exacerbation of cardiac problems; subcutaneous hematoma; asphyxiation; and death (Archea, McNeely, Martino-Saltzman, Hennessy, Whittington, & Myers, 1993; Landi et al., 2001; Robinson, Sucholeiki, & Schocken, 1993). Spreat et al. (1986) report a greater frequency of scratches and abrasions, cuts requiring or not requiring sutures, bruises and contusions, fractures, dental injury, respiratory distress, and tachycardia for those physically restrained as opposed to mechanically restrained. Additionally, data presented by Rapp and Miltenberger (2000) suggest that contingent restraint may actually reinforce SIB that has acquired mand function, when the intent of the practitioner is to decelerate the SIB with the restraint. It is clear that procedures involving restraint carry potential risk, and this risk must be careful analyzed relative to the potential risk of either not intervening or intervening differently, before a restraint procedure is used.

Summary

It has been said that the only treatments shown consistently effectively reducing SIB in the years prior to the advent of functional analysis and functional assessment were those that involved contingent aversive stimulation (Iwata, et al.,1982). Since this technology has brought greater attention to controlling contingencies of which particular self-injurious topographies are a part for individuals, however, there has been a sharp decline in reliance on "default procedures" (Mace, 1994), and greater use of reinforcement-based procedures in treating SIB (Pelios et al., 1999). Additionally, expanding functional analysis and functional assessment methodology to establishing operations appears to have further widened the scope of variables that can be addressed when developing function relevant treatment of this typically multiply determined behavior. Numerous interventions have been described in the literature over the past several years detailing effective implementation of multi-component treatment packages addressing various combinations of establishing operations, discriminative stimuli, and consequence operations, as well as examinations of parametric properties of these environmental events that produce greater treatment gains. The focus has shifted from intervention that merely superimposes contingencies atop maintaining contingencies in an effort to suppress SIB, to identifying and altering the variables maintaining SIB to render the behavior irrelevant, ineffective, and inefficient, and to promote functionally meaningful alternative behavior.

References

American Association on Mental Retardation (1992). *Mental retardation: Definition, classification, and systems of support (9th ed.)*. Washington, DC: Author.

American Association on Mental Retardation (2002). *Mental retardation: Definition, classification, and systems of support (10th ed.)*. Washington, DC: Author.

Anderson, L. T., & Ernst, M. (1994). Self-injury in Lesch-Nyhan Disease. *Journal of Autism and Developmental Disorders, 24,* 67-81.

Archea, C., McNeely, E., Martino-Saltzman, D., Hennessy, C., Whittington, F., & Myers, D. (1993). Restraints in long-term care. *Physical and Occupational Therapy in Geriatrics, 11,* 3-23.

Arntzen, E., & Werner, B. (1999). Water mist punishment for two classes of problem behavior. *Scandinavian Journal of Behavior Therapy, 28,* 88-93.

Bailey, J. S., & Pyles, D. A. M. (1989). Behavioral diagnostics. In E. Cipani (Ed.), *The treatment of severe behavior disorders: Behavior Analysis approaches* (pp. 85-107). Washington, D.C.: American Association on Mental Retardation.

Barton, L. E., Repp, A. C., & Brulle, A. R. (1985). Reduction of stereotypic behaviors using differential reinforcement procedures and momentary restraint. *Journal of Mental Deficiency Research, 29,* 71-79.

Berkson, G., Tupa, M., & Sherman, L. (2001). Early development of stereotyped and self-injurious behaviors: I. Incidence. *American Journal on Mental Retardation, 106,* 539-547.

Berney, T. P., Ireland, M., & Burn, J. (1999). Behavioral phenotype of Cornelia de Lange syndrome. *Archives of Disease in Childhood, 81,* 333-336.

Bird, F., Hepburn, S., Rhodes, K., & Moniz, D. (1991). Multiple reinforcement contingencies to reduce aggression, self-injury, and dysfunctional verbal behaviors in an adult who is sensory impaired. *Behavioral Residential Treatment, 6,* 367-383.

Bowman, L. G., Fisher, W. W., Thompson, R. H., & Piazza, C. C. (1997). On the relation of mands and the function of destructive behaviors. *Journal of Applied Behavior Analysis, 30,* 251-265.

Braithwaite, K. L., & Richdale, A. L. (2000). Functional communication training to replace challenging behaviors across two behavioral outcomes. *Behavioral Interventions, 15,* 21-36.

Brylewski, J., & Wiggs, L. (1999). Sleep problems and daytime challenging behaviour in a community-based sample of adults with intellectual disability. *Journal of Intellectual Disability Research, 43,* 504-512.

Carr, E. G. (1977). The motivation of self-injurious behavior: A review of some hypotheses. *Psychological Bulletin, 84,* 800-816.

Carr, E. G., & Smith, C. E. (1995). Biological setting events for self-injury. *Mental Retardation and Developmental Disabilities Research Reviews, 1,* 94-98.

Carr, E. G., Smith, C. E., Giacin, T. A., Whelan, B. M., & Pancari, J. (2003). Menstrual discomfort as a biological setting event for severe problem behavior: Assessment and intervention. *American Journal on Mental Retardation, 108,* 117-133.

Cooper, J.O., Heron, T.E., & Heward, W.L. (1987). *Applied behavior analysis.* Upper Saddle River, NJ: Prentice-Hall.

Crosland, K. A., Zarcone, J. R., Lindauer, S. E., Valdovinos, M. G., Zarcone, T. J., Hellings, J. A., et al. (2003). Use of functional analysis methodology in the evaluation of medication effects. *Journal of Autism and Developmental Disorders, 23,* 271-279.

DeLeon, I. G., Anders, B. M., Rodrigues-Catter, V., & Neidert, P. L. (2000). The effects of noncontingent access to single-versus multiple-stimulus sets on self-injurious behavior. *Journal of Applied Behavior Analysis, 34,* 623-626.

Derby, K. M., Fisher, W. W., & Piazza, C. C. (1996). The effects of contingent and noncontingent attention on self-injury and self-restraint. *Journal of Applied Behavior Analysis, 29,* 107-110.

Duncan, D., Matson, J. L., Bamburg, J. W., Cherry, K. E., & Buckley, T. (1999). The relationship of self-injurious behavior and aggression to social skills in persons with severe and profound learning disability. *Research in Developmental Disabilities, 20,* 441-448.

Durand, V. M., & Crimmins, D. B. (1988). Identifying the variables maintaining self-injurious behavior. *Journal of Autism and Developmental Disorders, 18,* 99-117.

Durand, V. M., & Crimmins, D. B. (1992). *The motivation assessment scale.* Topeka, KS: Monaco and Associates.

Durand, V. M., & Merges, E. (2001). Functional communication training: A contemporary behavior analytic intervention for problem behaviors. *Focus on Autism and Other Developmental Disabilities, 16,* 110-119.

Dykens, E. M., & Smith, A. C. M. (1999). Distinctiveness and correlates of maladaptive behavior in children and adolescents with Smith-Magenis syndrome. *Journal of Intellectual Disability Research, 42,* 481-489.

Favazza, A. R. (1996). *Bodies under siege: self-mutilation and body modification in culture and psychiatry (2nd ed.).* Baltimore: Johns Hopkins University Press.

Fischer, S. M., Iwata, B. A., & Mazaleski, J. L. (1997). Noncontingent delivery of arbitrary reinforcers as treatment for self-injurious behavior. *Journal of Applied Behavior Analysis, 30,* 239-249.

Frazier, J. A., Doyle, R., Chiu, S., & Coyle, J. T. (2002). Treating a child with Asperger's disorder and comorbid bipolar disorder. *American Journal of Psychiatry, 159,* 13-21.

Garcia, D., & Smith, R. G. (1999). Using analog baselines to assess the effects of naltrexone on self-injurious behavior. *Research in Developmental Disabilities, 20,* 1-21.

Grace, N. C., Thompson, R., & Fisher, W. W. (1996). The treatment of covert self-injury through contingencies on response products. *Journal of Applied Behavior Analysis, 29,* 239-242.

Hall, S., Oliver, C., & Murphy, G. (2001). Self-injurious behavior in young children with Lesch-Nyhan syndrome. *Developmental Medicine and Child Neurology, 43,* 745-749.

Healy, J. J., Ahearn, W. H., Graff, R. B., & Libby, M. E. (2001). Extended analysis and treatment of self-injurious behavior. *Behavioral Interventions, 16,* 181-195.

Horner, R. H., Day, H. M., & Day, J. R. (1997). Using neutralizing routines to reduce problem behaviors. *Journal of Applied Behavior Analysis, 30,* 601-614.

Iwata, B. A., Dorsey, M. F., Slifer, K. J., Bauman, K. E., & Richman, G. S. (1982). Toward a functional analysis of self-injury. *Analysis and Intervention in Developmental Disabilities, 2,* 3-20.

Iwata, B. A., Pace, G. M., Dorsey, M. F., Zarcone, J. R., Vollmer, T. R., Smith, R. G., et al. (1994). The functions of self-injurious behavior: An experimental-epidemiological analysis. *Journal of Applied Behavior Analysis, 27,* 215-240.

Iwata, B. A., Pace, G. M., Kissel, R. C., Nau, P. A., & Farber, J. M. (1990). The Self-Injury Trauma (SIT) Scale: A method for quantifying surface tissue damage caused by self-injurious behavior. *Journal of Applied Behavior Analysis, 23,* 99-110.

Jacobson, J. W. (1982) Problem behavior and psychiatric impairment within a developmentally disabled population I: Behavior frequency. *Applied Research in Mental Retardation, 3,* 121-139.

Kahng, S., Abt, K. A., & Wilder, D. (2001). Treatment of self-injury correlated with mechanical restraints. *Behavioral Interventions, 16,* 105-110.

Kahng, S., Iwata, B. A., & Lewin, A. B. (2002). Behavioral treatment of self-injury, 1964-2000. *American Journal on Mental Retardation, 107,* 212-221.

Kanfer, F. H., & Saslow, G. (1969). Behavioral diagnosis. In C. M. Franks (Ed.), *Behavior therapy: Appraisal and status.* New York: McGraw-Hill.

Kern, L., Carberry, N., & Haidara, C. (1997). Analysis and intervention with two topographies of challenging behavior exhibited by a young woman with autism. *Research in Developmental Disabilities, 18,* 257-287.

Kurtz, P. F., Chin, M. D., Huete, J. M., Tarbox, R. S. F., O'Connor, J. T., Paclawskyj, T. R., et al. (2003). Functional analysis and treatment of self-injurious behavior in young children: A summary of 30 cases. *Journal of Applied Behavior Analysis, 36,* 205-219.

Landi, F., Bernabei, R., Trecca, A., Marzi, D., Russo, A., Carosella, L., et al. (2001). Physical restraint and subcutaneous hematoma in an anticoagulated patient. *Southern Medical Journal, 94,* 254-255.

Lindauer, S. E., DeLeon, I. G., & Fisher, W. W. (1999). Decreasing signs of negative affect and correlated self-injury in an individual with mental retardation and mood disturbance. *Journal of Applied Behavior Analysis, 32,* 103-106.

Luiselli, J. K. (1992). Assessment and treatment of self-injury in a deaf-blind child. *Journal of Developmental and Physical Disabilities, 4,* 219-226.

Luiselli, J. K., & Waldstein, N. (1994). Evaluation of restraint-elimination interventions for students with multiple disabilities in a pediatric nursing care setting. *Behavior Modification, 18,* 352-365.

Mace, F. C. (1994). The significance and future of functional analysis methodologies. *Journal of Applied Behavior Analysis, 27,* 385-392.

Mace, F. C., Blum, N. J., Sierp, B. J., Delaney, B. A., & Mauk, J. E. (2001). Differential response of operant self-injury to pharmacologic versus behavioral treatment. *Journal of Developmental and Behavioral Pediatrics, 22,* 85-91.

Mace, A. B., Shapiro, E. S., & Mace, F. C. (1999). Effects of warning stimuli for reinforcer withdrawal and task onset on self-injury. *Journal of Applied Behavior Analysis, 31,* 679-682.

Matson, J. L., Bamburg, J. W., Mayville, E. A., Pinkston, J., Bielecki, J., Kuhn, D., et al. (2000). Psychotropic medications and developmental disabilities: A 10-year review. *Research in Developmental Disabilities, 21,* 263-296.

Matson, J. L., & Keyes, J. B. (1990). A comparison of DRO to movement suppression time-out and DRO with two self-injurious and aggressive mentally retarded adults. *Research in Developmental Disabilities, 11,* 111-120.

Matson, J. L., & Vollmer, T. R. (1995). *The Questions About Behavioral Function (QABF) User's Guide.* Baton Rouge, LA: Scientific Publishers, Inc.

McClintock, K., Hall, S., & Oliver, C. (2003). Risk markers associated with challenging behaviors in people with intellectual disabilities: A meta-analytic study. *Journal of Intellectual Disability Research, 47,* 405-416.

McCord, B.E., Thompson, R.J., & Iwata, B.A. (2001). Functional analysis and treatment of self-injury associated with transitions. *Journal of Applied Behavior Analysis, 34,* 195-210.

McGill, P. (1999). Establishing operations: Implications for the assessment, treatment, and prevention of problem behavior. *Journal of Applied Behavior Analysis, 32,* 393-418.

McKerchar, T. L., Kahng, S., Casioppo, E., & Wilson, D. (2001). Functional analysis of self-injury maintained by automatic reinforcement: Exposing masked social functions. *Behavioral Interventions, 16*, 59-63.

Michael, J. (2000). Implications and refinements of the establishing operations concept. *Journal of Applied Behavior Analysis, 33*, 401-411.

Mossman, D. A., Hastings, R. P., & Brown, T. (2002). Mediator's responses to self-injurious behavior: An experimental study. *American Journal on Mental Retardation, 107*, 252-260.

Murphy, G., Hall, S., Oliver, C. & Kissi-Debra, R. (1999). Identification of early self-injurious behaviour in young children with intellectual disability. *Journal of Intellectual Disability Research, 43*, 149-163.

Obi, C. (1997). Restraint fading and alternative management strategies to treat a man with Lesch-Nyhan syndrome over a two year period. *Behavioral Interventions, 12*, 195-202.

Oliver, C., Murphy, G.H., & Corbett, J.A. (1987). Self-injurious behaviour in people with mental handicap: A total population study. *Journal of Mental Deficiency Research, 31*, 147-162.

Oliver, C., Hall, S., Hales, J., Murphy, G., & Watts, D. (1998). The treatment of severe self-injurious behavior by the systematic fading of restraints: Effects on self-injury, self-restraint, adaptive behavior, and behavioral correlates of affect. *Research in Developmental Disabilities, 19*, 143-165.

O'Neill, R. E., Horner, R. H., Albin, R. W., Sprague, J. R., Storey, K., & Newton, J. S. (1997). *Functional assessment and program development for behavior problems.* Pacific Grove, CA: Brooks/Cole.

O'Reilly, M. F. (1996). Assessment and treatment of episodic self-injury: A case study. *Research in Developmental Disabilities, 17*, 349-361.

O'Reilly, M. F. (1997). Functional analysis of episodic self-injury correlated with recurrent otitis media. *Journal of Applied Behavior Analysis, 30*, 165-167.

O'Reilly, M. F., Lacey, C., & Lancioni, G. (2001). A preliminary investigation of the assessment and treatment of tantrums with two post-institutionalized Romanian adoptees. *Scandinavian Journal of Behavior Therapy, 16*, 127-135.

O'Reilly, M. F., & Lancioni, G. (2000). Response covariation of escape-maintained aberrant behavior correlated with sleep deprivation. *Research in Developmental Disabilities, 21*, 125-136.

O'Reilly, M. F., Lancioni, G.E., & Emerson, E. (1999). A systematic analysis of prior social context on aggression and self-injury within analogue analysis assessments. *Behavior Modification, 23*, 578-586.

Patel, M. R., Carr, J. E., Kim, C., Robes, A., & Eastridge, D. (2000). Functional analysis of aberrant behavior maintained by automatic reinforcement: Assessment of specific sensory reinforcers. *Research in Developmental Disabilities, 21*, 393-407.

Pelios, L., Morren, J., Tesch, D., & Axelrod, S. (1999). The impact of functional analysis methodology on treatment choice for self-injurious and aggressive behavior. *Journal of Applied Behavior Analysis, 32,* 185-195.

Persel, C. S., Persel, C. H., Ashley, M. J., & Krych, D. K. (1997). The use of noncontingent reinforcement and contingent restraint to reduce physical aggression and self-injurious behaviour in a traumatically brain injured adult. *Brain Injury, 11*, 751-760.

Rapp, J. T., & Miltenberger, R. G. (2000). Self-restraint and self-injury: A demonstration of separate functions and response classes. *Behavioral Interventions, 15*, 37-51.

Rapp, J. T., Miltenberger, R. G., Galensky, T. L., Ellingson, S. A., & Long, E. S. (1999). A functional analysis of hair pulling. *Journal of Applied Behavior Analysis, 32,* 329-337.

Roberts, M. L., Mace, F. C., & Daggett, J. A. (1995). Preliminary comparison of two negative reinforcement procedures to reduce self-injury. *Journal of Applied Behavior Analysis, 28,* 579-580.

Robey, K. L., Reck, J. F., Giacomini, K. D., Barabas, G., & Eddey, G. E. (2003) Modes and patterns of self-mutilation in persons with Lesch-Nyhan disease. *Developmental Medicine and Child Neurology, 45,*167-171.

Robinson, B. E., Sucholeiki, R., & Schocken, D. D. (1993). Sudden death and resisted mechanical restraint: A case report. *Journal of the American Geriatrics Society, 41,* 424-425.

Rojahn, J. (1986). Self-injurious behavior and stereotypic behavior in non-institutionalized mentally retarded people. *American Journal of Mental Deficiency, 91,* 268-276.

Rojahn, J., Borthwick-Duffy, S. A., & Jacobson, J. W. (1993). The association between psychiatric diagnoses and severe behavior problems in mental retardation. *Annals of Clinical Psychiatry, 5*, 163-170.

Rojahn. J., & Esbensen, A. J. (2002). Epidemiology of self-injurious behavior in mental retardation: A review. In: S. R. Schroeder, M. L. Oster-Granite, & T. Thompson (Eds.), *Self-injurious behavior: Gene-brain-behavior relationship* (pp. 41-77). Washington, DC: American Psychological Association.

Rojahn, J., Matson, J. L., Lott, D., Esbensen, A. J., & Smalls, Y. (1999). *Epidemiology and Topographic Assessment of SIB*. Invited address, Workshop on Self-Injurious Behavior, Rockville, MD, December 6.

Rojahn, J., Matson, J. L., Naglieri, J. A., & Mayville, E. (in press). Relationships between psychiatric conditions and behavior problems among adults with mental retardation. *American Journal on Mental Retardation.*

Romanczyk, R. G., Lockshin, S., & O'Conner, J. O. (1992). Psychophysiology and issues of anxiety and arousal. In J. K. Luiselli, J. L. Matson, & N. N. Singh (Eds.), *Self-injurious behavior: Analysis, assessment and treatment* (pp. 93-121). New York: Springer.

Romanczyk, R. G., & Matthews A. L. (1998). Physiological state as antecedent: Utilization of functional analysis. In J. K. Luiselli, & M. J. Cameron, (Eds.), *Antecedent control: Innovative approaches to behavioral support* (pp. 115-138). Baltimore: Brookes.

Rush, K.S., Crockett, J.L., & Hagopian, L.P. (2001). An analysis of the selective effects of NCR with punishment targeting problem behavior associated with positive affect. *Behavioral Interventions*, 16, 127-135.

Saunders, R.R., Saunders, M.D., Brewer, A., & Roach, T. (1996). Reduction of self-injury in two adolescents with profound mental retardation by the establishment of a supported routine. *Behavioral Interventions*, 11, 59-86.

Schroeder, S. R., Oster-Granite, M. L.& Thompson, T. (Eds.) (2002). *Self-injurious behavior: Gene-brain-behavior relationship*. Washington, DC: American Psychological Association.

Shore, B. A., Iwata, B. A., DeLeon, I. G., Kahng, S. W., & Smith, R. G. (1997). An analysis of reinforcer substitutability using object manipulation and self-injury as competing responses. *Journal of Applied Behavior Analysis, 30*, 21-41.

Sigafoos, J., & Meikle, B. (1996). Functional communication training for the treatment of multiply determined challenging behavior in two boys with autism. *Behavior Modification, 20*, 60-84.

Sigafoos, J., & Pennell, D. (1995). Noncontingent application versus contingent removal of tactile stimulation: Effects on self-injury in a young boy with multiple disabilities. *Behaviour Change, 12*, 139-143.

Sigafoos, J., Pennell, D., & Verslius, J. (1996). Naturalistic assessment leading to effective treatment of self-injury in a young boy with multiple disabilities. *Education and Treatment of Children, 19*, 101-123.

Spreat, S., Lipinski, D., Hill, J., & Halpin, M.E. (1986). Safety indices associated with the use of contingent restraint procedures. *Applied Research in Mental Retardation, 7*, 475-481.

Symons, F. J., Butler, M.G., Sanders, M.D., Feuer, I.D., & Thompson, T. (1999). Self-injurious behavior and Prader-Willi syndrome: Behavioral forms and body locations. *American Journal on Mental Retardation, 104*, 260-269.

Symons, F. J., Fox, N. D., & Thompson, T. (1998). Functional communication training and naltrexone treatment of self-injurious behavior: An experimental case report. *Journal of Applied Research in Intellectual Disabilities, 11,* 273-292.

Symons, F. J., Sutton, K. A., Walker, C., & Bodfish, J. W. (2003). Altered diurnal pattern of salivary substance P in adults with developmental disabilities and chronic self-injury. *American Association on Mental Retardation, 108,* 13-18.

Symons, F. J., & Thompson, T (1997). Self-injurious behavior and body site preference. *Journal of Intellectual Disability Research, 6,* 456-468.

Thompson, R.H., Iwata, B.A., Conners, J., & Roscoe, E.M. (1999). Effects of reinforcement of alternative behavior during punishment of self-injury. *Journal of Applied Behavior Analysis, 32,* 317-328.

Thompson, T., & Caruso, M. (2002). Self-injury: Knowing what we are looking for. In: S. R. Schroeder, M. L. Oster-Granite, & T. Thompson (Eds.): *Self-Injurious Behavior: Gene-Brain-Behavior Relationship* (pp. 3-21). Washington, DC: American Psychological Association.

Touchette, P. E., MacDonald, R. F., & Langer, S. N. (1985), A scatter plot for identifying stimulus control of problem behavior. *Journal of Applied Behavior Analysis, 18,* 343-351.

Treadwell, K., & Page, T.J. (1996). Functional analysis: Identifying the environmental determinants of severe behavior disorders. *Journal of Head Trauma Rehabilitation, 11,* 62-74.

Tsiouris, J. A., Mann, R., Patti, P. J., & Sturmey, P. (2003). Challenging behaviours should not be considered as depressive equivalents in individuals with intellectual disability. *Journal of Intellectual Disability Research, 47,* 14-21.

Van Camp, C. M., Vollmer, T. R., & Daniel, D. (2002). A systematic evaluation of stimulus preference, response effort, and stimulus control in the treatment of automatically reinforced self-injury. *Behavior Therapy, 32,* 603-613.

Van Houten, R. (1993). The use of wrist weights to reduce self-injury maintained by sensory reinforcement. *Journal of Applied Behavior Analysis, 26,* 197-203.

Vollmer, T. R., Progar, P. R., Lalli, J. S., Van Camp, C. M., Sierp, B. J., Wright, C. S., et al. (1998). Fixed-time schedules attenuate extinction-induced phenomena in the treatment of severe aberrant behavior. *Journal of Applied Behavior Analysis, 31,* 529-542.

Wacker, D. P., Harding, J., Cooper, L. J., Derby, K. M., Peck, S., Asmus, J., et al. (1996). The effects of meal schedule and quantity on problematic behavior. *Journal of Applied Behavior Analysis, 29,* 79-87.

Wilder, D.A., & Carr, J.E. (1998). Recent advances in the modification of establishing operations to reduce aberrant behavior. *Behavioral Interventions, 13,* 43-59.

Zarcone, J.R., Iwata, B.A., Hughes, C.E., & Vollmer, T.R. (1993). Momentum versus extinction effects in the treatment of self-injurious escape behavior. *Journal of Applied Behavior Analysis, 26,* 135-136.

Zhou, L., Goff, G.A., & Iwata, B.A. (2000). Effects of increased response effort on self-injury and object manipulation as competing responses. *Journal of Applied Behavior Analysis, 33,* 29-40.

9

STEREOTYPED ACTS

Lisa M. Noll, Ph.D., University of Chicago & Rowland P. Barrett, Ph.D., Emma Pendleton Bradley Hospital, Brown Medical School

Introduction

Stereotyped behavior is among the most perplexing forms of psychopathology in children with developmental disabilities. It is a highly conspicuous behavioral phenomenon that despite many years of clinical interest and dedicated research is not well understood. Theories abound as to the biological and motivational bases of this behavior. However, a true understanding as to why children with developmental disabilities engage in stereotyped acts remains a mystery. There is no single explanation that may be applied to stereotyped behavior. That it remains unexplained after years of devoted study contributes to the frustration experienced by clinicians attempting to provide treatment for a behavior that so clearly appears to unfavorably impact the quality of life. The purpose of this chapter will be to review the definition, taxonomy, and prevalence of stereotyped behavior, as well as the population of children most frequently affected by it. In addition, the chapter will review advances made toward understanding the biological and motivational bases for engaging in stereotyped behavior, discuss the indications for intervention, and review the latest empirically based treatment approaches.

What are stereotyped acts?

Stereotyped acts have been defined as repetitious, topographically invariant motor movements (or sequence of motor movements), where reinforcement is not apparent and the act of performing the behavior is considered pathological (Schroeder, 1970). Stereotyped acts also have been defined as voluntary, developmentally inappropriate, repetitive motor movements, which serve no apparent adaptive function

(Burkhart, 1987). Stereotyped behavior has been further characterized as possessing rhythmic and non-rhythmic qualities (Berkson, 1983). The American Psychiatric Association (1994) has defined stereotyped behavior as a movement disorder characterized by repetitive, seemingly driven, non-functional motor behavior. Common forms of stereotyped behavior (cf. Berkson, 1967; LaGrow & Repp, 1984) include hand flapping, finger twirling, gazing at complex hand/finger movements, body rocking, body posturing (tensing), jumping, spinning, toe-walking, light gazing, eye pressing, hair twirling, finger sucking, mouthing objects, and vocalizing. Twirling string, spinning objects, aligning or stacking objects also are commonly observed stereotyped acts. Each of these stereotypic forms may occur by itself or in combination with one or more other forms. In fact, observation of combinations of two or more stereotyped acts is not at all rare. For example, spinning an object, then jumping, hand flapping, and vocalizing while making facial grimaces and gazing intensely at the spinning object is not an unusual sequence of motor movements in certain children who engage in stereotyped behavior.

Stereotyped behavior typically is distinguished from self-injurious behavior (cf. Rojahn & Sisson, 1990; Schroeder, 1991). Certain forms of self-injurious behavior may be correctly viewed as voluntary, repetitious, developmentally inappropriate and topographically invariant. However, many forms of self-injurious behavior do not meet the criterion of appearing meaningless and serving no apparent adaptive function (Barrett, in press). Self-injurious behavior, in many instances, may be clearly identified either as a means of gaining social attention, escaping non-preferred circumstances, and/or communicating protest (Baumeister &Rollings, 1976; Carr, 1977). However, stereotyped behavior also may develop, evolve or incorporate a self-injurious component where the intent is not to gain social attention, escape from a non-preferred circumstance and/or communicate protest. In these instances, the self-injury is usually unintentional. For example, when repetitious hair twirling damages the hair follicle and results in hair loss or repeated eye pressing causes damage to the cornea. Other examples may occur when constant finger sucking damages the nail beds resulting in infection or when mouthing objects inadvertently results in the ingestion of a non-edible substance. Body rocking also may result in self-injury if it occurs while sitting on the palms of both hands. In this example, damage to the wrists as well as the soft tissue, knuckles and finger joints of the hands is common.

Who engages in stereotyped acts?

Prevalence estimates of stereotyped behavior coalesce at approximately 33% of the population of children diagnosed with mental retardation (Rojahn & Sisson, 1990). However, certain mental retardation syndromes, such as Cri du Chat, show markedly higher (82%) rates (Ross-Collins & Cornish, 2002). The vast majority of children manifesting stereotyped behavior are nonverbal with IQs below 50. In a 26-year longitudinal study, Thompson and Reid (2002) found stereotyped behavior in individuals with severe and profound mental retardation to be remarkably persistent across time with no evidence of significant abatement.

Stereotyped behavior also is a salient characteristic of children with pervasive developmental disorder. It is uniquely observed in the form of hand wringing and hyperventilation in virtually all (93%) children diagnosed with Rett syndrome (Hagberg, Aicardi, Dias, & Ramos, 1983; Mount, Hastings, Reilly, Cass, & Charman, 2003). Children within the so-called "autistic spectrum" (i.e., autistic disorder, Asperger disorder, pervasive developmental disorder, not otherwise specified) show varied prevalence. In this regard, the vast majority of children with autism manifest stereotyped acts prior to age 2. Stereotyped acts by children with PDD.NOS are less prevalent, while children with Asperger disorder demonstrate rates of about 30 percent, typically in the form of hand-flapping. However, it may be argued that individuals with Asperger Disorder engage in much higher rates of stereotypy if allowances are made for the consideration of a unique behavior that is characteristic of the disorder. Many individuals with Asperger Disorder display an exceptional ability to learn and recite facts about a particular topic. They also may collect things. In each case, what distinguishes these acts from normal hobbies is that they are obviously abnormal in intensity and focus. The extent of the facts is encyclopedic and the collections may fill an entire room. In many cases, the recitation of topical facts or collections of objects characteristic of individuals with Asperger' Disorder meets criteria for a stereotyped act, in that it is voluntary, repetitious, developmentally inappropriate, and serves no apparent adaptive function.

Why do they engage in stereotyped acts?

The etiology of stereotyped acts continues to be a controversial subject among researchers. Several explanations have been proposed and developed to account for the origin and maintenance of stereotyped behaviors. Explanations generally fall within one of three broad categories, depending on the degree to which environmental, biological, or behavioral factors are emphasized. These categories further relate to the theoretical orientation of the researchers' and, therefore, are subsumed within the realms of learning, homeostatic, neural oscillator, developmental, organic, and biological theories. The following discussion is both a review and analysis of the way in which these theories independently and interdependently relate to the current view of the origin and maintenance of stereotyped behaviors.

Learning Theory

The learning theory of stereotyped behavior posits that stereotypies result under schedules of reinforcement, either positive or negative. Within this perspective, stereotyped behaviors originate and are maintained by the interaction between the environment, the stereotyped behavior, and the resulting consequence. Thus, stereotypy is considered an instrumental or learned operant response maintained by stimuli that are either delivered or removed, dependent or independent, upon its elicitation (Carr, Newsom, & Binkoff, 1976), rather than as a spontaneous, random movement. Learning theory encapsulates two differing rationales to account for stereotyped behaviors, the positive reinforcement or discriminative stimulus hypothesis (Bachman, 1972; Skinner, 1953), and the negative reinforcement or avoidance hypothesis (Bucher & Lovaas, 1968; Skinner, 1953).

Positive Reinforcement (Discriminative Stimulus) Hypothesis

The positive reinforcement hypothesis is based on the notion that stereotyped acts may originate as superstitious behaviors (cf. Hollis, 1971b). Stereotyped behavior is created and produced by the individual and acquires reinforcing properties by the mere performance of the behavior (Lovaas, Freitag, Gold, & Kassorla, 1965; Lovaas & Simmons, 1969). Based on this premise, stereotyped behavior should decrease when the social and/or sensory contingencies in which the behavior is based are withdrawn.

Research has shown that for certain individuals contingent social attention may increase the rate of stereotypic self-injury, whereas withdrawal of attention may reduce or suppress repetitive self-injurious behavior (Bucher & Lovaas, 1968; Frankel & Simmons, 1976). These findings suggest that the behavior in question may serve as discriminative stimuli for gaining the social attention of others. According to this model, it is logical that stereotyped acts without a component of self-injury also can be brought under the stimulus control of positive reinforcement (Ayllon & Azrin, 1966; Baumeister & Forehand, 1973; Hollis, 1971a; Mulhern & Baumeister, 1969).

In this regard, Lovaas and colleagues (1987) proposed a perceptual reinforcement hypothesis, in which stereotyped behavior is thought to be reinforcing secondary to the resulting sensory input (Lovaas, Newsom, & Hickman, 1987). A recent study by Tang, Patterson, and Kennedy (2003) has provided support for this hypothesis with the finding that stereotyped behavior maintained by visual, auditory, or tactile sensory consequences may be decreased by providing competing sensory stimulation.

Skinner's (1953) initial discussions of the discriminative function of stereotyped behavior included the notion that aversive behaviors, such as self-injurious behaviors, could serve as conditioned positive reinforcement. This theory was based on the notion that such behavior would be selectively associated with positive reinforcement and maintained over long periods of time if exposed to intermittent schedules of reinforcement. This perspective has been further supported by research proposing that stereotypies are superstitious behaviors maintained by positive reinforcement (Spradlin, Girardeau, & Hom, 1966), irregular reinforcement (Baumeister & Forehand, 1971), or incompatibility between inward-directed response patterns which are reinforced by sensory stimuli that is discordant with outward-directed behaviors (Foxx & Azrin, 1973). Observations of stereotyped behaviors have suggested that the probability that these behaviors will be maintained across time is greatest if positively reinforcing stimuli occur at the time such behaviors are expressed. According to Hollis (1971a, 1978), as the rate and frequency of stereotyped behavior increases, there is a corresponding increase in the probability that reinforcing stimuli also will occur in the presence of these behaviors, serving to further strengthen their expression. In this regard, in certain individuals, self-injurious behaviors have been found to decrease when social consequences are removed (Ferster, 1961; Hamilton, Stephens, & Allen, 1967; Wolf, Risley, & Mees, 1964) or when the individual in question is isolated (Jones, Simmons, & Frankel, 1974; Lovaas & Simmons, 1969). Furthermore, research looking at the rates of self-injurious behavior in children has found that rates of self-injury may be low when children are alone, but increase when they are in the presence of adults (Bucher & Lovaas, 1968; Romanczyk & Goren, 1975).

Negative Reinforcement Hypothesis

According to the negative reinforcement hypothesis, stereotyped behavior is maintained through the termination, escape, or avoidance of an aversive stimulus (Carr, Newsome, & Binkoff, 1976). Research that has studied the development and maintenance of stereotyped behavior according to the negative reinforcement hypothesis has focused on the role of escape motivation, in which stimuli, associated with aversive consequences, develop conditioned aversive properties. Continual exposure to these conditioned situations may in time become as aversive as the initial exposure to the aversive stimulus (Burkhart, 1987). Thus, attempts to avoid or escape the aversive stimulus may result in repetitive patterns of responding (Skinner, 1953).

Additional research focusing on the escape or avoidance response includes associations between demand-related situations and self-injury (Jones et al., 1974; Myers & Deibert, 1971; Edelson, Taubman, & Lovaas, 1983; Wolf, Risley, Johnston, Davis, & Allen, 1967). The negative reinforcement hypothesis maintains that the placement of demands on an individual may result in self-injury, where self-injury is strengthened by the discontinuation of the aversive event (i.e., the demand), and becomes a learned escape/avoidance pattern of response (Burkhart, 1987). In support of this hypothesis, Carr (1977) found that incidences of self-injury were lower in a free play situation versus a classroom setting. Further research in the area of demands and increased self-injury also was revealed by Carr, Newsome, and Binkoff (1976), in their work with an 8-year old boy with schizophrenia who engaged in higher rates of self-injury in demanding versus nondemanding situations. Self-injury also has been found to increase following presentations of verbal demands, denials, and reprimands (Edelsen et al., 1983). Research also has suggested that the interruption of goal-directed behavior increases the rate of stereotypic responding (Baumeister & Forehand, 1971; Forehand & Baumeister, 1970b; Baumeister & Forehand, 1972).

Several researchers (Borrero, Vollmer, Wright, Lerman, & Kelley, 2002; Bucher & Lovaas, 1968; Green, 1967; Tate, 1972) have suggested a relationship between self-injurious behaviors and avoidance of an aversive situation. For example, Tate (1972) reported a frightened response associated with incidences of self-injury in a young female subject following removal of restraints. In support of this hypothesis, Carr (1977) proposed that restraints may represent "safety signals" when utilized over time, and removal of such restraints may signal placements of demands on the individual (e.g., bathing, working, etc.). Smith, Chethik, and Adelson (1969) extended the idea of safety to the presentation of stereotyped behavior. Smith and colleagues proposed that stereotyped behaviors are representations of regressive behaviors of a previous safe activity that accompanied demand-related situations or periods of frustration. In contrast, Silverman, Watanabe, Marshall, and Baer (1984) contended that self-injury may serve as a source of negative reinforcement, and that an individual's resistance to removal of restraints is maintained by the desire to avoid self-injury.

Additional support for the negative reinforcement model, in which an individual engages in stereotyped behavior because it has resulted in successful episodes of escape from or avoidance of unpleasant situations has been presented by Durand and Carr (1987). They reported that hand flapping and body rocking demonstrated in four children with developmental disabilities increased with the presentation of challenging academic tasks. Conversely, the removal of these tasks also increased the rate of the children's stereotyped behaviors.

Overall, the negative reinforcement (escape and avoidance) model appears to be more closely associated with repetitive patterns of self-injurious behavior as opposed to stereotyped behavior that occurs in the absence of self-injury (Rojahn & Sisson, 1990).

Homeostatic Theory

According to homeostatic theory, stereotyped responses are considered self-stimulatory in the form of arousal-inducing or arousal-reducing behaviors (Lewis & Baumeister, 1983). This perspective maintains that when the optimal level of environmental stimulation is not available to an individual, the individual will engage in compensatory activity in an attempt to generate an optimal of stimulation, often resulting in atypical movements (Baumeister & Forehand, 1973). Thus, the individual is seen as altering his or her level of arousal in relation to perceived changes in environmental stimuli (Johnson, Van Laarhoven, & Repp, 2002). Underlying this theory is the belief that individuals strive to maintain a balanced or homeostatic level of central nervous system (CNS) activation. There are several formulations of the origin and maintenance of stereotyped behaviors, according to homeostatic theory. Each formulation differs in the relative emphasis placed on environmental factors and intrinsic organismic variables. However, each formulation holds the notion that stereotyped behavior represents reflexive movements controlled within the central nervous system or sensory system of the individual (Burkhart, 1987).

Self-stimulation Hypothesis

The self-stimulation hypothesis is based on the notion that a certain minimum degree of stimulation is necessary. Stimulation, in the form of tactile, vestibular, and kinesthetic modalities must be balanced and maintained at a sufficient level by the individual. In this regard, when distal stimulation does not fulfill the needs of the individual, the under-aroused individual will engage in stereotyped acts of a proximal nature in an attempt to reach a balanced and sufficient level of sensory stimulation (Baumeister & Forehand, 1973; Cleland & Clark 1966; DeLissavoy, 1964; Green, 1967; Kulka, Fry, & Goldstein, 1960; Lourie, 1949). Conversely, stereotyped acts also function as self-stimulatory behaviors that regulate CNS activity when an individual is over-aroused. Engaging in proximal and monotonous self-stimulation is viewed as a means of effectively blocking external (distal) stimulation, and achieving a lower arousal level (Lovaas et al., 1987). The increased level of stereotyped behavior displayed by individuals with mental retardation and autism is hypothesized to be the result of striving to achieve this balance within the central nervous system (Rojahn & Sisson, 1990).

Similarly, Lovaas, Litrownic, and Mann (1971) proposed that in individuals with mental retardation, stereotyped acts may serve to increase sensory input, as compensation for a reduced capacity to respond in a meaningful way to the environment. In contrast, others have argued that individuals with mental retardation need more sensory input than cognitively intact individuals (Berkson & Mason, 1964b), because perceptual dysfunction mitigates against responding to normal levels of environmental stimulation (Cataldo & Harris, 1982; Metz, 1967). Usually, additional input is in the form of intense tactile self-stimulation, where the goal of the individual is to achieve sufficient awareness of sensory arousal (Edelson et al., 1983). In this regard, Buyer, Berkson, Winnega, and Morton (1987), investigated self-stimulatory behavior in nine children with severe and profound mental retardation across three stimulation conditions: stationary, passive, and active. Findings supported their proposal that self-stimulation was composed of at least two independent components, stimulation and control. Children preferred the active stimulation condition to the passive condition, and the passive condition over the stationary condition. This finding supported the notion of a stimulation component to the stereotyped response. However, as the specific stereotyped behavior and the level of stimulation differed across individuals and their resulting reaction, the notion that the individual preferred to control the stimulation associated with the stereotypy also was established.

Researchers over the past fifty years have investigated stereotyped behavior in terms of environmental conditions as well as emotional regulation. Specifically, the emergence of stereotyped behavior also has been linked to individuals being restrained against their will, reared in isolation, or exposed to monotony (Berkson, 1967; Berkson & Davenport, 1962; Berkson & Mason, 1964b; Kulka et al., 1960; Levy, 1944; Lourie, 1949). This research, too, has been based on the assumption that individuals require a certain level of stimulation, either though physical activity or variation within the their environment. Conversely, confinement which results in extreme alterations in emotionality and arousal (Evans, 1978), also has been attributed to the presentation of stereotyped behavior.

In this area, the animal-analogue research by Harlow and colleagues has been most instructive (Harlow & Griffin, 1965; Harlow & Harlow, 1962, 1971). Harlow found that when the level of interaction/contact with other monkeys was restricted for long periods of time, the development of stereotyped behavior, including repetitive self-injurious behavior, was likely. Even when social contact was no longer restricted, once-isolated monkeys tended to display withdrawal behaviors in the presence of others. Limitations in the isolate-reared monkeys' behavioral repertoire was proposed as resulting from a lack of stimulation associated with social contact, soothing, and relationships that emerge across the normal developmental trajectory. Similarly, Berkson and Mason (1964a) found that chimpanzees raised without their mothers developed abnormal stereotyped behavior not found in mother-raised animals. The work of Harlow and his colleagues (Cross & Harlow, 1965; Harlow & Griffin, 1965; Harlow & Harlow, 1962, 1971) and Berkson and Mason (1964a), further support the self-stimulatory hypothesis of stereotyped behavior. In each study, monkeys reared in the absence of social and sensory stimulation developed stereotyped behavior, while monkeys reared with contact from mothers and peers did not.

That an absence of interaction with others and a lack of stimulating activities for long periods of time may be responsible for the emergence of stereotyped behavior has been the subject of popular speculation for many years regarding individuals with mental retardation who have been institutionalized. It has been proposed that the high rates of repetitive self-injury and stereotyped behavior observed within the population placed in institutional settings may be related to an absence of social activities and stimulation (cf. Matson, 1989). Importantly, Matson (1989) pointed out that in order to advance the argument that diminished stimulation secondary to institutionalization results in the emergence of stereotyped behavior, certain historical factors must be taken into account and addressed. Most notably, that only individuals with severe and profound mental retardation and serious behavior problems were routinely admitted to institutions and that these were precisely the individuals who were most likely to engage in stereotypy and self-injury, regardless of institutionalized status. Nevertheless, it may be concluded that diminished stimulation and other environmental conditions present in such treatment centers, such as factors of isolation and decreased opportunities for activities, if they existed, were likely to play a part in the origin and maintenance of stereotyped behavior.

Additional research has suggested the following ecological conditions also may play a role in the origin and maintenance of stereotyped behaviors: food deprivation (Kaufman & Levitt, 1965), intense ambient noise (Forehand & Baumeister, 1970b), emotion producing restriction of location or movement (Berkson & Mason, 1963; Berkson, Mason, & Saxon, 1963), prior movement restraint (Forehand & Baumeister, 1970a), reduced sensory stimulation (Tizard, 1968), and contact with specific types of patients (Forehand & Baumeister, 1970b). "Frustration" was another topic of study found to be associated with stereotyped behaviors. Forehand and Baumeister (1970b) viewed "frustration" as a learned instrumental behavior, in that situations that evoked frustration and were paired with either non-reinforcement or an intermittent reinforcement schedule resulted in a high incidence of stereotyped behavior, as the individual viewed the absence and/or unpredictability of reward as aversive.

Vestibular stimulation, a closely related theoretical construct to the self-stimulatory hypothesis, also is believed to relate to the incidence of stereotyped behavior. Vestibular stimulation, a function of neurological development, is proposed to be an association between semicircular canal stimulation and maturation of synaptic conductivity in the cerebellum, as well as sequential dendritic elaboration (cf. Purpura & Reaser, 1974). An example of vestibular stimulation appears to be linked to crib confinement, which was found to be positively correlated in children with severe and profound mental retardation (Warren & Burns, 1970). Additional support for the notion that crib confinement reduces vestibular stimulation is found in the developmental literature. It is suggested that the amount of stereotypy is inversely related to the amount of vestibular stimulation provided by the caregivers (Thelen, 1979, 1981, 1996). Movements, such as spinning and rocking, have been associated with a reduction in stereotyped behavior (MacLean & Baumeister, 1981). Replacement theory, derived from cognitive psychology characterizes stereotypy as a replacement of unprocessed stimuli and/or responses. In this regard, unprocessed input is viewed by the individual as overwhelming. In an effort to cope, the individual engages in "overflow" movements that cause the excess stimulation to be dispersed.

Arousal Reduction and Filtering Hypothesis

In typically developing infants, stereotyped behavior indicates arousal states. For example, Berkson (1967) found that children engaged in stereotyped body rocking when they were bored or excited, but less so when they were in observed in other arousal states, suggesting that body rocking modulates general arousal (Berkson, 1983). Despite these findings, Berkson (1983) argued that it is difficult to ascertain any conclusion with certainty, as much research in this area utilizes "descriptive-correlational" approaches. Stereotyped behavior also has been inferred to relate to frustration (Forehand & Baumeister, 1970b), arousal (Berkson & Mason, 1964b), as well as anxiety and tension (Lourie, 1949). Several researchers in this area have suggested that pathological stereotypies are associated with increased central and peripheral nervous system activation. In this view, stereotyped behavior comes to represent a coping mechanism as the individual attempts to reduce excessive levels of arousal and/or stress (Hutt & Hutt, 1970; Kinsbourne, 1980; Stone, 1964). In contrast, other researchers have suggested that stereotyped behavior signals tension, discomfort, or unsatisfied needs (Klaber & Butterfield, 1968) and, therefore, are critical to the adaptive release of tension and anxiety (Lourie, 1949). Research compatible with this stance has supported the notion that repetitive and rhythmical stimulatory behavior acts as an arousal reducing or filtering system (Hutt & Hutt, 1965; Van den Daele, 1971). For example, Hutt and Hutt (1970) found evidence that children with autism engaged in increasing rates of stereotyped behavior during conditions associated with increased arousal levels, such as a novel context or social encounter, which was related to high levels of nonspecific activity in the ascending reticular activation system. Stereotyped behavior, therefore, served to decrease arousal from reaching critical levels (Hutt & Hutt, 1965). Brett and Levine (1979) found further support for this theory that suppression of activity in the pituitary-adrenal axis affected schedule-induced polydipsia. The pituitary-adrenal axis is an area believed to become activated in the presence of a perceived stressful situation (Mason, 1978). In contrast, Stone (1964) argued that stereotyped behavior, such as stimulating rhythmic activity, signals an attempt by the individual to cope with stressful stimuli, by producing a lowered state of consciousness, similar to that created during sleep.

Developmental Theory

Developmental theory takes into consideration the developmental sequence and timing during which stereotyped behavior emerges across the developmental trajectory. Developmental theory is based on the notion that stereotyped behavior occurs during the normal progression of early developmental stages and reflects the child's maturational process. It also is hypothesized that stereotyped behavior may serve adaptive functions. Lourie (1949) concluded that stereotyped behavior may promote motor and personality development. In support of this proposal, Sallustro and Atwell (1978) found that infants who engaged in bodyrocking and head banging, attained several developmental motor milestones earlier than children who had not, suggesting that repetitive behaviors may foster motor and cognitive development through the expansion of neural pathways. MacLean and Baumeister (1981) followed the development of an infant with severe developmental delays from 20 months of age across a four-week period. Their findings suggested an interaction between body position and the type of stereotyped behavior displayed. The authors proposed that a certain level of motoric control is necessary for the expression of certain stereotyped behavior when the body is in specific positions, such as supine versus prone. Their findings also lend further support to the argument that stereotypic movements are associated with adaptive motor development.

In contrast, several researchers have examined the repetitive nature of behaviors in infancy. It is the repetition of numerous behaviors and acts that is thought to be an important aspect of the child's behavioral repertoire and, ultimately, related to cognitive and motor development (Berkson, 1983). According to Thelen (1981) and Wolff (1968), repetitive behaviors exhibited during infancy may reflect innate "substrates" of more complex motor behaviors. It is through the maturational process that what was viewed during infancy as stereotyped behavior is replaced by more goal directed behavior, although the neural substrate remains during the first year of life (Thelen, 1979). If these behaviors do not meet their goal of promoting motor and cognitive development, then stereotyped behavior may remain in the infant's behavioral repertoire, and serve a stimulatory function that the infant otherwise would be expected to receive through interaction with the environment (Berkson, 1983; Thelen, 1981).

Based on the association between the emergence of particular rhythmical motor movements at particular ages during infancy, Thelen (1979) proposed that stereotyped behavior was associated with the onset of more organized and coordinated motor movements, signaling neuromuscular maturation. For example, the motor development of approximately 90 percent of typically developing infants includes body rocking. Higher Bayley Motor Scale scores, as indices of motor development, were predicted by the emergence of stereotyped body rocking during the first year of life. Thelen (1979) found that there was a significant effect of age and presentation of new motor behavior representing peak periods, further emphasizing the association between the emergence of these rhythmical events and neuromuscular development.

Specifically, infant motor movements were related to transitions between an absence of control over body and/or limb to adaptive and purposeful movement. The rate of kicking movements increased prior to the onset of crawling, rhythmical hand and arm movements presented prior to the onset of complex manual skills, and rhythmic movement was related to sitting and followed the development of smooth, coordinated motor movements (Thelen, 1981).

Research comparing the rates of stereotyped behavior in children with Trisomy-21 disorder and a matched same age control group found that both groups engaged in a similar developmental course of rhythmic behaviors. However, children with Trisomy-21 disorder performed significantly fewer rhythmic behaviors during each session and a greater proportion of head movements (MacLean, Ellis, Galbreath, Halpern, & Baumeister, 1991). This finding provides additional support to Thelen's argument that rhythmical stereotyped activity represents a transitional behavior that the infant performs with some level of control over the body parts involved in the specific movements. An infant seen flapping his arms turns into reaching with the activation of the appropriate "goal directed skills" (Thelen, 1996). In the absence of such skill, the adaptive behavioral pattern does not occur (Thelen, 1979) and what remains to be observed is the stereotyped act. According to this notion, stereotyped behavior may result when the voluntary control mechanism is interrupted, and the system thus oscillates, and continues to do so because it provides needed stimulation (Thelen, 1996).

Cognitive Development Hypothesis

Piaget (1952) and Wallon (1973), who viewed rhythmical motor movements to reflect early stages of cognitive development, also proposed a developmental nature of stereotyped behavior. Repetitive motor behavior was proposed to resemble infant behavior observed during the sensorimotor period of developmental (Piaget, 1952). For the infant, engagement in "circular reactions" emerged out of an innate propensity for repetition, allowing the infant to learn about his or her body during both early and later stages of development (Burkhart, 1987). For Thelen (1981), these circular reactions were seen when the infant was shaking and banging objects, as well as kicking when the mother appeared. During the first year of life, according to a normal developmental trajectory, the extent to which the child continued to engage in self-manipulation, impacted his or her ability to develop adaptive environment manipulation, which served to help the child come to understand the world (Piaget,

1952). During the normal course of development, stereotyped behavior is likely to decrease as the child learns more adaptive and mature behavior, such as communication, to interact in the world. However, as will be discussed, in children with disabilities, the onset of adaptive replacement behavior is slower (Berkson & Tupa, 2000). Piaget's (1952) studies on normal development during the first year of life also indicate that the extent to which the child continues to engage in self-manipulation, impacts the child's ability to develop additional adaptive environmental manipulations, which is essential to the child's continuing and growing understanding of the world.

For children not progressing in accordance with the normal developmental trajectory, engaging in repetitive body movements are said to have become "fixated" at levels of primary and secondary circular reactions (Inhelder, 1968). Repetitive motor mannerisms directed toward the self are said to represent primary circular reactions, while motor mannerisms directed toward the environment are said to represent secondary circular reactions (Inhelder, 1968). According to Inhelder, this fixation was not only a "slower" development, but also a "deceleration" and "termination" of progress in the latter stages of the developmental period, where a continued period of cognitive growth was anticipated (i.e., displays of old patterns of behavior were replaced by new coordinated skills). In summary, fixation is thought to occur during the course of the normal developmental sequence when a disruption occurs through inadequate learning experience, lack of appropriate stimuli, absence of critical role models, or physical and/or cognitive delays (Burkhart, 1987).

Motor Development Hypothesis

Motor development plays an important role in the emergence of stereotyped behavior. Based on developmental theory, stereotyped behavior may emerge when coordinated motor behavior has been delayed. This delay is thought to contribute to the emergence of repetitive self-injury and stereotyped acts in some individuals with mental retardation, and has been proposed to resemble infant patterns of behavior identified during the sensorimotor period (Piaget, 1952). Thus, repetitive behaviors identified as self-injurious and/or stereotypic may have a basis in delayed motor development and suggest, as well, a delay in general developmental functioning (Inhelder, 1968).

Kravitz and Boehm (1971) looked at the developmental gains of infants with Trisomy-21 disorder. Their findings revealed that when matched to a same age group of infants who were without a developmental disability, the onset of such developmental, rhythmical sequences as sucking were extremely delayed. Based on this notion of delayed onset, Field, Ting, and Shuman (1979) found that maturation, as opposed to age, was the distinguishing factor in assessing the developmental progression of rhythmic movements. This was based on their findings that the onset of rhythmic movements in a group of premature infants was behind that of postmature infants. However, when chronological age was corrected to reflect gestational age, there was no significant difference. Based on this notion of developmental theory, the typically developing child will replace repetitive early behaviors with more coordinated, functional behaviors, while less sophisticated, stereotyped behavior may persist in the delayed child (Matson, 1989).

While children with Trisomy-21 disorder continue to show a progression of motor development, albeit it delayed, congenitally blind infants show an uneven progression of motor development. This is believed to relate to an absence of visual motivation for mobility. Fraiberg (1977) found that blind infants' locomotor development was delayed, although the emergence of postural developmental milestones, such as sitting independently as well as standing, occurred within appropriate age ranges. In addition, both sighted and blind infants engaged in such behaviors as rocking while sitting, rocking on their hands and knees, and rocking while standing, although blind infants engaged in these behaviors for a longer period of time (Fraiberg, 1977). When looking at the developmental progression of crawling, while eight components of crawling were identified for both sighted and blind infants, ages 6-18 months, only blind infants rocked prior to the initiation of any movement (Maida & McCune, 1996).

In a similar finding to Thelen (1979), Berkson, Tupa, and Sherman (2001) reported that most infants with developmental delays in their study engaged in body rocking. The body position in which these infants demonstrated rocking behaviors differed, with 4-point and seated body rocking preferred over spine or standing rocking. They concluded that since positioning during body rocking was highly individual, associating it to the development of locomotion, as was suggested by Thelen (1979, 1981) was speculative, at best. Berkson (2002) continued to follow these infants until they were 3 years old. His findings did not support earlier claims of researchers that body rocking promoted adaptive motor development.

Organic Theory

Stereotyped behavior is frequently cited as presenting in individuals with mental retardation, autism, as well as schizophrenia. The organic theory characterizes stereotyped behavior as resulting from aberrant or abnormal physiological processes (Burkhart, 1987). Aberrations include those that are genetically based, such as Tourette disorder, or non-genetic aberrations such as those observed in children with mental retardation (Frith & Done, 1990; Ridley, 1994). While movement disorders such as tardive dyskinesia and akathisia have the outward appearance of a stereotyped behavior, they differ from such behavior because they occur exclusively following the administration of neuroleptic medication. It is noteworthy that previous literature reviews of the organic theory of stereotyped behavior have included discussions of disease models such Cornelia De Lange syndrome and Lesch-Nyhan syndrome, both genetic mental retardation syndromes, as well as discussions of the relationship of stereotyped behavior to pain in individuals with the mental retardation (cf. Burkhart, 1987; Matson, 1989).

Stereotyped behavior is likely to present among individuals characterized as mentally retarded, as defined by substandard intellectual (cognitive) and adaptive functioning (e.g., daily living skills, communication, social interactions) domains. Dura, Mulick and Rasnake (1987) found that among a sample of adults who were nonambulatory and profoundly mentally retarded, 34% exhibited at least one stereotyped behavior. An earlier study by Berkson and Davenport (1962) found the prevalence of stereotyped behavior among individuals with mental retardation to occur among two-thirds of a residential population. Specifically, the presence of stereotyped behavior was inversely correlated with IQ and directly correlated with length of residential placement. An implication of this study was that the presence of stereotyped behavior appeared to be associated to the proximity of others exhibiting such behavior (Shulman, Sanchez-Ramos, & Weiner, 1996).

Stereotyped behavior among individuals with autism may be present throughout the individual's lifetime and may assume a variety of forms, such as head banging, body rocking, and hair twirling. Within the population of children with autism, stereotypy is typically characterized as self-generated (Hermelin & O'Connor, 1963). Under the present diagnostic criteria for autism, questions have emerged regarding the relative prevalence of stereotyped and repetitive behaviors in children with autism in comparison to children with other neurodevelopmental disorders. In what has become a landmark study of children with developmental delays in England,

Wing and Gould (1979) found that stereotyped and repetitive behaviors were present in almost all of the children who were also characterized as socially impaired. In comparison, stereotyped and repetitive behaviors were found to a lesser extent in a group of children with developmental delays who were socially related. In a somewhat more recent study of 224 children with autism (Campbell et al., 1990), a majority were found to present with at least a mild form of stereotyped behavior. Stereotyped behavior, in this study, was specifically correlated with lower IQ as well as overall autistic symptomatology and severity of autistic symptoms. Matson et al. (1996) found stereotypy in over 75% of individuals with autism and severe/profound mental retardation in comparison to only 7% of a matched group without autism. In addition, stereotyped behavior also may be present in individuals with autism who present with both average and above average intelligence, such as in Asperger syndrome. Specifically, Turner (1997) found among a sample of individuals with autism who had either high or low IQ scores, that they engaged in significantly more stereotyped behavior than both psychiatric outpatients with average IQs and control subjects with developmental delays and low IQ scores. These studies lend support to the notion of a higher representation of stereotyped behavior among children with pervasive developmental disorders. Some research suggests, however, that stereotyped behavior in children diagnosed with Pervasive Developmental Disorder, Not Otherwise Specified (PDD.NOS) may be less severe than in children with autism and Asperger syndrome (Stella, Mundy, & Tuchman, 1999). Overall, the research differs on the extent to which the severity of social and communicative symptoms in children with autism relates to the severity of stereotyped behavior (cf. Campbell et al., 1990; Charman & Sweetenham, 2001; Lord & Pickles, 1996).

Stereotyped behavior in children with autism also has been thought to relate to arousal level, as previously discussed in this chapter. Hutt and Hutt (1968) looked at stereotyped behavior in autistic children as a function of both environmental complexity and the novelty of physical and social stimuli, where complexity and novelty generated an increase in physiological arousal leading to higher levels of stereotyped activity. This association was supported by electroencephalographic (EEG) studies where stereotyped behavior was associated with "desynchronized" EEG activity. This finding lent support to the hypothesis that stereotyped behavior may be categorized as a displacement activity that served to reduce the arousal the individual was experiencing by engaging in repetitive endogenous stimulation (Hutt & Hutt, 1968).

Multiple studies and reviews of the literature have documented the presence of behavioral stereotypy in both children with autism and schizophrenia (Friedman, 1969;

Hutt & Hutt, 1968; Kanner, 1943; Shulman et al., 1996). Specifically, findings have distinguished the two diagnostic categories by noting that children with schizophrenia engage in stereotyped acts suddenly with an accompanying decline in adaptive functioning, while the emergence of stereotyped behavior is very early (prior to age 2 years) in the course of the developmental trajectory of children with autism.

Stereotyped behavior also is well documented as co-occurring among individuals with schizophrenia prior to the introduction of neuroleptic medication. Stereotypy is most associated among individuals exhibiting catatonic forms of schizophrenia, and range from simple motor behaviors to complex or bizarre gestures that may hold some meaning for the particular individual (Shulman et al., 1996). Morrison (1973) found that among individuals with catatonic schizophrenia, 24 percent of 250 individuals demonstrated stereotyped behavior. Lovaas et al. (1965) analyzed childhood schizophrenia by investigating the variables which controlled self-destructive behaviors, specifically arm and head banging. Findings supported the functional relationship between specific environmental operations and self-injurious behaviors. Specifically they found an increase in frequency and severity of self-destructive behaviors in the presence of sympathetic comments, made contingent upon the presentation of such behaviors, while a decrease in stereotyped self-injury was observed when the behavior was placed on an extinction schedule. Frith and Done (1990) also noted the existence of perseveration among individuals with schizophrenia and cite these stereotypy-like behaviors to be consistent with the behaviors of other patients with frontal lobe damage. Specifically, research has suggested that individuals with schizophrenia tend to perform poorly on a neuropsychological measure, the Wisconsin card-sorting task, which taps issues associated with cognitive flexibility and the ability to respond to new information in a constructive (adaptive) manner (Kolb & Winshaw, 1983; Malmo, 1974).

Stereotyped behavior also may occur as a result of induction of pharmacologic agents targeting the dopaminergic pathways of the brain. For example, long term use of levodopa or dopamine receptor agonists, such as for Parkinson's Disease, is likely to result in the production of dyskinesias (Shulman, et al, 1996). Dyskinesias are characterized as involuntary movements, often generalized and choreiform in nature. Discontinuation and/or reduction of the dopaminergic agents reduce the dyskinesias at the expense of a return of Parkinsonian-like symptoms (Singer, Weiner, Sanchez-Ramos, 1992). Recent case studies have suggested an increased risk of neuroleptic withdrawal dyskinesia (NWD) in certain vulnerable children. Connor (1998) found that continuation of stimulant medication in a 9-year-old treated for nonpsychotic aggressive behavior and an ll-year-old male with moderate mental retardation, increased the risk for NWD when neuroleptic medication was discontinued. In a recent study, Connor, Fletcher, and Wood (2001) investigated neuroleptic drug-related dyskinesia in children and adolescents. Among the subjects, ages 7-21 years, who received neuroleptics, 5.9% presented with dyskinesia. The use of neuroleptic drugs was significantly associated with dyskinesia in comparison to those receiving non-neuroleptic medications. In addition, factors such as IQ, initial Abnormal Involuntary Movement Scale (AIMS) score, type of antipsychotic medication, and cumulative number of risk factors accounted for approximately almost 36% of the variance when predicting dyskinetic status.

Antipsychotic agents also have been found to result in additional side effects that mimic stereotyped behavior, one of which includes akathisia. Akathisia or behavioral activation characterized by constant leg movement and the inability to sit still, is often misdiagnosed in children given their difficulty in verbally describing difficulties, and may be thought to be associated with worsening psychotic symptoms (Gogtay, Sport, Alfaro, Mulqueent, & Rapoport, 2002). Gogtay et al. found clozapine-induced akathisia to be responsive to treatment with a beta-blocker and thus advised the consideration of akathisia in all cases of "apparent no response" to atypical antipsychotic treatment of stereotyped behavior in children. Akathisia has been distinguished from the stereotyped behavior present in children with autism as it appears to cause a subjective state of distress and sensation of inner restlessness (Brasic & Barnett, 1997). Additional research has suggested the presentation of akathisia within specific populations of children. Brasic et al. (1997) found a gradual decrease in several severe dyskinesias, including objective akathisia and tics, following the discontinuation of dopamine blockers used over a two-year period, and treatment with clomipramine, in a boy with autism and severe mental retardation. While the authors noted that a few stereotyped behaviors remained, the movement disorders (i.e., akathisia and tics), resolved over a two-year period.

As discussed above, children representing all developmental levels and individuals with a variety of psychiatric disorders may engage in a full range of stereotyped acts. However, certain abnormal motor movements exist that are similar to and, in some instances, may closely mimic stereotyped behavior. However, these abnormal movements are better defined by other diagnoses. For example, complex motor tics and Tourette syndrome may appear as stereotyped acts. An often misunderstood disorder (Shulman et al., 1996), Tourette syndrome consists of a combination of a variety of motor and vocal tics. Motor tics may include facial grimacing, twitching, licking, and eye blinking. Vocal tics may include sniffing, throat clearing, coughing, and grunting. While there may be some similarities among the behaviors presented, such as repetitive eye blinking and throat clearing, the etiology of the behavior differs and thus distinguishes Tourette disorder from general stereotyped behavior. One distinguishing factor relates to the importance of hereditary in tic disorders. Another distinguishing factor resides in the characterization of a tic. A tic is a recurrent, nonrhythmic movement that may be vocal or motoric, which occurs without warning (Phelps, Brown, & Power, 2002). Generally speaking, simple motor and vocal tics are accurately diagnosed and not confused with stereotyped behavior. However, the same is not true when complex motor and vocal tics are involved. Complex motor tics, which may include repetitive stomping of a foot or repetitive touching of an object or person and complex vocal tics, such as the repetition of words, mutterings and sounds, very closely mimic stereotyped behavior and require intense scrutiny by an experienced clinician to ensure an accurate differential diagnosis. Finally, there is evidence to suggest that Tourette disorder is related to alterations within the dopamine system, such that induction of dopamine agents precipitates or exacerbates the presentation of Tourette symptoms, whereas blockade of the dopamine pathways results in a decrease in both the frequency and severity of motor and vocal tics (Shulman et al., 1996).

Biological Theory

Stereotyped behavior, as characterized by the presentation of meaningless, purposeless activity is often taken as evidence of a dysregulated central nervous system (Lewis, Gluck, Bodfish, Beauchamp, & Mailman, 1996). Research examining the neurobiological mechanisms that underlie stereotyped behavior has stemmed from treatment studies aimed at decreasing such behavior within certain clinical populations. From this neurobiological stance comes the view that many stereotyped behaviors are mediated by action on certain neurotransmitters. According to the behavioral dopaminergic supersensitivity theory, stereotyped behavior results from a depletion of the neurotransmitter dopamine in the postsynaptic cells within the basal ganglia (cf. Rojahn & Sisson, 1990). This theory proposes that the receptor sites are "supersensitive" to dopamine and the receptors thus assume a compensatory response such that low levels of dopamine across the transmission sites cause an exaggerated response. Neuroleptic medication, neuronal degeneration, as well as high levels of stress can result in a block of dopamine receptor sites causing a depletion of dopamine within the postsynaptic sites (Rojahn & Sisson, 1990). One area of research considers stereotyped behavior to be elicited or enhanced by drugs that act on dopamine receptor sites either directly (e.g., apomorphines) or indirectly (e.g., amphetamines). Lewis and Baumeister (1983) proposed that individuals with mental retardation most likely have this supersensitivity of dopamine at the receptor sites resulting from lesions and/or discontinuance of dopaminergic pathways. Additional research also has suggested that amphetamine-inducted stereotypies are suppressed by postsynaptic dopamine receptor-blocking agents, such as that observed with neuroleptics (Iverson, 1977).

The dopamine hypothesis, upon which much of what is currently understood in terms of the neurobiological origins of stereotyped behavior, was first generated in 1968 (cf. Carlsson, 1995). Dopamine was identified and measured as a normal component of brain chemistry and considered an agonist involved in the control of psychomotor activity. Previous to this account, dopamine had been considered to play a role as a precursor to noradrenaline and adrenaline. Additionally, reserpine was noted to induce the depletion of dopamine, where the psychomotor inhibitory action could be restored with the induction of its precursor, levodopa (Fog & Randrup, 2002). Previous research revealed that neuroleptic drugs, specifically chlorpromazine and haloperidol, could have a stimulating impact on dopamine through the blockade of dopamine (and noradrenaline) receptors (Carlson & Lindquist, 1963). Randrup and Munkvad (1965) proposed that dopamine could be involved in schizophrenia, given the way in which dopamine agonists appeared to mimic schizophrenic-like states. In what is regarded as one of the landmark studies on dopamine, Randrup and Munkvad (1967) revealed, through numerous animal studies, that stereotyped activity might result from doses of amphetamine. Receiving amphetamine in doses above the therapeutic threshold, therefore, may facilitate a psychotic-like state in humans that closely resembles schizophrenia. Fog and Randrup (2002) and Carlsson (1995) note that while Randrup and Munkvad's research continues to hold an important place in psychopharmacological research, it rests on indirect pharmacological evidence, and anti-dopaminergic drugs appear to be the most efficacious treatment of the positive symptoms of schizophrenia.

Dopamine Agonist-Induced Stereotypy

Research has now established that stereotyped patterns of behavior can be induced though stimulant administration (cf. Lewis, et al, 1996), similar to the findings of early animal studies by Randrup and Mankvard (1967). The abuse of psychostimulants, such as amphetamines, has been characterized by highly stereo-typed sequences of behavior that appear to resemble aspects of schizophrenia. The presentation of stereotyped behavior in individuals abusing stimulants has been associated with a syndrome resembling paranoid psychosis (Lewis et al, 1996). CNS stimulants, such as amphetamines, pemoline, and methylphenidate may trigger repetitive motor behaviors through the release of dopamine from nerve terminals in the striatum. Specifically, this occurs through the activation of the nigostriatal dopaminergic system, originating in the substantia nigra and extending into the corpus striatum. Stereotyped behavior emerges because this tract is the largest of five dopaminergic systems in the brain and plays a primary role in the control of fine motor movements (Lloyd & Hornykiewicz, 1975), mediates afferent and efferent impulses, and processes proprioceptive and vestibular information (Iverson, 1977). Both high and low doses of amphetamines will induce repetitive motor behaviors in a variety of animals (Shulman et al., 1996). Studies have revealed that the behaviors present with induction of amphetamines are species specific (Klawans, Moses, & Beaulieu, 1974; Singer et al., 1992). Consequently, stereotyped behavior may result directly from amphetamine use by acting on dopamine receptors and dopamine precursors (Lewis et al., 1985). Similarly, use of cocaine also may increase the impact of repetitive motor mannerisms by inhibiting the synaptic uptake of dopamine and consequently increasing the synaptic concentration.

Researchers looking at the relationship between induction of stereotyped behavior and the resulting change and stimulation of dopamine receptors, led to investigations of receptor subtypes involved in this process. Research more than 30 years ago has revealed two different dopamine receptor types (Garau, Govani, Stefaninin, Trabucchi, & Spano, 1978; Kebabian & Calne, 1979). D_1-like receptors were believed to mediate dopamine-induced increases in adenylate cyclase activity, and D_2 like receptor activation likely inhibited the activity of this enzyme (Anderson et al., 1990; Clark & White, 1987). Furthermore, the D_2 receptor was noted to be the site of action of most psychopharmacologic agents, both dopamine agonists and antagonists, and thus likely involved in the induction and blockade of stereotyped behavior (Creese, Sibley, Hamblin, & Leff, 1983). More recent research has reveled that the cloned dopamine subtype D_5 is similar to D_1, whereas D_3 and D_4 are considered D_2 (Lewis et al., 1996). Interactions between D_1 and D_2, specifically related to the induction of a D_1 agonist to potently inhibit apomorphine-induced stereotyped behavior and amphetamine-inducted locomotion in rats, both D_2-receptor mediated behaviors, has been supported (Lewis, et al., 1984; Malloy & Waddington, 1984).

Another neurotransmitter known to mediate dopaminergic function, 5-hydrox-ytryptamine (a biochemical precursor to the production of serotonin), also has been found to impact stereotyped responding. Stereotyped behavior can be induced in animals from serotoninergic related compounds (Randrup & Munkvad, 1967). Ste-reotyped responding induced from amphetamine or apomorphine has been found to decrease with lesions in the raphe nuclei in the brain, which contain the serotonin neuronal system (Costall & Naylor, 1974). Post-mortem investigations of individu-als with Lesch-Nyhan syndrome have revealed increased serotonin and decreased dopamine levels, as well as decreased levels of the enzymes necessary for the synthesis of dopamine. These findings suggest a relationship between self-injurious behavior and Lesch-Nyhan syndrome based at the action of central neurotransmitters (Lloyd, et al., 1981).

Developmental disabilities research, specifically in the area of autism, has involved amphetamine-like drugs such as fenfluramine, which is similar in chemical structure to the amphetamines but the behavioral manifestations are considered to be more vari-able (Campbell, Deutsch, Perry, Wolsky, & Palij, 1986). Fenfluramine is described as an anorexigenic amine (i.e., an appetite suppressant) that has been used to treat obesity in adults. The use of fenfluramine with children with autism resulted after it was found that one-third of a sample of individuals with autism had elevated peripheral serotonin levels (Ritvo, Yuwiler, Geller, Ornitz, Saeger, & Plotkin, 1970). While fenfluramine was originally approved solely for the treatment of obesity in adults, its initial use in the treatment of three patients with autism resulted in significant increases in IQ and an overall reduction in symptoms associated with the disorder (Geller, Ritvo, Freeman, & Yuwiler, 1983). A multicenter study of the effects of fenfluramine on children with autism found mixed results (Ho, Lockitch, Eaves, & Jacobson, 1986; Klykylo, Feldis, O'Grady, Ross, & Holloran, 1985; Ritvo, Freeman, Geller, & Yuwiler, 1983; Stubbs, Budden, Jackson, Teredal, & Ritvo, 1986). Overall results suggested a relationship be-tween fenfluramine and serotonin, with blood serotonin levels falling an average of 57 percent while the children were on fenfluramine. Baseline serotonin levels were in-versely related to good clinical response, including performance IQ. Furthermore, results indicated that there was a significant decrease in motor disturbances, such as stereotyped responding, during fenfluramine treatment.

Additional independent studies on the effects of fenfluramine on children with au-tism by Campbell and colleagues also were conducted (Campbell et al., 1986). Among their sample of 10 children, with a mean average age of 4 years, significant reduction in symptoms were revealed in the areas of hyperactivity, withdrawal, and uncooperative behavior, as well as stereotyped behavior. However, additional research did not confirm the initial positive results with fenfluramine pertaining to IQ and serotonin levels (Geller et al., 1983), and also revealed concerns about neurotoxicity (Gualtieri, 1986; Harvey & McMaster, 1975; Schuster, Lewis, & Seiden, 1986) and side effects (Piggott, Gdowski, Villaneuva, Fischoff, & Frohman, 1986; Realmuto et al., 1986). In a double-blind study by Leventhal, Cook, Morford, Ravitz, Heller, and Freedman (1993), 15 children with autism were treated with fenfluramine over the course of 62 weeks. Results of the study did not reveal any significant advantages to using fenfluramine. Specifically, changes in Verbal and Performance IQs of 2.6 to 4 points were not specific to drug treatment given that the changes were sustained during the placebo period. In addition, favorable changes in hyperactivity and sensory motor abnormalities reported by parents of children receiving fenfluramine were not confirmed by teacher report. Finally, fenfluramine was found to be related to both acute and chronic changes in catecholamine regulation, which was believed to be related to long-term changes in serotonergic regulation. These catecholomic/serotonergic changes were proposed as underlying reported improvements in social relationships and affective responses over time. Overall, this study was consistent with findings of other double-blind studies of fenfluramine on children with autism and mental retardation.

Dopamine agents have been found to both induce as well as enhance stereotyped behavior. Dextro-amphetamine significantly increased rocking behaviors in isolation-reared monkeys (Berkson & Mason, 1964; Fitz-Gerald, 1967) and changed cage-specific stereotypy in canaries (Keiper, 1969). Attempts to generalize animal-based research to human subjects have revealed mixed results. In one case example, Berkson (1965) varied doses of amphetamine, ranging from 10 to 15 mg/100 pounds, which did not impact presentation of stereotyped behavior in a population of individuals who were blind and mentally retarded. Similarly, Hollis (1967) did not find any significant changes in the frequency of rocking behavior in individuals with severe mental retardation administered dextro-amphetamine in 2, 4, and 8 mg doses. Furthermore, Davis, Sprague, and Werry (1969), in their comparison of rocking behavior in nine individuals with severe mental retardation, did not find a difference in occurrence of the target behavior across treatment with methylphenidate (0.44 mg/kg), placebo, and no-drug. In response to the discrepancy in the research with amphetamine induction and humans versus nonhuman subjects, Lewis and Baumeister (1983) proposed that differences may be a result not only of different etiologies and functions between human and nonhuman subjects, but it also may be a result of varying degrees of drug dosages.

Specifically, human subjects typically received lower dosages, in the range of 0.38 mg/kg and 0.44 mg/kg, in comparison to the 1 to 2 mg/kg typically administered to nonhuman primates (Lewis & Baumeister, 1983)

While the dopamine hypothesis has accounted for a great deal of the research in the area of the neurobiology of stereotyped behavior, complex behaviors, such as those typified by stereotypy, usually involve multiple neurotransmitters (Lewis et al., 1996). Lewis and Baumeister (1983) found that nondopaminergic receptors, such as opioids, serotonin, gamma amino butyric acid (GABA), acetylcholine, and adesoine, have been shown to induce stereotyped behavior. For example, the nucleus accumbens, a dopamine terminal, located near the striatum, also has been suggested to be involved in stereotyped behavior. The nigostriatal dopamine system, a loop containing dopamine terminals, act upon cells, which then act upon cells containing GABA, located within the striatum. This loop extends to terminals within the striatum, where they synapse with dopamine (Groves, Wilson, Young, & Rebec, 1975). Anticholinergic drugs, acetylcholine antagonists, produce stereotyped responses that are considered to be less severe and less continuous than those resulting from dopamine antagonists (Lewis & Baumeister, 1983).

Pierce and Courchesne (2001) compared the relationship between visuospatial exploration, stereotyped motor movement, and magnetic resonance imaging measures of the cerebellar vermis, whole brain volume and frontal lobes in 14 children with autism and 14 children with normal development. Findings revealed that rates of stereotyped behavior were significantly negatively correlated with area measures of cerebellar vermis lobules VI-VIII and positively correlated with frontal lobe volume in the autism sample. Marazziti (2002) cites research in which his colleagues have found support for the link between autism, cerebellum and serotonin (Marazziti, Nardi, & Cassano, 1999; Pasqualetti, Ori, Nardi, Cassano, & Marazziti, 1999). Specifically, Marazziti and colleagues have found high levels of 5-HT$_{5A}$ mRNA expression in the Purkinje cell perikarya, granule layer, and the dentate nucleus. Based on the wide distribution of 5-HT$_{5A}$ mRNA in the cerebellum, Marazziti and his colleagues have proposed that the receptor may be involved in such functions as cognition and emotion. Further support for this proposal is based on the notion that when the motor control function of the cerebellum is impaired, ataxia results. Marazziti (2002) further proposed that when the emotional and cognitive aspects of the cerebellum are impaired, a type of 'cognitive and emotional' ataxia may result, which may be expressed as autism.

The effect of dopamine blockers or antagonists also has been investigated. Overall, research has suggested that lower doses of antipsychotic agents that block dopamine receptors, such as thiorizidazine, 1.3-2.5 mg/kg each day, reduce stereotyped responding (Davis, 1971; Davis et al., 1969; Singh & Aman, 1981); whereas higher does of thiorizidazine, above 2.5 mg/kg each day, have caused an increased occurrence of stereotypy (Singh & Aman, 1981).

Opioid Theory of Stereotypy

A neurochemical theory also has been proposed for autism, which includes the origination and maintenance of stereotyped behavior. Panksepp (1979) proposed that autism is caused by "endogenous overactivity" of the opiate system in the brain. He based his argument on the on the fundamental deficits of autism in the realm of social interaction and the absence of social interaction in animals following doses of morphine, an opiate based drug. This theory relates to stereotyped behavior given that morphine in young animals has been found to lead to unusual body posturing as well as what Panksepp describes as "unusual motor flurries." The opioid system is also implicated in our responsivity to pain. This is believed to account for those children with autism who do not appear to experience pain in the course of stereotyped behavior that results in self-injury. Opioid systems are found throughout the brain and have been implicated as modulators of emotional and motivational states (Frecska & Arato, 2002; Panksepp, Herman, & Vilberg, 1978; Panksepp, Vilberg, Bean, Coy, & Kastin, 1978). Watson, Akil, Sullivan, and Barchas (1977) found that the opioid system is located within several areas of the brain implicated in the integration of sensation and affect. Based on this opioid hypothesis, autism has been proposed to result from an oversaturation of opioids within the neonatal brain caused by an inability of certain cleavage enzymes to appear (Panksepp & Sahley, 1987). Furthermore, research suggests that endogenous opiates control the developmental process (Zagon & McLaughlin, 1978; Zagon, McLaughlin, Weaver, & Zagon, 1982) and long-term treatment with opiate antagonists effects physical and social development (Zagon & McLaughlin, 1984). The endogenous opiate system also has been found to have a close functional relationship to serotonin which, as previously discussed, is also believed to play a critical role in the presentation of stereotyped behavior.

When should stereotyped acts be modified?

While stereotyped behavior, for the most part, appears relatively harmless, forceful treatment is mandatory under certain conditions. For example, stereotyped head banging, knee-to-head striking, and other forms of life-threatening behavior require immediate intervention. Even less obvious forms of self-injury, such as stereotyped self-pinching or self-scratching and skin picking should be modified, regardless of whether the individual appears to be distressed or in pain as the result of the behavior. The accumulation of seemingly minor damage to soft tissue can result in the development of a life-threatening infection (cellulitis), if not properly managed. Stereotyped behavior that involves pushing others, throwing objects, or finding open doors and slamming them shut also needs to be modified because of the potential danger that it represents to others. Even stereotyped behavior as benign as hand flapping or body rocking may require modification, if it interferes with the individual's availability to learn in the classroom, be productive in the work setting, engage in age appropriate activities of daily living, or if it serves to stigmatize the person and set them apart from others in society (Rojahn, Hammer, & Kroeger, 2001).

Generally speaking, indications for the modification of stereotyped behavior are limited to four conditions. These conditions include:

1. the stereotyped act has the potential to harm the individual

2. the stereotyped act has the potential to harm someone else

3. the stereotyped act interferes with the individual's potential to learn or work or otherwise interact adaptively with the environment and/or

4. the stereotyped act is socially odd or bizarre and serves as a "Scarlet Letter" of exceptionality that compromises potential for normalization within the community.

What treatments are available to modify stereotyped acts?

Behavior modification accounts for a majority of the research as well as the interventions utilized with individuals who engage in stereotyped behavior (Repp, Felce, & Barton, 1988). With the advance of psychopharmacology, psychotropic medications also are being utilized to decrease the incidence of stereotypy (cf. American Academy of Child and Adolescent Psychiatry, 1999). An additional intervention includes physical exercise (Rojahn & Sisson, 1990).

Behavior Modification

Behavior modification includes both direct and indirect paths in terms of reducing the incidence of stereotyped behavior. Specifically, behavior modification decreases the incidence of stereotypy by directly manipulating the antecedents and consequences surrounding the behavior and indirectly reduces stereotypy by increasing the incidence of other appropriate behavior (Rojahn, Hammer, & Kroeger, 2001).

Indirect Strategies

Environmental modification

Stereotyped behavior has been known to vary with situational factors, such as room size, the number of people present in a room, and noise level. Stereotyped behavior also may vary in accordance with the availability of a preferred activity within a particular setting. Environmental modification (cf. Smith & Churchill, 2002) is an example of an indirect strategy that involves making systematic changes within the environment aimed at reducing the incidence of stereotyped behavior, while not completely eliminating it. Structural analysis can provide a means for assessing the environment in which the stereotyped behavior is occurring and implicate structural rearrangements, which can be employed as a first line intervention. Touchette, MacDonald, and Langer (1985), through systematic behavioral observation found that an 18-year old female with autism would scream and hold her ears during certain scheduled activities, particularly those that were poorly structured and loud. By rescheduling her participation in a smaller group and gradually increasing her involvement across longer periods of time, stereotyped screaming was reduced by 60 to 70%. In other studies, Gallagher and Berkson (1986) significantly reduced hand gazing in two boys who were developmentally disabled and nearsighted through the use of corrective lenses and Mulick, Hoyt, Rojahn, and Schroeder (1978) decreased the incidence of nail biting and finger picking by increasing access to toys.

Gaylord-Ross, Weeks, and Lipner (1980) also employed an environmental change for the purpose of reducing escape-motivated stereotyped behavior by altering specific aversive aspects of the situation. Through a functional analysis, they found that a 20-year-old young man with autistic-like features engaged in stereotyped body rocking, hand-flapping, and loud humming when he found a situation to be aversive (such as riding a bus with large crowds of people) and wanted to escape. By modifying the environment, in this case, by changing the time when he rode the bus to a time when fewer people were aboard, decreased stereotyped behavior was observed.

Positive reinforcement

The use of positive reinforcement is another means of indirectly reducing an individual's stereotyped behavior, which includes training adaptive behavior and differential reinforcement procedures. Training adaptive behavior refers to the notion that by increasing a person's adaptive functioning, there is a systematic reduction in maladaptive behavior, such as stereotyped responding. This approach includes teaching the individual purposeful ways of interacting with the environment such as play skills, which can replace stereotyped behavior being maintained through self-stimulation as well as boredom (Rojahn et al., 2001).

Researchers have observed a decrease in stereotyped behavior when novel objects are made available (Davenport & Berkson, 1963; Berkson & Mason, 1964b). Eason, White, and Newsom (1982) extended this finding to the treatment setting by training six children with mental retardation and autism to play with a variety of toys followed by rewards in the form of edibles, tickles, or music. Results revealed that stereotyped behavior decreased to negligible rates, while appropriate toy play increased across multiple settings, including in the absence of the trainer and during a two-month follow-up. While extrinsic reinforcement has been noted to account for the initial changes in rates of maladaptive behavior, the sustained results were suggested by Eason et al. (1982) to be related to "natural maintaining contingencies of reinforcement" (Stokes & Baer, 1977). According to this proposal, playing with toys was likely to result in positive interactions with caretakers, as well as sensory reinforcement which may have been experienced as more rewarding than the sensory reinforcement presumed inherent to stereotyped behavior.

Functional communication training

Functional communication training (FCT) is an additional form of adaptive training and an appropriate means of intervention when stereotyped behavior is escape-motivated or maintained by positive social reinforcement (Rojahn et al., 2001). In the presence of functional communication, the individual is able to utilize adaptive communication skills (e.g., signs, gestures) to attract appropriate attention or to effect a leave from an aversive situation (Day, Horner, & O'Neill, 1994). For example, Durand and Carr (1987) were able to substitute hand flapping and body rocking for signing for assistance.

Differential reinforcement (DRO, DRI, DRL)

Differential reinforcement is a form of positive reinforcement, which acts indirectly to decrease the rate of stereotyped behavior. Differential reinforcement procedures consist of differential reinforcement of other behavior (DRO), incompatible behavior (DRI), and low rates (DRL) of stereotyped behavior. Differential reinforcement of other behavior (DRO) refers to the delivery of a reward after a certain period of time has elapsed during which stereotyped behavior has not occurred. This strategy reinforces the occurrence of the behavior immediately preceding the reward and, indirectly, reinforces the omission of the stereotyped behavior. The amount of time may vary from approximately 5 to 30 seconds to more than an hour, depending upon the child's level of functioning and the frequency with which the stereotyped behavior occurs. In the initial treatment stages of treatment utilizing DRO, the intervals for reinforcement are short and then gradually increased as the intervention phase continues. Early research utilizing DRO for mediating stereotyped behavior revealed mixed results with some studies revealing no meaningful change in target behaviors (Luiselli, 1975), while some revealed marginal results (Mulhern & Baumeister, 1969), and others reported significant reductions in behaviors (Repp, Deitz, & Speir, 1974). Despite discrepant results, DRO generally is considered to be useful in the treatment of stereotyped responding when included as part of a comprehensive behavior management plan (LaGrow & Repp, 1984).

The research of Luiselli and colleagues (Luiselli, Colozzi, & O'Toole, 1980; Luiselli, Myles, Evans, & Boyce, 1985) is credited for illustrating the effectiveness of DRO in managing self-stimulatory behavior, and incorporating fading phases to facilitate maintenance of appropriate behaviors. In their initial study, tokens were provided to a child with moderate mental retardation contingent upon the absence of stereotyped behavior. The tokens, in turn, allowed the child to gain access to a play area. Tokens were delivered according to intervals established by a timer. Once the stereotyped behavior was suppressed, maintenance procedures followed, which included removal of the tokens, timer, and increasingly longer periods of access to the play area. Follow-up at two months indicated maintenance of results. In their second study, a child with severe mental retardation and multiple handicaps was allowed access to a toy in the absence of stereotyped behavior according to changing criterion in the form of increasing intervals. Treatment gains were significant and maintained at 3-month follow-up. In another study, Kennedy, Meyer, Knowles, and Shukla (2000) found decreases in stereotyped behavior associated with the use of differential reinforcement contingencies involving the use of alternative forms of communication.

DRO is considered to be a labor-intensive means of intervention. It requires a great deal of professional time and effort to closely observe an individual across designated intervals, as well as to accurately maintain the timing procedure, and deliver rewards in a timely manner according to established criteria (Rojahn & Sisson, 1990). Given the difficulty in maintaining such a treatment, momentary DRO has been proposed, which is based on a modified DRO procedure involving less caregiver monitoring. According to a momentary DRO model, reinforcement is delivered if the behavior does not occur at a particular observational time period (Repp, Barton, & Brulle, 1983). The research with momentary DRO illustrates variable responses. For example, Harris and Wolchik (1979) found momentary DRO was only moderately effective in suppressing the rate of self-stimulatory behavior exhibited in one boy with autism and mental retardation, while it did not result in rates of change in two other subjects, and increased stereotyped behavior in a fourth child. Despite inconsistent results, research has suggested that momentary DRO may play a role in sustaining suppression of behaviors initially achieved through traditional DRO procedures (Barton, Brulle, & Repp, 1986).

Another differential reinforcement procedure involves rewarding rates of a targeted behavior that appear to be lower than baseline. Differential reinforcement of low rates of behavior or DRL was employed by Singh, Dawson, and Manning (1981) with three teenaged boys with profound mental retardation. In their study, praise was delivered contingent upon a targeted response if it followed stereotyped behavior by at least 12 seconds. Once the stereotyped behavior was decreased, the inter-response time was increased from 12 seconds to 30 seconds and, finally, to 180 seconds. Results of the study indicated that DRL procedures decreased stereotyped responding, but did not suppress it completely.

A final form of differential reinforcement is DRI or differential reinforcement of incompatible behavior. In this procedure, a specific behavior that competes with the stereotyped behavior is shaped through contingent reinforcement. DRI has been used successfully to increase adaptive behavior and reduce stereotyped behavior in children with mental retardation (Favell, 1973). For example, differentially rewarding the use of a hand switch decreased stereotyped hand mouthing in a boy with multiple handicaps (McClure, Moss, McPeters, & Kirkpatrick, 1986). However, a review of the literature also has revealed inconsistent results. Differential reinforcement of toy play remediated stereotyped behavior in one of three subjects, while the remaining children required aversive strategies to suppress targeted behaviors (Denny, 1980).

There are several possible explanations for the variability in responses across the research utilizing DRO, DRI and DRL procedures. Mainly, however, unsuccessful applications are attributed to the absence of a truly potent reward for any particular individual (Rojahn & Sisson, 1990), as well as the difficulty inherent to learning that a reward will be delivered in the absence of a response (Berkson & Mason, 1964b; Davenport & Berkson, 1963).

Direct Strategies

Extinction

Stereotyped behavior that has been determined through functional analysis to be maintained by positive reinforcement is an indication for the use of extinction as a viable course of treatment. An extinction procedure, in clinical terms, refers to the withholding of the reward identified as previously or currently reinforcing the occurrence of the targeted stereotyped response.

Given that poor environmental conditions and decreased sensory stimulation typically increase stereotyped behavior, withdrawal of rewards from the environment has not been utilized to decrease non-self-injurious stereotyped behavior. Research in support of this approach was employed by Foxx and McMorrow (1984) who evaluated the effects of a novel program incorporating reinforcement and extinction procedures in the reduction of stereotyped behaviors in two women with profound mental retardation. Results revealed that the continuous presentation of external consequences (rewards) identified as maintaining stereotyped behavior, did not change the rate of stereotyped behavior, although temporary rates of change were observed when the consequences (rewards) were halted. Utilization of a FR-5 schedule of positive reinforcement resulted in a marked increase in stereotyped behavior and large, but transitory reductions in stereotyped behavior when access to reward was withheld (extinction). While the results were promising in terms of treatment programming, the authors advised against intentionally rewarding stereotyped behavior in order to gain stimulus control followed by extinction because the desired effect of suppression was not a durable result. Consequently, extinction or time-out from positive reinforcement alone is not likely to be effective in the treatment of stereotyped behavior (Schroeder, 1991). However, extinction with the addition of reinforcement of alternative activities (DRO, DRI) has been shown to be effective in decreasing stereotyped behavior (Baumeister & Forehand, 1971; Favell, 1973).

Avoidance Extinction

Avoidance extinction (e.g., Patel, Piazza, Martinez, Volkert, & Santana, 2002) is a variation of the extinction principle that can be applied to stereotyped behavior when it is sustained by negative reinforcement. In other words, stereotyped behavior that is rewarded because it results in the avoidance or escape from an aversive stimulus. Avoidance extinction is achieved through a disruption in the association between the target behavior (stereotypy) and the reinforcement (escape), such that by disrupting the negative reinforcement paradigm, the stereotyped behavior ceases (Rojahn et al., 2001). For example, if a child engages in stereotyped behavior such as body rocking or vocalizing to avoid classroom tasks found to be aversive, ignoring the stereotyped behavior will act as avoidance extinction. By not allowing the child to avoid the tasks, the child will come to learn that engaging in stereotyped behavior will not result in a discontinuation of (or escape from) the aversive activity. Consequently, stereotyped behavior should decrease and, eventually, become extinct because it is no longer being rewarded (negatively reinforced) as an effective means of escape.

Sensory Extinction

Sensory extinction relates to the notion that stereotyped behavior may be sustained through the self-stimulatory or sensory consequences that the individual experiences while engaged in the response. Effective treatment using sensory extinction methods relies on accurate identification of the source of internal reinforcement. Stereotyped object dropping by a blind, 26-year-old male with profound mental retardation was decreased with the elimination of auditory feedback (Dalrymple, 1989). In addition, use of contingent auditory stimulation for correct object placement (DRO, DRI) increased appropriate behavior.

Maag, Wolchik, Rutherford, and Parks (1986) conducted two experiments to assess sensory extinction procedures on the self-stimulatory behaviors of boys with autism, aged 7 and 12. Overall findings suggested that a reduction occurred only across those stereotyped behaviors that were topographically similar and thus maintained by the same sensory modality, while dissimilar behaviors continued. A similar finding was supported by Aiken and Salzberg (1984), in which a sensory extinction procedure resulted in the suppression of topographically similar stereotypy but did not impact topographically dissimilar stereotyped behavior. Specifically, the use of white noise to mask stereotyped vocalizations resulted in suppression of this behavior, while clapping and object-dropping behaviors continued, probably because they included additional and dissimilar sensory components (kinesthetic, visual) by comparison to vocalizations.

Facial or visual screening is a form of sensory extinction that refers to interventions in which the individual's face and eyes are temporarily covered with a cloth or a therapist's hand contingent upon the occurrence of stereotyped behavior. This procedure has a long history of being utilized successfully as a means of intervening with repetitive self-injurious behavior, especially with young children with autism and severe mental retardation (McGonigle, Duncan, Cordisco, & Barrett, 1982). Its usefulness with older children, regardless of level of functioning, is suspect. Facial screening, involving the brief vision blocking of a 16-year-old with profound mental retardation, was employed as a means of decreasing stereotyped spitting behaviors (Dura, 1990). Results revealed that both planned ignoring and facial screening increased the rate of spitting behaviors.

Punishment

Currently, punishment procedures generally are not utilized to reduce stereotyped behavior, unless self-injury or aggression is involved (Schroeder, 1991). Hamilton and Standahl (1969) utilized contingent faradic electrical stimulation to decrease stereotyped growling in a woman with profound mental retardation. Research comparing treatment of stereotyped and self-injurious behaviors, using meta-analytic procedures and rule out criteria, revealed that in comparison to punishment, DRO was the most effective treatment to decrease the incidence of stereotyped behavior in individuals with profound mental retardation who were 16 years of age and older (Gorman-Smith & Matson, 1985). In contrast, Barrett and colleagues (Barrett, Matson, Shapiro, & Ollendick, 1981) treated two children with mental retardation, ages 5 and 9, who engaged in high rates of stereotyped responding with alternate conditions of no treatment, mild punishment and DRO. Results indicated that mildly aversive procedures, such as contingent brief immobilization of hands, were most effective in suppressing stereotyped behavior in both subjects. These results continued across a six-month follow-up.

Mayhew and Harris (1978) utilized punishment procedures with two adolescents with profound mental retardation when they engaged in repetitive self-stimulatory behavior. Results revealed that both subjects appeared to experience negative side effects of the punishment condition, in the form of experimenter directed aggression and decrease in social behavior. The authors proposed that the use of punishment procedures may result in negative side effects and that the potential for decreased social behavior should be closely monitored when response cost or punishment is the treatment of choice.

Response Prevention

Response prevention or response blocking is a procedure that may be viewed alternately as punishment or extinction. Masaleski, Iwata, Rodgers, Vollmer, and Zarcone (1994) looked at the use of protective equipment in decreasing stereotyped hand mouthing for two women with profound mental retardation. Results indicated that non-contingent use of oven mitts produced a large decrease in the rate of hand mouthing for one subject. However, the second subject responded favorably only when the oven mitts were applied as a punishment contingent upon engaging in stereotyped hand mouthing.

In either form, extinction or punishment, response prevention (blocking) can be used effectively to reduce stereotyped behaviors (Barrett, Ackles, Burkhart, & Payton, 1987; Lerman & Iwata, 1996; MacDonald, Wilder, & Dempsey, 2002; Smith, Russo, & Le, 1999; Tarbox, Wallace, & Tarbox, 2002; Thompson, Iwata, Conners, & Roscoe, 1999). However, results of most response blocking studies usually contain a caveat. For example, Hagopian and Adelinis (2001) used response blocking successfully in the treatment of pica where the individual was prompted to secure an alternative substance. However, increased aggression was a noted side effect during the course of treatment. In a recent study, Lerman and colleagues expanded upon the work of Hagopian and Adelinis to evaluate the use of response blocking treatment to address stereotyped behaviors of head and tooth tapping (Lerman, Kelley, Vorndran, & Van Camp, 2003). These behaviors were determined as resulting in hair loss and decreases in adaptive functioning in an 18-year-old female with severe mental retardation and autism. Four treatment protocols were employed with the first providing environmental enrichment in the form or offering beads and bells. This was followed by a response blocking procedure, a conditioned response block, a prompted item interaction, and finally response blocking and item interaction. Results across the conditions revealed that blocking of the stereotyped behavior of head and tooth tapping was related to decreased interaction with beads and bells and increases in stereotyped hand wringing.

Overcorrection

Overcorrection refers to the use of several treatment modalities to remediate difficult behavior. One such treatment is positive practice overcorrection, which refers to engaging the child in a program of repeated motor movements following the demonstration of the problem behavior (Rojahn et al, 2001). The use of both verbal and graduated physical prompts can be implemented to cue the child to engage in positive practice activities. Macfarlane, Young, and West (1987) investigated the effects of an overcorrection procedure with two female students, ages 11 and 12 years old, with multiple handicaps. The procedure was implemented within the context of a school/home program. A multiple-probe variation of several baseline designs was used to validate experimental control. Results supported the use of overcorrection as an intervention to reduce longstanding stereotyped behavior in both home and school settings.

The duration of an overcorrection procedure also has been an area of research when examining its effectiveness in reducing stereotyped behavior. Luiselli (1984) evaluated the effectiveness of brief overcorrection procedures with two girls (ages 12 and 18) with severe mental retardation. In the first experimental design, stereotyped finger sucking and saliva rubbing was followed by having the girls clean and dry their hands each time the behavior occurred. Findings revealed that the behaviors terminated during the course of two classroom sessions and the overcorrection procedure was found to be more effective than the alternative response of praise and touch for more appropriate behavior. In a second experimental design, tongue protrusion was suppressed during speech therapy sessions through the combined intervention of 15 seconds of overcorrection (wiping lips and mouth with a tissue). Significant results were maintained at follow-up and supported the use of brief duration overcorrection procedures to produce effective results while maintaining effective use of teaching time. Maag, Rutherford, Wolchik, and Parks (1986) also assessed the effects of a brief overcorrection procedure on two boys with autism, ages 7 and 12 years. Results showed near total suppression of stereotyped behavior occurred for one subject under a 20-second overcorrection design, while the other child required a 60-second procedure to achieve suppression. The authors proposed that there appears to be variability in responding across children regarding rates of reduction under specific time durations, with longer durations being necessary for some children.

The use of overcorrection procedures has long been accompanied by the notion that a longer procedural duration is better. In a recent study comparing the effectiveness of three positive practice overcorrection (PPOC) treatments (30 seconds, 2 minutes, and 8 minutes) on stereotyped hand movements of adults with severe to profound developmental disabilities, Cole, Montgomery, Wilson, and Milan (2000) looked specifically at the role of PPOC duration in response suppression. Using an alternating treatment, multiple baseline design, Cole and colleagues found that the different durations were of equal effectiveness in reducing stereotyped behavior to near-zero levels. Thus, the study did not support previously held convictions on PPOC that longer durations produce greater clinical significance.

The use of overcorrection procedures that include the presentation of appropriate alternative behavior also has been proposed in the remediation of stereotyped behavior. In a case study presentation, Powers and Crowel (1985) utilized a positive practice overcorrection procedure with an 8-year-old boy with autism that included the incorporation of specific learning objectives in the treatment protocol that purposely focused on reducing stereotyped vocalizations. Their results demonstrated that not only were the boy's vocalizations reduced, but that he also acquired, maintained and generalized 24 social questions to replace the inappropriate behaviors. The authors proposed that topographically similar learning objectives should be considered when implementing an overcorrection procedure to increase the therapeutic value of the intervention.

Research also has looked at the effectiveness of overcorrection in comparison to other interventions. Harris, Handleman, and Fong (1987) compared the impact of overcorrection and adult imitation on the stereotyped behavior of three children with autism, ranging in age from six to eight years. Results showed that the rates of stereotyped responding for two of the three subjects systematically changed. Specifically, mean levels of self-stimulation decreased during the overcorrection phase but increased during imitation, with parallel changes in both mood and attention during imitation. The authors proposed that adult imitation may serve as a means of establishing a reinforcing relationship with children with autism.

Multiple interventions

Sisson, Van-Hasselt, Hersen, and Aurand (1988) developed an intervention to take place within a classroom laboratory to reduce stereotyped behavior in three 4-year-old children with multiple handicaps. Preferred stimuli were identified and utilized as rewards in a differential reinforcement of other (DRO) program. Behavioral interventions were implemented and evaluated in multiple-baseline designs. Findings of decreased stereotyped responding and destructive behavior was associated with the combined use of momentary DRO plus immobilization time-out, as well as momentary DRO combined with overcorrection. Efficacy of the treatment was further substantiated through implementation of the intervention in a regular classroom environment and results were maintained at 5-month follow-up.

Psychopharmacology

Pharmacotherapy or drug treatment has been widely used for the purpose of behavior modification (Silva, 1979; Sprague, 1977), despite significant associated side effects (Aman & Singh, 1980; Gualtieri, Quade, Hicks, Mayo, & Schroeder, 1984).

Neuroleptic drugs have a long history of being used with individuals with mental retardation (Aman & Singh, 1986; Aman, White, & Field, 1984) and autism (Aman, Van Bourgondien, Wolford, & Sarphare, 1995; McDougle, 1997) with mixed results (Matson, Bielecki, Mayville, & Matson, 2003). In one study, Singh and Aman (1981) found that both low and high does of thioridazine were equally effective in reducing the rate of stereotyped behavior. However, this finding was unable to be generalized to all neuroleptic medications. For example, haloperidol, in lower doses than delivered with other medications, such as thioridazine, promoted increased levels of stereotypy in certain cases (Aman, Teehan, White, Turbott, & Vaithiananthan, 1989). Furthermore, it was noted that individuals with higher rates of stereotyped behavior showed a more favorable response to haloperidol, while individuals with lower levels of stereotyped behavior showed a less favorable response to the medication. Several additional studies with D2 antagonists, such as haloperidol, at doses of 0.25-4mg day (Anderson, Campbell, Adams, Small, Perry, & Shell, 1989; Campbell, et al., 1978; Joshi, Capozzoli, & Coyle, 1988) resulted in decreased stereotyped responding, as well as decreased social withdrawal, hyperactivity, angry affect and negative attitude.

However, the presence of significant adverse effects is reported to occur in children with developmental disabilities treated with neuroleptics (i.e., chlorpromazine, thioridazine, and haloperidol). Findings of associated untoward effects has prompted the exploration of newer, alternative medications. Phelps and colleagues (2002) note the recent use of so-called atypical antipsychotic medication, such as risperidone and olanzapine, to address stereotyped behavior. Unfortunately, very few controlled studies (e.g., Aman, DeSmedt, Derivan, Lyons, & Findling, 2002; McCracken, McGough, Shah, Cronin, & Hong, 2002; Snyder, Turgay, Aman, Binder, Fisman, & Carroll, 2002) have been conducted. Moreover, these studies have not focused very clearly on stereotypy as a dependent measure. Promise of the efficacy of new classes of medication rests in the absence of any negative impact on cognition as well as fewer other types of adverse effects typically associated with the use of older neuroleptic medications (Werry & Aman, 1999). In this regard, the results of early studies (e.g., McAdam, Zarcone, Hellings, Napolitano, & Schroeder, 2002) are favorable.

The use of opiate antagonists also has been proposed as a psychopharmacological intervention in the treatment of stereotyped behavior, particularly repetitive forms of self-injurious behavior (cf. Sandman et al., 1998). Barrett, Feinstein, and Hole (1989) examined the effect of naltrexone, an opiate antagonist, on repetitive, intractible self-injury in a young girl with autism and severe mental retardation. Results of the double-blind, placebo-controlled study showed lawful decreases and increases in rates of self-injurious responding depending upon the presence or absence, respectively, of the drug. Zero rates of once life-threatening behavior was observed on 22-month follow-up. The authors argue for the use of opiate antagonists in the treatment of stereotyped and self-injurious behaviors, as well as for individuals with developmental disabilities who present with decreased social responsiveness (Smith, Gupta, & Smith, 1995; Walters, Barrett, Feinstein, Mercurio, & Hole, 1990).

Selective serotonin reuptake inhibitors (SSRIs) also represent a newer class of drugs that have been investigated as treatment for stereotyped behavior, in part because of the similarity of stereotypy with compulsive behavior and also because of the fewer side effects associated with these medications. Fluoxetine is one such SSRI that has been studied in several open clinical trials and, subsequently, found to decrease perseverative, compulsive, and stereotyped behavior (Cook, Rowlett, Jaselskis, & Leventhal, 1992; Ricketts, Goza, Ellis, Singh, & Singh, 1993). Fatemi, Realmuto, Khan, and Thuras, (1998) also found that fluoxetine resulted in decreased rates of stereotyped behavior as well as inappropriate speech, mood lability, and lethargy.

Despite the potential of benefits that may be derived from pharmacotherapy in any particular case, Rojahn and Sisson (1990) have noted the continued concerns expressed by parents and professionals regarding the use of medication, particularly with children. Beyond the obvious worry related to side effects, concern also was expressed about the confines that drug treatment places on other forms of intervention. Aman, Singh, and White (1987) found that direct care staff members responsible for the day-to-day management of various behavioral difficulties, considered behavior modification to be a viable alternative for many of the stereotyped behaviors exhibited by individuals with developmental disabilities, including repetitive forms of self-injury. In another study, Singh, Watson, and Winton (1987) found that mothers seeking behavior management training for their children with mild to moderate mental retardation preferred positive reinforcement procedures as opposed to medication and punishment. Although the opinions of parents and paraprofessionals are valid and worthy of consideration, research has supported the efficacy of combining medication with a variety of behavioral interventions in order to achieve a desired treatment effect. For example, Schalock, Foley, Toulouse, and Stark (1985) conducted a combined behavioral-drug intervention addressing stereotyped behavior in a group of adults with mental retardation. Results of the study supported the use of the combined behavioral-drug intervention, which resulted in a decrease in targeted behaviors as well as lower dosages of medication. The utility of pharmacotherapy likely rests in its combination with direct and indirect behavioral strategies.

Exercise

A review of interventions used to suppress the rate of stereotyped behavior in individuals with autism and/or mental retardation includes the use of physical exercise (Baumeister & MacLean, 1984; Kern, Koegel, Dyer, Blew, & Fenton, 1982; Watters & Watters, 1980). Schroeder, Bickel, and Richmond (1986) have proposed that exercise may reduce stereotyped behavior by acting upon dopamine receptors. Exercise may promote an increase in the dopamine metabolite norepinephrine which, in turn, may cause to counterbalance the absence of dopamine in the brain and decrease stereotyped behavior. However, the reduced rates associated with exercise also may simply be due to extraneous factors, such as fatigue (Baumeister & MacLean, 1984).

Summary

Stereotyped behavior is among the most perplexing forms of psychopathology in persons with developmental disabilities. Stereotyped acts are defined as voluntary, repetitive motor movements that serve no apparent adaptive purpose. Approximately 33% of the population of children with mental retardation engage in stereotyped responding, the vast majority of whom are non-verbal and present with IQs below 50. Stereotyped behavior also is a salient characteristic of children with autism. A majority of children with autism present with stereotyped behavior prior to age 2 years. The etiology of stereotyped behavior is a controversial subject. Several explanations have been proposed to account for the origin and maintenance of stereotyped acts, including learning, homeostatic, neural oscillator, developmental, organic and biological theories. Controversy also exists as to whether stereotyped behavior, which appears harmless, should be treated. Four indications for clinical intervention were reviewed. Available treatment in the form of behavior modification utilizing direct (extinction, sensory extinction, punishment, response prevention) and indirect (DRO, DRI, DRL) strategies was reviewed, as well as advances in pharmacotherapy.

References

Aiken, J. M., & Salzberg, C. (1984). The effects of a sensory extinction procedure on stereotypic sounds of two autistic children. *Journal of Autism and Developmental Disorders, 14,* 291-299.

Aman, M. G., DeSmedt, G., Derivan, A., Lyons, B., & Findling, R. L. (2002). Double- blind, placebo-controlled study of risperidone for the treatment of disruptive behaviors in children with subaverage intelligence. *American Journal of Psychiatry, 159,* 1337-1346.

Aman, M. G., & Singh, N. N. (1980). The usefulness of thioridazine for treating childhood disorders—fact or folklore? *American Journal of Mental Deficiency, 84,* 331-338.

Aman, M. G., & Singh, N. N. (1986). A critical appraisal of recent drug research in mental retardation: The Coldwater studies. *Journal of Mental Deficiency Research, 30,* 203-216.

Aman, M. G., Singh, N. N., & White, A. J. (1987). Caregiver perceptions of psychotropic medication in residential facilities. *Research in Developmental Disabilities, 8,* 449-465.

Aman, M. G., Teehan, C. J., White, A. J., Turbott, S. H., & Vaithiananthan, C. (1989). Haloperidol treatment with chronically medicated residents: Dose effects on clinical behavior and reinforcement contingencies. *American Journal of Mental Retardation, 93,* 452-460.

Aman, M. G., Van Bourgondien, M. E., Wolford, P. L., & Sarphare, G. (1995). Psychotropic and anticonvulsant drugs in subjects with autism: Prevalence and patterns of use. *Journal of the American Academy of Child and Adolescent Psychiatry, 34,* 1672-1681.

Aman, M. G., White, A. J., & Field, C. (1984). Chlorpromazine on stereotypic and conditioned behavior of severely retarded patients: A pilot study. *Journal of Mental Deficiency Research, 28,* 253-260.

American Academy of Child and Adolescent Psychiatry (1999). Practice parameters for the assessment and treatment of children, adolescents, and adults with mental retardation and comorbid mental disorders. *Journal of the American Academy of Child and Adolescent Psychiatry, 38* (Suppl. 1), 5-31.

American Psychiatric Association (1994). *Diagnostic and statistical manual of mental disorders. Fourth edition.* Washington, DC: Author.

Anderson, L. T., Campbell, M., Adams, P., Small, A. M., Perry, R., & Shell, J. (1989). The effects of haloperidol discrimination learning and behavioral symptoms in autistic children. *Journal of Autism and Developmental Disorders, 19,* 227-239.

Anderson, J., Gingrich, J., Bates, M., Dearry, A., Faladeau, P., Senopgles, S., et al. (1990). Dopamine receptor subtypes: Beyond the D1/D2 classification. *Trends in Pharmacological Sciences, 22,* 231-236.

Ayllon, T., & Azrin, N. H. (1966). Punishment as a discriminative stimulus and conditioned reinforcer with humans. *Journal of the Experimental Analysis of Behavior, 9,* 411-419.

Bachman, J. (1972). Self-injurious behavior: A behavioral analysis. *Journal of Abnormal Psychology, 80,* 221-248.

Barrett, R. P. (in press). Self-injurious behavior. In S. Lee (Ed.), *Encyclopedia of school psychology. Volume 6.* New York: Macmillan.

Barrett, R. P., Ackles, P. K., Burkhart, J. E., & Payton, J. (1987). Behavioral treatment of chronic aerophagia. *American Journal of Mental Retardation, 91,* 620-625.

Barrett, R. P., Feinstein, C., & Hole, W. (1989). Effects of naloxone and naltrexone on self-injury: A double-blind, placebo-controlled analysis. *American Journal on Mental Retardation, 96,* 644-651.

Barrett, R.P., Matson, J. L., Shapiro, E. S., & Ollendick, T. H. (1981). A comparison of punishment and DRO procedures for treating stereotypic behavior of mentally retarded children. *Applied Research in Mental Retardation, 2,* 247-256.

Barton, L. E., Brulle, A. R., & Repp, A. C. (1986). Maintenance of therapeutic changes by momentary DRO. *Journal of Applied Behavior Analysis, 19,* 227-282.

Baumeister, A. A., & Forehand, R. (1971). Effects of extinction of an instrumental response on stereotyped rocking in severe retardates. *Psychological Record, 21,* 235-240.

Baumeister, A. A., & Forehand, R. (1972). Effects of contingent shock and verbal command on body rocking of retardates. *Journal of Clinical Psychology, 28,* 586-590.

Baumeister, A. A., & Forehand, R. (1973). Stereotyped acts. In N. R. Ellis (Ed.), *International review of research in mental retardation. Volume 6* (pp. 55-96). New York: Academic Press.

Baumeister, A. A., & MacLean, W. E. (1984). Deceleration of SIB and stereotypic responding by exercise. *Applied Research in Mental Retardation, 5,* 385-394.

Baumeister, A. A., & Rollings, J. P. (1976). Self-injurious behavior. In N. R. Ellis (Ed.), *International review of research in mental retardation. Volume 8* (pp. 1-34). New York: Academic Press.

Berkson, G. (1965). Stereotyped movements of mental defectives. VI. No effect of amphetamine or a barbiturate. *Perceptual and Motor Skills, 21,* 68.

Berkson, G. (1967). Abnormal stereotyped acts. In J. Zubin & H. Hunt (Eds.), *Comparative psychopathology-Animal and human* (pp. 74-84). New York: Grune & Stratton.

Berkson, G. (1983). Repetitive stereotyped behaviors. *American Journal of Mental Deficiency, 88,* 239-246.

Berkson, G. (2002). Early development of stereotyped and self-injurious behaviors: II. Age trends. *American Journal on Mental Retardation, 107,* 468-477.

Berkson, G., & Davenport, R .K. (1962). Stereotyped Movements in mental defectives: I. Initial survey. *American Journal of Mental Deficiency, 66,* 849-852.

Berkson, G., & Mason, W., (1963). Stereotyped movements of mental defectives: III. Situation effects. *American Journal of Mental Deficiency, 68,* 409-412.

Berkson, G., & Mason, W. (1964a). Stereotyped behaviors of chimpanzees' relation to general arousal and alternative activities. *Perceptual and Motor Skills, 19,* 635-652.

Berkson, G., & Mason, W. A. (1964b). Stereotyped movements of mental defectives: IV. The effects of toys and the character of the acts. *American Journal of Mental Deficiencies, 68,* 511-524.

Berkson, G., Mason, W., & Saxon, S. V. (1963). Situation and stimulus effects on stereotyped behaviors of chimpanzees. *Journal of Comparative and Physiological Psychology, 56,* 786-792.

Berkson, G., & Tupa, M. (2000). Early development of stereotyped and self-injurious behavior. *Journal of Early Intervention, 23,* 1-19.

Berkson, G., Tupa, M., & Sherman, L. (2001). Early development of stereotyped and self-injurious behaviors: I. Incidence. *American Journal on Mental Retardation, 106,* 539-547.

Borrero, J. C., Vollmer, T. R., Wright, C. S., Lerman, D. C., & Kelley, M. E. (2002). Further evaluation of the role of protective equipment in the functional analysis of self-injury. *Journal of Applied Behavior Analysis, 35,* 69-72.

Brasic, J. R., & Barnett, J. Y. (1997). Hyperkinesias in a prebutertal boy with autistic disorder treated with haloperidol and valproic acid. *Psychological Reports, 80*(1), 163-170.

Brasic, J. R., Barnett, J. Y., Aisemberg, P., Ahn, S. C., Nadrich, R. H, Kaplan, D., et al. (1997). Dyskinesias subside off all medication in a boy with autistic disorder and severe mental retardation. *Psychological Reports, 1* (3 Pt 1), 755-767.

Brett, L. P., & Levine, S. (1979). Schedule induced polydipsia suppresses pituitary-adrenal activity in rats. *Journal of Comparative and Physiological Psychology, 93*, 946-956.

Bucher, B., & Lovaas, O. I. (1968). Use of aversive stimulation in behavior modification. In M. R. Jones (Ed.), *Miami symposium on the prediction of behavior-aversive stimulation* (pp. 77-145). Coral Gables, FL: University of Miami Press.

Burkhart, J. (1987). Theories on the etiology and maintenance of stereotypic behaviors. In R. P. Barrett & J. L. Matson (Eds.), *Advances in developmental disorders. Volume 1* (pp. 41-76). Greenwich, CT: JAI Press Inc.

Buyer, L. S., Berkson, G., Winnega, M. A., & Morton, L. (1987). Stimulation and control as components of stereotyped body rocking. *American Journal of Mental Deficiency, 91*, 543-547.

Campbell, M., Adams, P., Small, A., Curren, E. L., Overall, J. E., Anderson, L. T., et al. (1978). Efficacy and safety of fenfluramine in autistic children. *Journal of the American Academy of Child and Adolescent Psychiatry, 27*, 434-439.

Campbell, M., Deutsch, S. I., Perry, R., Wolsky, B. B., & Palij, M. (1986). Short-term efficacy and safety of fenfluramine in hospitalized preschool-age autistic children: An open study. *Psychopharmacology Bulletin, 22*, 141-147.

Campbell, M., Locascio, J. J., Choroco, M. C., Spencer, E. K., Malone, R. P., Kafantaris, V., et al. (1990). Stereotypies and tardive dyskinesia: Abnormal movements in autistic children. *Psychopharmacological Bulletin, 26*, 260-266.

Carlsson, A. (1995). The dopamine theory revisited. In S. Hirsch, & D. Weinberger (Eds.), *Schizophrenia* (pp. 379-400). Oxford: Blackwell.

Carlsson, A., & Lindquist, M. (1963). Effect of chlorpromazine and haloperidol on the formation of 3-methoxytyramine and normetanephrine in mouse brain. *Acta Pharmacologica Toxicologica, 20*, 140-144.

Carr, E. G. (1977). The motivation of self-injurious behavior: A review of some hypotheses. *Psychological Bulletin, 84*, 800-816.

Carr, E. G., Newsome, C. D., & Binkoff, J. A. (1976). Stimulus control of self-destructive behavior in a psychotic child. *Journal of Abnormal Child Psychology, 4*, 139-153.

Cataldo, M. F., & Harris, J. (1982). The biological basis for self-injury in the mentally retarded. *Analysis and Intervention in Developmental Disabilities, 2*, 21-39.

Charman, T., & Swettenham, J. (2001). Repetitive behaviors and social-communicative impairments in autism: Implications for developmental theory and diagnosis. In J. Aurack, T. Charman, N. Yirmiya, & P. R. Zelazo (Eds.), *The development of autism: Perspectives from theory and research* (pp. 325-345). Mahwah, NJ: Lawrence Erlbaum Associates.

Clark, D., & White, F. J. (1987). D1 dopamine receptor: The search for a function. A critical evaluation of the D1/D2 dompamine receptor classification and its functional implications. *Synapse, 1,* 347-388.

Cleland, C. C., & Clark, C. M. (1966). Sensory deprivation and aberrant behavior among idiots. *American Journal of Mental Deficiency, 71,* 213-225.

Cole, G. A., Montgomery, R. W., Wilson, K. M., & Milan, M. A. (2000). Parametric analysis of overcorrection duration effects: Is longer really better than shorter? *Behavior Modification, 24,* 359-378.

Connor, D. F. (1998). Stimulants and neuroleptic withdrawal dyskinesia. *Journal of the American Academy of Child and Adolescent Psychiatry, 37,* 247-248.

Connor, D. F., Fletcher, K. E., & Wood, J. S. (2001). Neuroleptic-related dyskinesias in children and adolescents. *Journal of Clinical Psychiatry, 62,* 967-974.

Cook, E. H., Rowlett, R., Jaselskis, C., & Leventhal, B. L. (1992). Fluoxetine treatment of children and adults with autistic disorder and mental retardation. *Journal of American Academy of Child and Adolescent Psychiatry, 31,* 739-745.

Costall, B., & Naylor, R. J. (1974). Stereotyped and circling behavior induced by dopamine-like agents after lesions of the mid-brain raphe nuclei. *European Journal of Pharmacology, 29,* 206-222.

Creese, I., Sibley, D. R., Hamblin, M. W., & Leff, S. E. (1983). The classification of dopamine receptors: Relationship to radioligand binding. *Annual Review of Neuroscience, 6,* 43-71.

Cross, H. A., & Harlow, H. F. (1965). Prolonged and progressive effects of partial isolation on the behavior of Macaque monkeys. *Journal of Experimental Research in Personality, 1,* 39-49.

Dalrymple, A. J. (1989). Sensory extinction of stereotyped object-dropping: Identification of a reinforcer for skill training. *Behavioral Residential Treatment, 4,* 99-111.

Davenport, R. K., & Berkson, G. (1963). Stereotyped movements of mental defectives: II. Effects of novel objects. *American Journal of Mental Deficiency, 67,* 879-882.

Davis, K. V. (1971). The effect of drugs on stereotyped and non-stereotyped operant behaviors in retardates. *Psychopharmacologia, 22,* 195-213.

Davis, K. V., Sprague, R. L., & Werry, J. S. (1969). Stereotyped behavior and activity level in severe retardates: The effect of drugs. *American Journal of Mental Deficiency, 73,* 721-727.

Day, H. M., Horner, R. H., & O'Neill, R. E. (1994). Multiple functions of problem behaviors: Assessment and intervention. *Journal of Applied Behavior Analysis, 27,* 279-289.

DeLissavoy, V. (1964). Head banging in early childhood: Review of empirical studies. *Pediatrics Digest, 6,* 49-55.

Denny, M. (1980). Reducing self-stimulatory behavior of mentally retarded persons by alternative positive practice. *American Journal of Mental Deficiency, 84,* 610-615.

Dura, J. (1990). Facial screening fails in the treatment of stereotypy. *Psychological Reports, 67*(3, Pt 2), 1171-1174.

Dura, J. R, Mulick, J. A., & Rasnake, L. K. (1987). Prevalence of stereotypy among institutionalized nonambulatory profoundly mentally retarded people. *American Journal of Mental Deficiency, 91,* 548-549.

Durand, V. M., & Carr, E. G. (1987). Social influences on "self-stimulatory" behavior: Analysis and treatment application. *Journal of Applied Behavior Analysis, 20,* 119-132.

Eason, L. J., White, M. G., & Newsom, C. (1982). Generalized reduction of self-stimulatory behavior: An effect of teaching appropriate play to autistic children. *Analysis and Intervention in Developmental Disabilities, 2,* 157-169.

Edelson, S. M., Taubman, M. T., & Lovaas, O. I. (1983). Some social contexts of self-destructive behavior. *Journal of Abnormal Child Psychology, 11,* 299-312.

Evans, G. W. (1978). Human spatial behavior: The arousal mode. In A. Baum & Y. Epstein (Eds.), *Human response to crowding* (pp. 41-87). Hillsdale, NJ: LEA.

Fatemi, S. H., Realmuto, G. M., Khan, L., & Thuras, P. (1998). Fluoxetine in the treatment of adolescent patients with autism: A longitudinal open trial. *Journal of Autism and Developmental Disorders, 28,* 303-307.

Favell, J. E. (1973). Reduction of stereotypies by reinforcement of toy play. *Mental Retardation, 11,* 21-23.

Ferster, C. B. (1961). Positive reinforcement and behavioral deficits of autistic children. *Child Development, 32,* 437-456.

Field, T., Ting, G., & Shuman, H. H. (1979). The onset of rhythmic activities in normal and high-risk infants. *Developmental Psychobiology, 12,* 97-100.

Fitz-Gerald, F. (1967). Effects of d-amphetamine upon behavior in young chimpanzees reared under different conditions. In H. Brill & J. Cole (Eds.), *Neuropsychopharmacology, 5* (pp. 37-57). Amsterdam: Elsevier.

Fog, R., & Randrup, A. (2002). Commentary on: "Stereotyped activities by amphetamine in several animal species and man." *Psychopharmacology, 164,* 349-350.

Forehand, R., & Baumeister, A. A. (1970a). Body rocking and activity level as a function of prior motion restraint. *American Journal of Mental Deficiency, 74,* 608-610.

Forehand, R., & Baumeister, A. A. (1970b). Effect of frustration on stereotyped body rocking of severe retardates as a function of frustration of goal-directed behavior. *Journal of Abnormal Psychology, 78,* 35-42.

Foxx, R. M., & Azrin, N. H. (1973). The elimination of autistic self-stimulatory behavior by overcorrection. *Journal of Applied Behavior Analysis, 6,* 1-14.

Foxx, R. M., & McMorrow, M. J. (1984). The effects of continuous and fixed ratio schedules of external consequences on the performance and extinction of human stereotyped behavior. *Behavior Analysis Letters, 3*(6), 371-379.

Fraiberg, S. (1977). *Insights from the blind: Comparative studies of blind and sighted children.* New York: Basic Books.

Frankel, F., & Simmons, J. Q. (1976). Self-injurious behavior in schizophrenic and retarded children. *American Journal of Mental Deficiency, 80,* 512-522.

Frecska, E., & Arato, M. (2002). Opiate sensitivity test in patients with stereotypic movement disorder. *Progress in Neuropsychopharmacology and Biological Psychiatry, 26,* 909-912.

Friedman, E. (1969). The "autistic syndrome" and phenylketonuria. *Schizophrenia, 1*(4), 249-261.

Frith, C. D., & Done, D. J. (1990). Stereotyped behavior in madness and in health. In S. J. Cooper & C. T. Dourish (Eds.), *Neurobiology of stereotyped behavior* (pp. 232-259). Oxford, UK: Oxford University Press.

Gallagher, R. J., & Berkson, G. (1986). Effect of intervention techniques in reducing stereotypic hand gazing in young severely disabled children. *American Journal of Mental Deficiency, 91,* 170-177.

Garau, L., Govoni, S., Stefanini, E., Trabucchi, M., & Spano, P. F. (1978). Dopamine receptors: Pharmacological and anatomical evidences indicate that two distinct dopamine receptor populations are present in rat striatum. *Life Sciences, 23,* 1745-1750.

Gaylord-Ross, R. J., Weeks, M., & Lipner, C. (1980). An analysis of antecedent and response , and consequence events in the treatment of self-injurious behavior. *Education and Training of the Mentally Retarded, 15*, 35-42.

Geller, E., Ritvo, E. R., Freeman, B. J., & Yuwiler, A. (1983). Preliminary observations on the effect of fenfluramine on blood serotonin and symptoms in three autistic boys. *New England Journal of Medicine, 307*, 165-169.

Gogtay, N., Sporn, A., Alfaro, C. L., Mulqueent, A., & Rapoport, J. L (2002). Clozapine-induced akathisia in children with schizophrenia. *Journal of Child and Adolescent Psychopharmacology, 12*(4), 347-349.

Gorman-Smith, D., & Matson, J. L. (1985). A review of treatment research for self-injurious and stereotyped responding. *Journal of Mental Deficiency Research, 29*, 295-308.

Green, A. H. (1967). Self-mutilation in schizophrenic children. *Archives of General Psychiatry, 17,* 234-244.

Groves, A. M., Wilson, C. J., Young, S. J., & Rebec, G. V. (1975). Self-inhibition by dopamine neurons. *Science, 190,* 522-529.

Gualtieri, C. T. (1986). Fenfluramine and autism: Careful reappraisal is in order. *Journal of Pediatrics, 108,* 417-419.

Gualtieri, C. T., Quade, D., Hicks, R .E., Mayo, J. P., & Schroeder, S. R. (1984). Tardive dyskinesia and other clinical consequences of neuroleptic treatment in children and adolescents. *American Journal of Psychiatry, 141,* 20-23.

Hagberg, B., Aicardi, J., Dias, K., & Ramos, O. (1983). A progressive syndrome of autism, dementia, ataxia, and loss of purposeful hand use in girls: Rett's syndrome: Report of 35 cases. *Annals of Neurology, 14,* 471-479.

Hagopian, L. P., & Adelinis, J. D. (2001). Response blocking with and without redirection for the treatment of pica. *Journal of Applied Behavior Analysis, 34,* 527-530.

Hamilton, J., & Standahl, J. (1969). Suppression of stereotyped screaming behavior in a profoundly retarded institutionalized female. *Journal of Experimental Child Psychology, 7,* 114-121.

Hamilton, H., Stephens, L., & Allen, P. (1967). Controlling aggressive and destructive behavior in severely retarded institutionalized residents. *American Journal of Mental Deficiency, 71,* 852-856.

Harlow, H. F., & Griffin, G. (1965). Induced mental and social deficits in Rhesus monkeys. In S. F. Osler & R. E. Cooke (Eds.), *The biosocial basis of mental retardation* (pp. 121-139). Baltimore: Johns Hopkins Press.

Harlow, H. F., & Harlow, M. K. (1962). Social deprivation in monkeys. *Scientific American, 207,* 136-146.

Harlow, H. F., & Harlow, M. K. (1971). Psychopathology in monkeys. In H. D. Kimmel (Ed.), *Experimental psychopathology* (pp. 51-78). New York: Academic Press.

Harris, S. L., & Wolchik, S. A. (1979). Suppression of self-stimulation: Three alternative strategies. *Journal of Applied Behavior Analysis, 12,* 185-198.

Harris, S. L., Handleman, J. S., & Fong, P. L. (1987). Imitation of self-stimulation: Impact on the autistic child's behavior and affect. *Child and Family Behavior Therapy, 9,* 1-21.

Harvey, J. A., & McMaster, S. E. (1975). Fenfluramine: Evidence for a neurotoxic action on midbrain and a long-term depletion of serotonin. *Psychopharmacology Communications, 1,* 217-228.

Hermelin, B. & O'Connor, N. (1963). The response of self-generated behavior of severely disturbed children and severely subnormal controls. *British Journal of Social Clinical Psychology, 2,* 37-43.

Ho, H. H., Lockitch, G., Eaves, L., & Jacobson, B. (1986). Blood serotonin concentrations and fenfluramine therapy in autistic children. *Pediatric Pharmacology and Therapeutics, 108,* 465-469.

Hollis, J. H. (1967). Direct measurement of the effect of drugs and alternate activity on stereotyped behavior. Parsons Research Center, Paper No. 168, Parsons, Kansas.

Hollis, J. H. (1971a). Body rocking: Effects of sound and reinforcement. *American Journal of Mental Deficiency, 75,* 642-644.

Hollis, J. H. (1971b). "Superstition": A systematic study of independent and contingent events on human free operant responses. *American Journal of Mental Deficiency, 75,* 645-649.

Hollis, J. H. (1978). Analysis of rocking behavior. In C. E. Meyers (Ed.), *Quality of life in severely and profoundly mentally retarded people: Research foundations for improvement* (pp. 1-53). Washington, DC: American Association on Mental Deficiency.

Hutt, C., & Hutt, J. S. (1965). Effects of environmental complexity on stereotyped behavior of children. *Animal Behavior, 13,* 1-4.

Hutt, C., & Hutt, J. S. (1970). Stereotypies and their relation to arousal: A study of autistic children. In J. S. Hutt & C. Hutt (Eds.), *Behavior studies in psychiatry* (pp. 110-136). New York: Pergamon Press.

Hutt, S. J., & Hutt, C. (1968). Stereotypy, arousal and autism. *Human Development, 11,* 277-286.

Inhelder, B. (1968). *The diagnosis of reasoning in the mentally retarded (2nd ed.).* New York: Chandler Publishing.

Iversen, S. D. (1977). Striatal function and stereotyped behavior. In A. R. Cools, A. H. M. Lohman, & J. H. L. Van den Bercken (Eds.), *Psychobiology of the striatum* (pp.198-211). Amsterdam: Elsevier/North-Holland Biomedical Press.

Johnson, J. W., Van Laarhoven, T. V., & Repp, A. C. (2002). Effects on stereotypy and other challenging behavior of matching rates of instruction to free-operant rates of responding. *Research in Developmental Disabilities, 23,* 266-284.

Jones, F. H., Simmons, J. Q., & Frankel, F. (1974). An extinction procedure for eliminating self-destructive behavior in a 9-year-old autistic girl. *Journal of Autism and Childhood Schizophrenia, 4,* 241-250.

Joshi, P. T., Capozzoli, J. A., & Coyle, J. T. (1988). Low dose neuroleptic therapy for children with childhood onset pervasive developmental disorder. *American Journal of Psychiatry, 145,* 335-338.

Kanner, L. (1943). Autistic disturbances of affective contact. *Nervous Child, 2,* 217-250.

Kaufman, M. E., & Levitt, H. (1965). A study of three stereotyped and social behaviors in mental defectives. *American Journal of Mental Deficiency, 80,* 231-233.

Kebabian, J. W., & Calne, D. B. (1979). Multiple receptors for dopamine. *Nature, 277,* 93-96.

Keiper, R. R. (1969). Causal factors of stereotypes in caged birds. *Animal Behavior, 17,* 114-119.

Kennedy, C. H., Meyer, K. A., Knowles, T., & Shukla, S. (2000). Analyzing the multiple functions of stereotypical behavior for students with autism. Implications for assessment and treatment. *Journal of Applied Behavior Analysis, 33,* 559-571.

Kern, L., Koegel, R. L., Dyer, K., Blew, P. A., & Fenton, L. R. (1982). The effect of physical exercise on self-stimulation and appropriate responding in autistic children. *Journal of Autism and Developmental Disabilities, 12,* 399-419.

Kinsbourne, M. (1980). Do repetitive movement patterns in children and animals serve a dearousing function? *Developmental and Behavioral Pediatrics, 1,* 39-42.

Klaber, M. M., & Butterfield, E. C. (1968). Stereotyped rocking: A measure of institution and ward effectiveness. *American Journal of Mental Deficiency, 73,* 13-20.

Klawans, H. L., Moses, H., & Beaulieu, D. M. (1974). The influence of caffeine on d-amphetamine and apomorphine-induced stereotyped behavior. *Life Sciences, 14,* 1493-1500.

Klykylo, W. M., Feldis, D., O'Grady, D., Ross, D. L., & Holloran, C. (1985). Clinical effects of fenfluramine in ten autistic subjects. *Journal of Autism and Developmental Disorders, 15,* 417-423.

Kolb, B., & Winshaw, I. Q. (1983). Performance of schizophrenic patients on tests sensitive to left or right frontal, temporal or parietal function in neurological patients. *Journal of Nervous and Mental Disorders, 171,* 435-443.

Kravitz, H., & Boehm, J. J. (1971). Rhythmic habit patterns in infancy: Their sequence, age of onset, and frequency. *Child Development, 42,* 339-413.

Kulka, A., Fry, C., & Goldstein, F. J. (1960). Kinesthetic needs in infancy. *American Journal of Orthopsychiatry, 30,* 561-571.

LaGrow, S. J., & Repp, A. C. (1984). Stereotypic responding: A review of intervention research. *American Journal of Mental Deficiency, 88,* 595-609.

Lerman, D. C., & Iwata, B. A. (1996). A methodology for distinguishing between extinction and punishment effects associated with response blocking. *Journal of Applied Behavior Analysis, 29,* 231-234.

Lerman, D. C., Kelley, M. E., Vorndran, C. M., & Van Camp, C. M. (2003). Collateral effects of response blocking during the treatment of stereotypic behavior. *Journal of Applied Behavior Analysis, 36,* 119-123.

Leventhal, B. L., Cook, E. H., Morford, M., Ravitz, A. J., Heller, W., & Freedman, D. X. (1993). Clinical and neurochemical effects of fenfluramine in children with autism. *Journal of Neuropsychiatry and Clinical Neurosciences, 5,* 307-315.

Levy, D. M. (1944). On the problem of movement restraint: Tics, stereotyped movements and hyperactivity. *American Journal of Orthopsychiatry, 14,* 644-671.

Lewis, M. H., & Baumeister, A. A. (1983). Stereotyped mannerisms in mentally retarded persons: Animal models and theoretical analyses. In N. R. Ellis (Ed.), *International review of research on mental retardation. Volume II.* (pp. 123-161). New York: Academic Press.

Lewis, M. H., Baumeister, A. A., McCorkle, D. L., & Mailman, R. B. (1985). A computer supported method for analyzing behavioral observations: Studies with stereotypy. *Psychopharmacology, 85,* 204-209.

Lewis, M. H., Gluck, J. P., Bodfish, J. W., Beauchamp, A. J., & Mailman, R. B. (1996). Neurobiological basis of stereotyped movement disorder. In R. L. Sprague & K. M. Newell (Eds.), *Stereotyped movements: Brain and behavior relationships* (pp. 37-67). Washington, DC: American Psychological Association.

Lewis, M. H., MacLean, W. E., Bryson-Brockman, W., Arendt, R., Beck, B., Fidler, P., et al. (1984). Time-series analysis of stereotyped movements: The relationship of body rocking to cardiac activity. *American Journal of Mental Deficiency, 89,* 287-294.

Lloyd, K. G., & Hornykiewicz, O. (1975). Catecholamines in regulation of motor function. In A. J. Friedhoff (Ed.), *Catecholamines and behavior. Volume I.* New York: Plenum Press.

Lloyd, K. G., Hornykiewicz, O., Davidson, L., Shannak, R., Farley, I., Goldstein, M., et al. (1981). Biochemical evidence of dysfunction of brain neurotransmitters in the Lesch-Nyhan syndrome. *New England Journal of Medicine, 305,* 1106-1111.

Lord, C., & Pickles, A. (1996). Language level and nonverbal social-communicative behaviors in autistic and language-delayed children. *Journal of the American Academy of Child and Adolescent Psychiatry, 35,* 1542-1550.

Lourie, R. S. (1949). The role of rhythmic patterns in childhood. *American Journal of Psychiatry, 105,* 653-660.

Lovaas, O. I., Freitag, G., Gold, V. J., & Kassorla, I. C. (1965). Experimental studies in childhood schizophrenia: Analysis of self destructive behavior. *Journal of Experimental Child Psychology, 2,* 67-84.

Lovaas, O.I ., Litrownik, A., & Mann, R. (1971). Response latencies to auditory stimuli in autistic children engaged in self-stimulatory behavior. *Behavior Research and Therapy, 1,* 39-59.

Lovaas, O. I., Newsome, C., & Hickman, C. (1987). Self-stimulatory behavior and perceptual reinforcement. *Journal of Applied Behavior Analysis, 20,* 45-68.

Lovaas, O. I., & Simmons, J. Q. (1969). Manipulation of self-destruction in three retarded children. *Journal of Applied Behavior Analysis, 2,* 143-157.

Luiselli, J. K. (1975). The effects of multiple contingencies on the rocking behavior of a retarded child. *Psychological Record, 25,* 559-565.

Luiselli, J. K. (1984). Effects of brief overcorrection on stereotypic behavior of mentally retarded students. *Education and Treatment of Children, 7*(2), 125-138.

Luiselli, J. K., Colozzi, G. A., & O'Toole, K. M. (1980). Programming response maintenance of differential reinforcement effects. *Child Behavior Therapy, 2,* 65-73.

Luiselli, J. K., Myles, E., Evans, T. P., & Boyce, D. A. (1985). Reinforcement control of severe dysfunctional behavior of blind, multihandicapped students. *American Journal of Mental Deficiency, 90,* 328-334.

Maag, J. W., Rutherford, R. B., Wolchik, S. A , & Parks, B. T. (1986). Comparison of two short overcorrection procedures on the stereotypic behavior of autistic children. *Journal of Autism and Developmental Disorders, 16*(1), 83-87.

Maag, J. W., Wolchik, S. A., Rutherford, R. B., & Parks, B. T. (1986). Response covariation on self-stimulatory behaviors during sensory extinction procedures. *Journal of Autism and Developmental Disorders, 16*(2), 119-132.

MacDonald, J. E., Wilder, D. A., & Dempsey, C. (2002). Brief functional analysis and treatment of eye-poking. *Behavioral Interventions, 17,* 261-270.

Macfarlane, C. A., Young, K. R., & West, R. P. (1987). An integrated school/home overcorrection procedure for eliminating stereotypic behavior in students with severe multiple handicaps. *Education and Training in Mental Retardation, 22*(3), 156-166.

Maclean, W. E. Jr., & Baumeister, A. A. (1981). Observational analysis of the stereotyped mannerisms of a developmentally delayed infant. *Applied Research in Mental Retardation, 2,* 257-262.

Maclean, W. E., Jr., Ellis, D. N., Galbreath, H. N., Halpern, L. F., & Baumeister, A. A. (1991). Rhythmic motor behavior of perambulatory motor impaired Down syndrome and nondisabled children: A comparative analysis. *Journal of Abnormal Child Psychology, 19,* 319-330.

Maida, S. O., & McCune, L. (1996). A dynamic systems approach to the development of crawling by blind and sighted infants. *RE:view, 28*(3), 119-134.

Malloy, A. G., & Waddington, J. L. (1984). Dopaminergic behavior stereospecifically promoted by the D_1 agonist R-SK&F38393 and selectively blocked by the D_1 antagonist SCH23390. *Psychopharmacology, 82,* 409-410.

Malmo, H. P. (1974). On frontal lobe functions: Psychiatric patient controls. *Cortex, 10,* 231-237.

Marazziti, D. (2002). A further support to the hypothesis of a link between serotonin, autism, and the cerebellum. *Biological Psychiatry, 50,* 50.

Marazziti, D., Nardi, I., & Cassano, G. B. (1999). Autism, seretonin, and cerebellum: Might there be a connection? *CNS Spectrums, 3,* 80-82.

Masaleski, J. L., Iwata, B., Rodgers, T. A., Vollmer, T. R., & Zarcone, J. R. (1994). Protective equipment as treatment for stereotyped hand mouthing: Sensory extinction or punishment? *Journal of Applied Behavior Analysis, 27,* 345-355.

Mason, J. W. (1978). A review of psychoendocrine research on the pituitary adrenal cortical system. *Psychosomatic Medicine, 30,* 576-607.

Matson, J. L. (1989). Self-injury and stereotypies. In T. O. Ollendick, & M. Hersen (Eds.). *Handbook of child psychopathology* (2nd ed., pp. 265-275). New York: Plenum.

Matson, J. L., Bielecki, J., Mayville, S. B., & Matson, M. L. (2003). Psychopharma-cology research for individuals with mental retardation: Methodological issues and suggestions. *Research in Developmental Disabilities, 24,* 149-157.

Matson, J., Baglio, C., Smiroldo, B., Hamilton, M., Packlowskyi, T., Williams, D., et al. (1996). Characteristics of autism as assessed by the Diagnostic Assessment for the Severely Handicapped-II (DASH-II). *Research in Developmental Disabilities, 17,* 135-143.

Mayhew, G. L., & Harris, F. C. (1978). Some negative side effects of a punishment procedure for stereotyped behavior. *Journal of Behavior Therapy and Experi-mental Psychiatry, 9,* 245-251.

McAdam, D. B., Zarcone, J. R., Hellings, J., Napolitano, D. A., & Schroeder, S. R. (2002). Effects of risperidone on aberrant behavior in persons with develop-mental disabilities: II. Social validity measures. *American Journal on Mental Retardation, 107,* 261-269.

McClure, J. T., Moss, R. A., McPeters, J. W., & Kirkpatrick, M. A. (1986). Reduc-tion of hand mouthing by a boy with profound mental retardation. *Mental Retardation, 24,* 219-222.

McCracken, J. T., McGough, J., Shah, B., Cronin, P., & Hong, D. (2002). Risperidone in children with autism and serious behavior problems. *New England Journal of Medicine, 347,* 314-321.

McDougle, C. J. (1997). Psychopharmacology. In D. J. Cohen & F. R. Volkmar (Eds.), *Handbook of autism and pervasive developmental disorders* (2nd ed., pp. 169-194). New York: Wiley.

McGonigle, J. J., Duncan, D., Cordisco, L., & Barrett, R. P. (1982). Visual screen-ing: An alternative method for reducing stereotypic behavior. *Journal of Applied Behavior Analysis, 15,* 461-467.

Metz, J. R. (1967). Stimulation level preferences of autistic children. *Journal of abnormal Psychology, 72,* 529-535.

Morrison, J. R. (1973). Catatonia: Retarded and excited types. *Archives of General Psychiatry, 28,* 957-962.

Mount, R. H., Hastings, R. P., Reilly, S., Cass, H., & Charman, T. (2003). Towards a behavioral phenotype for Rett's syndrome. *American Journal on Mental Retardation, 108,* 1-12.

Mulhern T., & Baumeister, A. A. (1969). An experimental attempt to reduce stereotypy by reinforcement procedures. *American Journal of Mental Defi-ciency, 74,* 69-74.

Mulick, J. A., Hoyt, P., Rojahn, J., & Schroeder, S. R. (1978). Reduction of a "nervous" abit in a profoundly retarded youth by increasing toy play. *Journal of Behavior Therapy and Experimental Psychiatry, 9, 381*-185.

Myers, J., & Deibert, A. (1971). Reduction of self-abusive behavior in a blind child by using a feeding response. *Journal of Behavior Therapy and Experimental Psychiatry, 2,* 141-143.

Panksepp, J. (1979). A neurochemical theory of autism. *Trends in Neurosciences, 2,* 174-177.

Panksepp, J., & Sahley, T.L. (1987). Possible brain opioid involvement in disrupted social intent and language development of autism. In E. Schopler & G.B. Mesibov (Eds.), *Neurobiological issues in autism* (pp. 357-372). New York: Plenum Press.

Panksepp, J., Herman, B., & Vilberg, T. (1978). An opiate excess model of autism. *Neuroscience Abstract, 4,* 500.

Panksepp, J., Vilberg, T., Bean, N. J., Coy, D. H., & Kastin, A. J. (1978). Reductions of distress vocalizations in chicks by opiate-like peptides. *Brain Research Bulletin, 3,* 663-667.

Pasqualetti, M., Ori, M., Nardi, I., Cassano, G.B., & Marazziti, D. (1999). Distribution of seretonin 5A receptors in the human brain. *Molecular Brain Research, 56,* 1-8.

Patel, M. R., Piazza, C. C., Martinez, C.J ., Volkert, V. M., & Santana, C. M. (2002). An evaluation of two differential reinforcement procedures with escape extinction to treat food refusal. *Journal of Applied Behavior Analysis, 35,* 363-374.

Phelps, L., Brown, R. T., & Power, T. J. (Eds.). (2002). *Pediatric psychopharmacology.* Washington, DC: American Psychological Association.

Piaget, J. (1952). *The origins of intelligence in children.* New York: International Universities Press.

Pierce, K., & Courchesne, E. (2001). Evidence for a cerebellar role in reduced exploration and stereotyped behavior in autism. *Biological Psychiatry, 49,* 655-664.

Piggott, L. R., Gdowski, C. L., Villaneuva, D., Fischoff, J., & Frohman, C. F. (1986). Side effects of fenfluramine in autistic children. *Journal of the American Academy of Child Psychiatry, 25,* 287-289.

Powers, M. D., & Crowel, R. L. (1985). The educative effects of positive practice overcorrection: Acquisition, generalization, and maintenance. *School Psychology Review, 14,* 360-372.

Purpura, D. P., & Reaser, G. P. (1974). *Methodological approaches to the study of brain maturation and its abnormalities.* Baltimore: University Park Press.

Randrup, A., & Munkvad, I. (1965). Special antagonism of amphetamine-induced abnormal behavior. Inhibition of stereotyped activity with increase of normal activities. *Psychopharmacologia, 7,* 416-422.

Randrup, A., & Munkvad, I. (1967). Stereotyped activities produced by amphetamines in several animal species and men. *Psychopharmacology, 11,* 300-310.

Realmuto, G. M., Jensen, B. J., Klykylo, W., Piggott, L., Stubbs, G., Yuwiler, A., et al. (1986). Untoward effects of fenfluramine in autistic children. *Journal of Clinical Psychopharmacology, 6,* 350-355.

Repp, A. C., Barton, L. E., & Brulle, A. (1983). A comparison of two procedures for programming the differential reinforcement of other behaviors. *Journal of Applied Behavior Analysis, 16,* 435-445.

Repp, A. C., Deitz, S. M., & Speir, N. (1974). Reducing stereotypic responding of retarded persons by the differential reinforcement of other behavior. *American Journal of Mental Deficiency, 78,* 279-284.

Repp, A. C., Felce, D., & Barton, L. E. (1988). Basing the treatment of stereotypic and self-injurious behaviors on hypotheses of their causes. *Journal of Applied Behavior Analysis, 21*(3), 281-289.

Ricketts, R. W., Goza, A. B., Ellis, C. R., Singh, Y. N., & Singh, N. N. (1993). Fluoxetine treatment of severe self-injury in young adults with mental retardation. *Journal of the American Academy of Child and Adolescent Psychiatry, 32,* 865-869.

Ridley, R. M. (1994). The psychology of perseverative and stereotyped behavior. *Progress in Neurobiology, 44,* 221-231.

Ritvo, E. R., Freeman, B. J., Geller, E., & Yuwiler, A. (1983). Effects of fenfluramine on 14 outpatients with the syndrome of autism. *Journal of the American Academy of Child and Adolescent Psychiatry, 22,* 549-558.

Ritvo, E. R., Yuwiler, A., Geller, E., Ornitz, E. M., Saeger, K., & Plotkin, S. (1970). Increased blood serotonin and platelets in early infantile autism. *Archives of General Psychiatry, 23,* 566-572.

Rojahn, J., Hammer, D., and Kroeger, T. L. (2001). Stereotypy. In N. N. Singh (Ed.), *Prevention and treatment of severe behavior problems: Models and methods in developmental disabilities* (pp. 199-216). Pacific Grove, CA: Brooks/Cole.

Rojahn, J., & Sisson, L. A. (1990). Stereotyped acts. In J.L. Matson (Ed.), *Handbook of behavior modification with the mentally retarded 2nd ed.* (pp. 181-223). New York: Plenum Press.

Romanczyk, R., & Goren, E. (1975). Severe self-injurious behavior: The problem of clinical control. *Journal of Clinical Psychology, 43,* 730-739.

Ross-Collins, M. S., & Cornish, K. (2002). A survey of the prevalence of stereotypy, self-injury, and aggression in children and young adults with Cri du Chat syndrome. *Journal of Intellectual Disability Research, 46,* 133-140.

Sallustro, F., & Atwell, C. (1978). Body rocking, head banging, and head rolling in normal children. *Journal of Pediatrics, 93,* 704-708.

Sandman, C., Thompson, T., Barrett, R. P., Verhoven, W., McCubbin, J., Schroeder, S. R., et al. (1998). Opiate blockers. In S. Reiss & M. G. Aman (Eds.), *Psychotropic medications and developmental disabilities: The international consensus handbook* (pp. 291-302). Columbus, OH: The Ohio State University Press.

Schalock, R. L., Foley, J. W., Toulouse, A., & Stark, J. A. (1985). Medication and programming in controlling the behavior of mentally retarded individuals in community settings. *American Journal of Mental Deficiency, 89,* 503-509.

Schroeder, S. R. (1970). Usage of stereotypy as a descriptive term. *Psychological Record, 29,* 457-464.

Schroeder, S. R. (1991). Self-injury and stereotypy. In J. L. Matson & J. A. Mulick (Eds.), *Handbook of mental retardation (2nd ed.)* (pp. 382-396). New York: Pergamon.

Schroeder, S. R., Bickel, W. A., & Richmond, G. (1986). Primary and secondary prevention of self-injurious behaviors: A life-long problem. In K. D. Gadow (Ed.), *Advances in learning and behavioral disabilities. Volume 5* (pp. 63-85). Greenwich, CT: JAI Press.

Schuster, C. R., Lewis, M., & Seiden, S. S. (1986). Fenfluramine: neurotoxicity. *Psychopharmacology Bulletin, 22,* 148-151.

Shulman, L. M., Sanchez-Ramos, J. R., & Weiner, W. J. (1996). Defining features, clinical conditions, and theoretical constructs of stereotyped movements. In R. L. Sprague & K. M. Newell (Eds.), *Stereotyped movements: Brain and behavior relationships* (pp. 17-34). Washington, DC: American Psychological Association.

Silva, D. A. (1979). The use of medication in a residential institution for mentally retarded persons. *Mental Retardation, 17,* 285-288.

Silverman, K., Watanabe, K., Marshall, A. M., & Baer, D. M. (1984). Reducing self-injury and corresponding self-restraint through the strategic use of protective clothing. *Journal of Applied Behavior Analysis, 17,* 545-552.

Singer, C., Weiner, W. J., & Sanchez-Ramos, G. (1992). Autonomic dysfunction in men with Parkinson's disease. *European Neurology, 32,* 134-140.

Singh, N. N., & Aman, M. G. (1981). Effects of thioridazine dosage on the behavior of severely mentally retarded persons. *American Journal of Mental Deficiency, 85,* 588-595.

Singh, N. N., Dawson, M. J., & Manning, P. (1981). Effects of spaced responding DRL on the stereotyped behavior of profoundly retarded persons. *Journal of Applied Behavior Analysis, 14,* 521-526.

Singh, N. N., Watson, J. E., & Winton, A. S. W. (1987). Parents' acceptability ratings of alternative treatments for use with mentally retarded children. *Behavior Modification, 1,* 17-26.

Sisson, L. A., Van-Hasselt, V. B., Hersen, M., & Aurand, J. C. (1988). Tripartite behavioral intervention to reduce stereotypic and disruptive behaviors in young multihandicapped children. *Behavior Therapy, 19,* 503-526.

Skinner, B. F. (1953). *Science and human behavior.* New York: Macmillan Company.

Smith, M. A., Chethik, M., & Adelson, E. (1969). Differential assessment of "blindisms". *American Journal of Orthopsychiatry, 39, 807-817.*

Smith, R. G., & Churchill, R. M. (2002). Identification of environmental determinants of behavior disorders through functional analysis of precursor behaviors. *Journal of Applied Behavior Analysis, 35,* 125-136.

Smith, R. G., Russo, L., & Le, D. D. (1999). Distinguishing between extinction and punishment effects of response blocking: A replication. *Journal of Applied Behavior Analysis, 32,* 367-370.

Smith, S. G., Gupta, K. K., & Smith, S. H. (1995). Effects of naltrexone on self-injury, stereotypy, and social behavior of adults with developmental disabilities. *Journal of Developmental and Physical Disabilities, 7*(2), 137-146.

Snyder, R., Turgay, A., Aman, M. G., Binder, C., Fisman, S., & Carroll, A. (2002). Effects of risperidone on conduct and disruptive behavior disorders in children with subaverage IQs. *Journal of the American Academy of Child and Adolescent Psychiatry, 41,* 1026-1036.

Spradlin, J. E., Giradeau, F. L., & Hom, G. L. (1966). Stimulus properties of reinforcement during extinction of a free operant response. *Journal of Experimental Child Psychology, 4,* 369-380.

Sprague, R. L. (1977). Overview of psychopharmacology for the retarded in the U.S. In P. Mittler (Ed.), *Research to practice in mental retardation: Biomedical aspects-Volume 3* (pp. 350-364). Baltimore: University Park Press.

Stella, J., Mundy, P., & Tuchman, R. (1999). Social and nonsocial factors in the childhood autism rating scale. *Journal of Autism and Developmental Disorders, 29,* 307-317.

Stokes, T. F., & Baer, D. M. (1977). An implicit technology of generalization. *Journal of Applied Behavior Analysis, 10,* 349-367.

Stone, A. A. (1964). Consciousness: Altered levels in blind retarded children. *Psychosomatic Medicine, 26,* 14-19.

Stubbs, E., Budden, S., Jackson, R., Teredal, L., & Ritvo, E. (1986). Effects of fenfluramine on eight outpatients with the syndrome of autism. *Developmental Medicine and Child Neurology, 28,* 229-235.

Tang, J. C., Patterson, T. G., & Kennedy, C. H. (2003). Identifying specific sensory modalities maintaining the stereotypy of students with multiple profound disabilities. *Research in Developmental Disabilities, 24,* 433-451.

Tarbox, J., Wallace, M. D., & Tarbox, R. S. F. (2002). Successive generalized parent training and failed schedule thinning of response blocking for automatically maintained object mouthing. *Behavioral Interventions, 17,* 169-178.

Tate, B. G. (1972). Case study: Control of chronic self-injurious behavior by conditioning procedures. *Behavior Therapy, 3,* 72-83.

Thelen, E. (1979). Rhythmical stereotypies in normal human infants. *Animal Behavior, 27,* 699-715.

Thelen, E. (1981). Kicking, rocking, and waving: Contextual analysis of rhythmical stereotypies in normal human infants. *Animal Behavior, 29,* 3-11.

Thelen, E. (1996). Normal infant stereotypies: A dynamic systems approach. In R.L. Sprague, & K.M. Newell (Eds.), *Stereotyped movements: Brain and behavior relationships* (pp. 130-165). Washington, DC: American Psychological Association.

Thompson, C. L., & Reid, A. (2002). Behavioural symptoms among people with severe and profound intellectual disabilities: A 26-year follow-up study. *British Journal of Psychiatry, 181,* 67-71.

Thompson, R. H., Iwata, B. A., Conners, J., & Roscoe, E. M. (1999). Effects of reinforcement for alternative behavior during punishment of self-injury. *Journal of Applied Behavior Analysis, 32,* 317-328.

Tizard, B. (1968). Observations in overactive imbecile children in controlled and uncontrolled environments: II. Experimental studies. *American Journal of Mental Deficiency, 72,* 548-553.

Touchette, P. E., MacDonald, R. F., & Langer, S. N. (1985). A scatter plot for identifying stimulus control of problem behaviors. *Journal of Applied Behavior Analysis, 18,* 343-351.

Turner, M. (1997). Towards an executive dysfunction account of repetitive behavior in autism. In Russell (Ed.), *Executive functioning and autism* (pp. 57-100). New York: Oxford University Press.

Van den Daele, L. D. (1971). Infant reactivity to redundant proprioceptive and auditory stimulation: A twin study. *Journal of Psychology, 45,* 269-276.

Wallon, H. (1973). The psychological development of the child. *International Journal of Mental Health, 1,* 29-39.

Walters, A. S., Barrett, R. P., Feinstein, C., Mercurio, A., & Hole, W. (1990). A case report of naltrexone treatment of self-injury and social withdrawal in autism. *Journal of Autism and Developmental Disorders, 20,* 169-176.

Warren, S. A., & Burns, N. R. (1970). Crib confinement as a factor in repetitive and stereotyped behavior in retardates. *Mental Retardation, 8,* 25-29.

Watson, S. J., Akil, H., Sullivan, S., & Barchas, J. D. (1977). Immunocytochemical localization of methionine enkephalin: Preliminary observations. *Life Sciences, 21,* 733-738.

Watters, R. W., & Watters, W. E. (1980). Decreasing self-stimulatory behavior with physical exercise in a group of autistic boys. *Journal of Autism and Developmental Disabilities, 10,* 378-387.

Werry, J. S., & Aman, M. G. (Eds.). (1999). *Practitioner's guide to psychoactive drugs for children and adolescents (2nd ed.).* New York: Plenum Press.

Wing, L., & Gould, J. (1979). Severe impairments of social interaction and associated abnormal behavior in children: Epidemiology and classification. *Journal of Autism and Developmental Disorders, 11,* 11-29.

Wolf, M. M., Risley, T. R., Johnston, M., Davis, F., & Allen, K. E. (1967). Application of operant conditioning procedures to the behavior problems of an autistic child: A follow-up and extension. *Behavior Research and Therapy, 5,* 103-111.

Wolf, M. M., Risley, T. R., & Mees, H. (1964). Application of operant conditioning procedures to the behavior problems of an autistic child. *Behaviour Research and Therapy, 1,* 302-312.

Wolff, P. H. (1968). Stereotypic behavior and development. *Canadian Psychologist, 9,* 474-483.

Zagon, I. S., & McLaughlin, P. J. (1978). Perinatal methadone exposure and brain development: A biochemical study. *Journal of Neurochemistry, 31,* 49-54.

Zagon, I. S., & McLaughlin, P. J. (1984). Perinatal exposure to methadone alters sensitivity to drugs in adult rats. *Neurobehavioral Toxicology and Teratology, 6,* 319-323.

Zagon, I. S., McLaughlin, P. J., Weaver, D. J., & Zagon, E. (1982). Opiates, endorphins, and the developing organism: A comprehensive bibliography. *Neuroscience and Biobehavioral Reviews, 6,* 439-479.

10

Treatment of Aggression and Related Disruptive Behaviors in Persons with Intellectual Disabilities and Mental Health Issues

William I. Gardner, Ph.D.
Emeritus Professor, University of Wisconsin-Madison

Dorothy M. Griffiths, Ph.D.
Professor, Brock University, St. Catharines, Ontario

Introduction

Aggression and related disruptive behaviors represent the most frequently occurring behavior problems presented by persons with intellectual disabilities. Prevalence rates vary greatly across studies depending on the diagnostic criteria, sampling procedures, and measures used, and range from 2% to 50%. To illustrate, Harris (1993) reported rates of up to 50% in studies of adults with intellectual disabilities who were receiving specialist services and up to 40% among children who were viewed as more challenging who attended special schools (Kiernan & Kiernan, 1994). In studies that included only high impact behaviors involving aggression (those that caused more than minor injury or judged to be seriously disruptive or threatening (Kiernan & Quereshi, 1993) or caused injury that required immediate medical attention (Borthwick-Duffy, 1994), a rate of 2% was reported. In a more recent study, O'Brien

(1998, 2000) reports a rate of 15% in a group of young adults with moderate and severe impairments. The problem becomes even more acute in persons who have a concurrent mental disorder. Jacobson (1982), in a survey of a large number of persons receiving developmental disabilities services, reported that aggression occurred in 19.5% of persons with a diagnosis of a psychiatric disorder and in only 10.5% of persons not so diagnosed. Reiss and Rojahn (1993), in a study involving a large number of persons presenting problems of aggression, found those persons to be 4 times as likely to meet criteria for depression than those without aggression. Borthwick-Duffy (1994) noted in study of over 90,000 persons "two or three serious forms of destructive behaviors were more prevalent among persons with a dual diagnosis than among those with only a mental retardation diagnosis (p. 15)".

In view of the high prevalence and the related numerous and major personal and social implications of recurring acts of aggression and related disruptive behaviors (Gardner, 2002a), effective diagnostic and treatment approaches are needed to reduce the impact of these socially and personally disruptive acts. This chapter provides description of the clinical process for selection of treatment procedures and offers a rationale for determination of effectiveness of treatments used.

Chapter Overview

Brief description is provided initially of the interrelated topics of treatment targets, treatment objectives, and treatment efficacy. This is followed by description of a number of assumptions and related observations about the nature of aggressive responding that impact on treatment selection, treatment implementation, and subsequently on treatment efficacy. Following examination of these, brief description and evaluation of frequently used clinical case formulation approaches reflecting behavioral, psychological, and biomedical explanatory systems are provided. The chapter concludes with discussion of an integrative psychological case formulation approach that utilizes central features of each of the individual approaches described.

The reader will recognize that the specific suppositions held by a clinician influence his or her selection of the case formulation model used to determine assessment targets, assessment procedures, and the interpretations given to assessment results. The assessment results obtained and interpretation of these in turn influence the specific treatment and management procedures selected to address the conditions identified as controlling various features of a person's aggressive behavior, that is, those conditions that influence frequency of aggression, its severity, the variability in frequency and severity across time and conditions, and its persistent recurrence. As illustrations, under the assumption that information about current reinforcement contingencies is central to an understanding of acts of aggression, the case formulation model used by a behavior analyst may result in use of such assessment procedures as the Motivational Assessment Scale (Durand & Cummins, 1992) or the Questions About Behavior Function scale (Matson & Vollmer, 1995) to identify these behavioral functions. A second clinician may use a case formulation approach compatible with his or her supposition that a person's aggressive acts reflect the mediating effects of cognitive distortions. Diagnostic procedures such as a personal interview or exposure to video vignettes may be used to identify the specific distortions present. A third clinician may use a case formulation approach compatible with his or her supposition that a person's aggressive acts reflect the effects of a mental illness. Diagnostic procedures such as a mental status examination and observational procedures for obtaining sleep patterns and related symptoms may be selected (Lowry, 1994). In each case, results obtained from the diagnostic assessment process would influence selection of the specific treatment procedures used to reduce or eliminate the conditions presumed to control a person's aggressive responding.

In the first illustration, the behavior analyst would likely use environmental interventions to eliminate or modify the presumed maintaining reinforcement contingencies (Luiselli, Benner, Stoddard, Kisowski, & Weiss, 2000). In contrast, cognitive behavior therapy procedures would likely be selected in the second illustration to reduce or eliminate the cognitive distortions presumed to influence the aggressive acts (Lindsay, Marshall, Neilson, Quinn, & Smith, 1998). In the third instance, drug therapy would likely be selected to reduce or eliminate the mental illness symptoms presumed to influence the aggressive acts (Davanzo, Berlin, Widawski, & King, 1998).

Treatment Targets, Treatment Objectives, and Treatment Efficacy

Treatment Targets

A review of studies comprising the clinical and empirical literatures on approaches undertaken to reduce features of aggressive and related disruptive acts reveals a broad potpourri of interventions (Allen, 2000; Whitaker, 1993). Writers have noted that a significant percentage of persons with persistent problems of aggression become the targets of psychotropic medication administered for the person's "behavior" rather than for specific psychiatric or psychological symptoms that are presumed to serve as controlling influences (Matson et al., 2000; Reiss & Aman, 1998). Although a reduction in frequency or severity of aggressive responding may be observed with some persons, the question of "what is being treated" and the controlling relationship between these drug targets and acts of aggression is seldom addressed.

The same question of "what is being treated" may be raised relative to a number of behavioral interventions when used in the absence of person specific diagnostic hypotheses that suggest specific interventions to address specific hypothesized controlling conditions. These interventions include such procedures as noncontingent reinforcement, differential reinforcement procedures, punishment procedures involving overcorrection, time out, response cost and related behavior reduction techniques, providing choices, and general social skills training.

Each of these interventions of course could be selected to address diagnostically-identified controlling conditions. As one example, studies have demonstrated reduction in aggressive behaviors following implementation of a noncontingent reinforcement procedure that matches the motivational basis for the behavior. Following demonstration of the controlling influence of physical contact with a caregiver (handholding) on aggressive responding in a 41-year-old male with profound intellectual disabilities, this reinforcing experience was provided on a noncontingent basis during treatment, that is, independent of the aggressive responding. The treatment target in this case became the motivational condition controlling the aggression rather than the acts of aggression. Aggressive acts involving grabbing, hair pulling, and biting were eliminated during treatment that matched the motivational requirements of the adult (Britton, Carr, Kellum, Dozier, & Weil, 2002).

Selection of intervention procedures continue nonetheless to be reported without the guidance of diagnostic information to address specific antecedent, personal, or maintaining conditions relevant to a specific person. Baker and Thyer (2000) provide illustration of this case formulation deficiency in their use of a DRO procedure to address problems of aggression and related disruptive acts in a man with cognitive impairment who attended a vocational center. Even though frequency of aggressive responding reduced following implementation of a procedure of providing a reinforcer following periods of time during which these aggressive and related disruptive behaviors were absent, no assessments of the motivational bases of the acts were conducted. Further, the program did not teach alternative means of coping with the unidentified antecedent instigating conditions controlling these aggressive and disruptive acts or to change the motivational basis for these responses. Maintenance and generalization of treatment effects following withdrawal of the DRO procedures, while not reported by the writers, seems highly unlikely.

As specific acts of aggression represent the end result of a complex of antecedent (instigating and mediating) and maintaining events that differ from one person to another, there can be no specific treatments for aggression. Rather, treatment and associated management procedures are selected to address the specific environmental and personal conditions identified during individual diagnostic analysis as significant controlling influences on occurrence, severity level, variation across time in occurrence and severity, and durability or strength of aggressive responding (Allen, 2000; Gardner, 2002a; Taylor, 2002). Individualization is required in this selection process. As suggested by Nezu and Nezu (1994), "clinical interventions for aggression are more likely to be conceptualized as strategies based on an idiographic assessment of a particular individual, rather than as simple techniques uniformly and inflexibly applied for all aggressive patients (p. 39)."

This individual assessment is sensitive to the possibility that antecedent conditions that set the occasion for occurrence of aggressive acts may differ from those that influence severity and variability of these acts. Thus, the interventions selected to address frequency of acts of aggression may differ from those selected to address conditions that influence severity levels. To illustrate, an adolescent's low intensity acts of verbal aggression following attempts by peers residing in his group home to use his personal property without permission may become high intensity acts of physical aggression when these intrusions occur during periods of heightened states of personal agitation associated with the recent cancellation of an anticipated and valued parental visit. In this instance, the stimulus feature of peer intrusion, that is, its level of aversiveness, was modified by the presence of a heightened emotional state (Baker, Blumberg, Freeman, & Wieseler, 2002; Gardner, Cole, Davidson, & Karan, 1986; Gardner, 2002a). To be effective, treatments would address the manner in which the adolescent responds to peer intrusion as well as his manner of coping with disappointment.

As a result of these potentially multiple and individually unique biomedical and psychosocial sources of influence on the aggressive responding of any specific person, multiple interrelated interventions may be required to address multiple sets of controlling influences (Allen, 2000; Gardner, 2002a; Nezu & Nezu, 1994). Treatment and management approaches will be effective in influencing various features of aggressive responding to the extent that these potentially multiple controlling conditions reflecting possible biomedical and psychosocial sources are identified and altered.

Treatment Objectives

Treatments are provided to accomplish three interrelated objectives. The primary objective of treatments is to eliminate or reduce the specific conditions identified as having a controlling influence on features of aggressive responding. In the example of the adolescent described in the previous section, attention would be given to teaching him alternative prosocial ways of expressing his disapproval of peer intrusions and of expressing his personal disappointment following unmet expectations. Additionally, appropriate motivational supports would be developed to insure timely use of these newly acquired skills. Attainment of these primary objectives will in turn accomplish the second objective of reducing or eliminating acts of aggression as the person had acquired functional alternatives means of coping with the conditions of instigation. Finally, treatments are selected to support maintenance and generalization of treatment effects following termination of treatment. As described in the following section, evaluation of treatment efficacy requires consideration of each of these objectives.

Treatment Efficacy

The question of efficacy of treatments for aggression thus becomes a broader question of the efficacy of specific interventions that address specific instigating, mediating, and maintaining conditions identified during the diagnostic assessment process as having potential influence on features of aggressive responding in a particular person. That is, are there effective treatments for the multiple medical, psychiatric, psychological, and environmental conditions that may represent controlling influences over aggressive responding?

If a controlling influence consists of a psychiatric symptom such as delusional ideation, irritability, anxiety associated with flashbacks, or a hypomanic mood state (Ryan, 2000; Sovner & Fogelman, 1996), efficacy of drug treatment for the psychiatric condition producing the psychiatric symptoms would represent the target of evaluation. The reader will note that aggressive acts do not represent the primary drug target. If heightened levels of anger were presumed to influence aggressive acts (Benson, 2002; Taylor, 2002), efficacy of treatments in reducing anger in anger arousing situations or in teaching ways of coping with heightened levels of anger as alternatives to aggression would represent the focus of evaluation. If these controlling influences reside in personal distress arising from a medical illness or medication side effects (Kalachnik, Hanzel, Harder, Bauernfeind, & Engstromn, 1995; Peine, Darvish, Adams, Blakelock, Jenson, & Osborne, 1995), evaluation would be made of the efficacy of medical treatments for the medical conditions producing the pain, discomfort, irritability, or related forms of personal distress. If a person's interpretation of the intent of the actions of others were presumed to influence a person's aggressive acts (Benson, 2002), the effectiveness of an intervention to modify this cognitive set would be assessed. If aggression were hypothesized to reflect communication skill deficits (Bailey, McComas, Benavides, & Lovascz, 2002; Bird, Dores, Moniz, & Robinson, 1989; Reichle & Wacker, 1993), the usefulness of specific methods of teaching alternative functional communication skills would be assessed.

In each case, if the selected treatments are successful in removing or reducing these presumed controlling conditions that render a person at heightened risk for acts of aggression, the frequency of aggressive responding as well as severity levels and variability of these acts would be influenced to the extent that these treated conditions in fact served as controlling influences over these features of aggressive responding. It is possible of course that an intervention might be highly effective in modification of presumed controlling influences (e.g., elimination of anxiety associated with flashbacks, reduction in heightened levels of irritability associated with delusions, reduction in contingent staff attention following aggressive acts, reduction in anger following taunts from peers, increase in socially-appropriate alternative communication skills, increase in conflict resolution skills, modification of a social information processing set) but have minimal or no effects on features of aggressive responding. In this event, either the presumed relationships did not exist, that is, the diagnostic hypotheses used to select the specific interventions used were incorrect or other untreated conditions were present that continued to be influential in producing the aggressive acts.

To summarize, the primary treatment target becomes the controlling conditions rather than a person's acts of aggression. The question "Are effective treatments available for aggression?" becomes "Are effective treatments available for the range of conditions of a biomedical and psychosocial nature that influence various features of aggressive responding?" In the final analysis, the question of efficacy also becomes an exercise in evaluating the accuracy and completeness of the clinical hypotheses concerning controlling conditions. Thus, a case formulation approach is required that is most useful to the clinician (a) in identification of these potentially multiple sources of influences, (b) in speculating about the role(s) served by each (i.e., instigating, mediating, maintaining), (c) in hypothesizing about the relative magnitude of effects of the separate and joint influences on features of aggressive responding, and (d) in providing direction to selection of those interventions that address the potentially multiple controlling conditions and also maximize continuation and generalization across situations of treatment effects following termination of treatments.

Features of Aggression Influencing Selection of Case Formulation Model

Social Learning Nature of Aggression

A premise requiring consideration by the case formulation approach selected to guide the assessment and treatment selection process is that habitual acts of aggression, including those involving severe forms of violence, predominately reflect a person's unique history of social learning experiences (Bandura, 1969, 1973, 1977, 1986; Staats, 1996). These aggressive acts have been shaped and strengthened into functional means of reducing, delaying, terminating, or avoiding experiences of personal distress. These activating experiences of psychological distress that initiate and provide direction to the aggressive actions may represent states of aversive affective over arousal (e.g., fear, anxiety, irritability, anger, boredom) or states of deprivation (e.g., sexual contact, social attention, sensory stimulation) (Gardner, 2002a; Repp, 1999). A case formulation model thus is required that addresses the social environmental nature of aggressive responding.

Psychiatric and Related Biomedical Influences

In assuming a social learning view of the origin and habitual continuation of aggressive behaviors, it nonetheless is recognized that the instigation as well as the reinforcing experiences that follow the occurrence of aggressive acts reflect the influences of various aspects of the person's biomedical, including psychiatric and neurological, features (Barnhill, 1999; Gardner, 2002a; Sheard, 1984; Sovner & Fogelman, 1996). Prevalence studies report in fact, as noted earlier, that persons with intellectual disabilities who also have a diagnosis of a mental disorder present an increased rate of occurrence of aggression and related disruptive acts (Borthwick-Duffy, 1994; Jacobson, 1982; Reiss & Rojahn, 1993). Seldom, however, can it be assumed that recurring aggressive acts represent reflexive or involuntary behaviors that are the direct and sole result of antecedent biomedical influences. Matson and Mayville (2001) demonstrated the influence of environmental or physical contingencies in understanding aggression even in persons with intellectual disabilities and a co-occurring psychiatric disturbance. Using the Questions About Behavior Function scale (Matson &

Vollmer, 1995), the writers found that 75% of the sample studied of persons identi-fied as presenting a dual diagnosis showed an environmental or physical function for their aggression. These writers concluded that, even though all persons studied had a diagnosed mental disorder, factors other than the mental illness represented major contributions to the functionality of the aggressive acts. The potential multiple sources of biomedical and psychosocial influence on aggressive responding thus require a transactional case formulation approach that recognizes these influences and the potential interactions among these.

Uniqueness of Antecedent Controlling Conditions

A third consideration in selection of a case formulation model to guide diagnosis and treatment of aggression involves the recognition that acts of aggression occur selec-tively under specific and individually unique antecedent conditions. These antecedent events may reflect biomedical (medical, psychiatric, neuropsychiatric) and psycho-logical features of the person occurring independent of or in interaction with social and physical environmental events. As illustrations of the transactions between bio-medical and environmental influences, Lowry (1994), Lowry and Sovner (1992), and Sovner, Foxx, Lowry, and Lowry (1993) provide descriptions of the possible contributing roles of anxiety, irritability, and fluctuating mood states and the man-ner in which these interact with specific features of the social environments in influencing occurrence of aggression and self-injury. In persons with intellectual dis-abilities and a mood disorder, occurrence of problem behavioral symptoms was noted to be dependent on the presence of the specific mood states plus occurrence of various staff prompts. Different kinds of prompts served as components of the instigating stimulus complex depending on the nature of the person's mood state. During mood states of dysphoria, staff prompts intended to get the person involved in activities that typically were enjoyed produced the problem behavior. During episodes of hy-pomania, prompts to slow the person down or focus attention produced the behavioral symptoms.

Tsiouris (2001), in describing the antecedent events for occurrence of aggression in persons with severe intellectual disabilities and mood disorders, noted, "usually it was directed towards noisy consumers who invaded the isolation of others. It was also directed at staff who urged individuals to do different chores, to get ready for their programme in the morning, or to participate in activities which they had previously enjoyed" (p. 118). The disruptive behaviors represented the end result of the interactive influences of personal affective states and specific environmental events. Lindsay et al.

(1998) provide illustration of the role of individually unique psychological features in determination of the influence of antecedent stimulus conditions over aggressive responding. These writers evaluated the cognitive distortions of persons with intellectual disabilities who engaged in sexually aggressive activities. Men who had been charged with exhibitionism were found to have the distorted beliefs that their victims did not object to but rather actually enjoyed the exposure experience.

Further demonstrations of the idiosyncratic nature of these instigating antecedent conditions are provided by Berg et al. (2000), Carr, Langdon, and Yarbrough (1999), O'Reilly (1995), and Taylor, Sisson, McKelvey, and Trefelner (1993). Berg et al. (2000), in a study involving a 9-year-old boy with developmental disabilities and autism, demonstrated that a teacher prompt to complete academic tasks that previously had been completed set the occasion for aggressive acts of hitting and pinching. Aggressive acts seldom occurred following directives to complete tasks that previously had not been completed.

Carr et al. (1999) observed that some children with autism are quite reactive to loud noises. A child with this sensitivity may cover her ears to reduce the personal discomfort or distress produced by a noisy classroom. A teacher's prompt to uncovered her ears in order to hear the classroom instruction may result in an aggressive act toward the teacher as a means of communicating her discomfort. The aggressive response in this instance resulted from a combination of the noise-produced personal discomfort in a child with excessive noise sensitivity and the teacher's prompt. Neither the noise nor the prompt in isolation was sufficient to produce the aggressive act. A more complete analysis of this action would include, as one component, an assessment of deficits in alternative means of communicating her concern to the teacher.

O'Reilly (1995) observed that rates of aggression of a 31-year-old man with intellectual disabilities, when provided directives from family members and staff in both home and vocational settings, were higher following periods of sleep deprivation than following periods of no sleep deprivation. The antecedent personal distress associated with sleep deprivation combined with the social directives to increase the likelihood of the aggressive acts.

Finally, Taylor et al. (1993) noted that low levels of adult attention sometimes occasioned problem behavior in a young girl with a diagnosis of intellectual disabilities. Further analysis revealed that problem behaviors did not occur in the social context in which an adult limited her attention by speaking to another child. In a second context, problems behaviors did occur when the adult limited her attention to the girl by speaking to another adult. An identification of the controlling antecedent conditions could be fully understood only when the specifics of the triadic social context were examined.

These and similar illustrations emphasize that social and physical environmental as well as cognitive and emotional features of the person may represent vital components of antecedent controlling conditions. A recent clinical experience provides further illustration of these personal antecedent influences. During a visit by the author to an inpatient forensic mental hospital unit, a young adult with intellectual disabilities was observed assaulting a nursing staff supervisor. The assault was sudden, unexpected, and, upon antecedent analysis of potential environmental triggers for the episode, occurred in the absence of any apparent environmental provocation. A subsequent interview with the young man revealed that the assault was motivated by anger toward the nursing supervision generated by the man's cognitive assumption that the supervisor had come on the unit to reassign a specific staff with whom the man had developed a positive attachment. In the absence of this information, meaningful interventions to (a) correct the person's faulty assumption, (b) teach alternative means of expressing his anxieties and related emotions, (c) teach alternative problem solving strategies, and (d) provide the personal motivational basis for selecting a prosocial coping response would have been overlooked. The behavioral intervention program in effect at the time of the incident resulted in a time out and related response costs of loss of privileges. These reactive behavioral punishment procedures neither addressed the motivational basis for the aggressive act nor the alternative functional skills required for appropriate expression of personal concerns.

In summary, these examples illustrate that the instigating events that signal occurrence of aggressive behaviors have been shown to have their origin in the external physical, social, and/or program environments and in covert or internal psychological, medical, and psychiatric conditions. Stimulus states emanating from any of the sources, in isolation and in combination with other conditions, may influence occurrence, severity, or variability over time in each of these measures. Depending on the number of these controlling events and the person's mediating reactivity to these conditions, occurrence of any specific stimulus states may place the person at risk of heightened levels of personal distress or discomfort. This distress level may serve a major instigating role for occurrence and severity levels of aggressive acts in a person inclined to use aggression as a coping attempt to reduce the noxious personal experience. Thus, the type and magnitude of control of the various antecedent influences over aggressive responding is unique to each person and thus requires a case formulation process (diagnostic activities and resulting interventions) that is individualized and also addresses controlling antecedents of both biomedical and psychosocial origins.

Uniqueness of Personal Characteristics

The case formulation selected also must attend to those personal features of a biomedical and psychological nature that place a person at increased risk for aggressive behaviors. These features determine the influence on occurrence, severity, and variability of aggressive acts of specific antecedent conditions such as a threatening peer, a painful headache, auditory hallucinations, a distressful level of irritability, a state of deprivation relating to valued activities or experiences, or a demanding work supervisor. These mediating central processing influences address the question of why one person would be at increased risk for aggressive and related disruptive responding when another person would be at minimal or no risk when both are exposed to similar antecedent conditions such as peer provocation, staff instructional demands, an environment that provides insufficient social attention or opportunities for social interactions, or heightened levels of anger arousal.

Two classes of vulnerability features that place the person at increased risk for aggressive responding are of significance. A person's level of risk for aggressive responding when exposed to individually unique conditions of instigation is related to the type, number, and strength of these central processing vulnerability features. The initial class consists of *psychobiological* features involving (a) neurological and related neurochemical abnormalities (Barnhill, 1999), (b) psychiatric disorders and symptoms (Tuinier & Verhoeven, 1993), (c) medical abnormalities (Gedye, 1997), and (d) genetic syndromes (Dykens, Hodapp, & Finucane, 2000) that influence the manner in which antecedent activating events are mediated or processed by an individual and the transactions that may occur between these (Gardner, 2002a). More specifically, features such as an inclination for generalized affective overarousal (hyperexcitability, hyperirritability) even to seemingly minor conditions of threat or provocation, impairments in the processes of modulating states of overarousal with the result that the person remains in an overaroused state for extended periods, and impairments in skills of inhibiting exaggerated impulsive aggressive reactions are present with increased frequency and severity among persons with more severe cognitive and adaptive behavior impairments (Sovner & Fogelman, 1996). Additionally, similar personal features are reported in persons with intellectual disabilities who present with various psychiatric and personality disorders (Bradley, 2000; Mavromatis, 2000; Reiss, 1994).

Persons with psychiatric disorders also present with other more discrete features that may serve as mediating risk influences on aggressive responding. Various mood/affective (e.g., irritability, dysphoria, anxiety, emotional agitation), cognitive (e.g. delusional thought processes, flights of ideas), perceptual (e.g., auditory and visual hallucinations), and related symptoms associated with major mental disorders and various personality disorders and traits may influence the meaning or function of instigating stimulus events. To illustrate, a person may have a tendency to view the actions of others in a paranoid or hostile manner. Others and their actions or intent are viewed with suspicion and mistrust. These and similar paranoid traits are reported to occur with some frequency in persons with intellectual disabilities who engage in disruptive behaviors (Bouras & Drummond, 1992; Reiss, 1990). This cognitive view of the actions of others will influence the information-processing activities involved in encoding and interpreting social events. This impaired cognitive-perceptual set interferes with the selection and evaluation of alternative means of coping with the perceived sources of threat. These in combination with a strong habit of aggressive responding are likely to be processed into an impulsive aggressive act in an effort by the person to reduce or remove the presumed source of threat. This scenario emphasizes the dynamic transactions between instigating and central processing features.

The second class of risk conditions for aggressive responding consists of two subclasses of *psychological* features. The initial psychological subclass, consisting of personal features of a cognitive, emotional/motivational, and behavioral nature, represents vulnerabilities for aggressive responding due to their *presence or excessive* nature. This initial subclass is illustrated by such personal features as (a) presence of a strong habit of aggressive responding, (b) a cognitive hostile attributional bias (Baker & Bramston, 1997), (c) cognitive distortions (Lindsley et al., 1998), and (d) a motivational inclination to enjoy sexual contact with children (Griffiths, 2002).

A person's habit strength of aggressive responding provides one illustration of the role that personal characteristics assumes in mediating antecedent events, as well as the manner in which assessment information about these personal characteristics influences clinical decisions concerning treatment selection. The effectiveness of interventions, whether a specific procedure such as extinction or a treatment package with multiple components, will be influenced by the habit strength of acts of aggression and the presence and relative strength of functional alternatives in the person's repertoire. Specific interventions may be quite effective when used with an individual with low habit strength of aggressive acts and who also has behavioral alternatives to address the instigating motivational condition. These same intervention procedures or packages of procedures may be relative ineffective when used with a person whose habit strength is quite high and who has minimal functional alternatives available for use. Bradley (2000) suggested that, following repeated use of aggressive responding, neural circuits are changed and thus are more resistant to treatment effects. Vitiello, Behar, Hunt, Stoff, and Ricciuti (1990) offered similar observations in their supposition that impulsive aggression associated with emotional states of fear or anger toward conditions of provocation may be more neurologically "hardwired" and become more automatic and habitually utilized. As a result, more powerful interventions provided over repeated therapy sessions would be required for significant and enduring reduction in habit strength and successful replacement of acts of aggression with functionally appropriate behaviors.

MacLean, Stone, and Brown (1994) noted that although intensive interventions may result in reduction in frequency and intensity of aggressive and destructive behaviors in persons with long standing aggressive habits "…such intervention efforts have been largely ineffective in eliminating destructive behaviors. In many cases the behavior rebounds when intervention efforts are terminated" (p. 68). An examination of the literature on which this conclusion was based suggests that treatments used had not modified critical personal motivational and alternative functional skills to the extent that these would become predominate over the habitual aggressive response if exposed again to pretreatment instigating and reinforcement contingencies. Thus, consideration of habit strength, the presence and strength of functional alternatives, related motivational features, and similar present psychological features require a case formulation approach that gives consideration to these in selection of interventions and in speculation both about the potential effectiveness of specific interventions as well as the number of treatment experiences required prior to expecting durable treatment effects.

The second subtype of psychological central processing features places a person at risk for aggressive responding as a result of the *functional absence or low strength* of these. These include such personal features as (a) deficits in skills of anger management (Benson, Rice, & Miranti, 1986; Cole, Gardner, & Karan, 1985), (b) communication skill deficits (Bird et al., 1989; Carr, Levin, McConnachie, Carlson, Kemp, & Smith, 1994), (c) problem solving skill deficits (Benson, 2002), (d) deficits in prosocial skill alternatives to aggression (Fredericks & Nishioka-Evans, 1999) and deficits in skills to self-manage prosocial skill alternatives (Gardner, 1998b). These functional deficits increase the risk of aggressive responding when a person with an inclination to use aggression as a coping response is exposed to conditions of provocation that require the deficit psychological features for alternative socially appropriate action.

Singh, Wahler, Adkins, and Myers (2003) provide an illustration of reduction of risk factors for aggressive responding in a person by teaching a mediating behavior that interrupted the aggressive sequence. These clinicians taught a self-controlling strategy to an adult with intellectual disabilities and mental illness whose aggression had precluded successful community placement. Treatment consisted of teaching a simple meditation technique that required the adult to shift his attention and awareness from an anger-producing situation to the soles of his feet. After learning this technique, he was guided to use it in situations that normally would have resulted in aggressive acts. This self-controlling technique resulted in 6 months of aggression-free behavior at which time the man was transitioned to the community. No aggressive behavior was reported during a one-year follow-up after community placement.

As a second illustration of a treatment focus on psychological deficits, a person with a communication skill deficit who is inclined to use aggression to cope with distress-producing conditions is at increased risk for aggressive responding when exposed to situations that require some form of expressive communication. Under these conditions, acts of aggression may serve a substitute communicative function in producing valued consequences (Carr & Durand, 1985; Schroeder, Reese, Hellings, Loupe, & Tessel, 1999). A large number of studies have demonstrated reduction in acts of aggression following acquisition and use of alternative communicative and related functional replacement behaviors (Matson & Duncan, 1997; Repp & Horner, 1999; Scotti & Meyer, 1999).

It is not unusual for a number of different central processing features to contribute to a person's aggressive acts. As an illustration, when an intrusive peer violates his personal space, an adult with severe cognitive impairments may respond immediately with a sudden surge in emotional and motor agitation followed by impulsive acts of physical aggression. Under these conditions of instigation, the adult has a number of psychological and psychobiological characteristics that place him at high risk for aggressive and related disruptive responding. These include such features as an inclination to become hyperaroused under minor conditions of instigation, limited effective socially appropriate communicative means of expressing his distress, an impaired emotional modulation system that is nonfunctional in reducing his states of emotional overarousal, a strong habit of aggressive responding under conditions of hyperarousal and related distress states, and limited cognitive and affective skills to inhibit the motivational conditions controlling aggressive acts (Gardner, 2002b). In view of the major influence on aggressive responding of these central processing features, a case formulation approach is needed to guide the assessment and related treatment selection process.

Case Formulations Models

Review of current conceptual, empirical, and clinical literatures devoted to treatment of conditions presumed to control aggressive responding reflects use of a range of case formulation paradigms to guide research and clinical activities (Gardner, 2002a, 2002b; Rush & Frances, 2000; Whitaker, 1993). As noted, in clinical settings these paradigms are used to offer guidance in selection both of the diagnostic targets and related assessment procedures as well as the resulting interventions derived from the diagnostic findings. Close review of these paradigms, however, reveals that the most frequently used paradigms involving behavioral and psychiatric interventions address only selective components of the complex biomedical and psychosocial matrix of potential influences. As suggested by Singh, Wahler, Adkins, and Myers (2003), "Aggressive behaviors are typically treated with psychotropic medication, behavioral interventions or their combination; but often the behaviors persist at a level that is problematic for the individual as well as care providers (p. 158)." As background for description of a contrasting view of specifying the specific instigating, mediating, and maintaining roles that may be assumed by each of multiple sets of influences and the possible resulting significant interactive effects of these on aggressive responding, brief description is provided of both biomedical and behavioral case formulations paradigms.

Biomedical Case Formulation Paradigms

To address possible biomedical influences on aggressive responding, two case formulation approaches, the Medical Illness and the Psychiatric Disorders paradigms, are used to provide direction to medical interventions for conditions presumed to influence aggressive responding. A *Medical Illness* case formulation is used to guide selection of treatment for a wide range of medical illnesses presumed to produce personal discomfort or distress levels that in turn combines with physical and social environmental events to influence aggressive acts in those persons prone to use aggression as a means of coping with conditions experienced as noxious. The presence of medical conditions that produce headaches, menstrual discomfort, middle ear infections, sleep difficulties, allergic reactions, skin disorders, gastrointestinal abnormalities, seizure activity, and tooth infections have been described as correlated with an increased likelihood of aggressive responding (Didden, Korzilius, van Aperlo, van Overloop, & de Vries, 2002; Gardner & Whalen, 1996; Kastner, Walsh, & Fraser, 2001; Mikkelsen & McKenna, 1999). Each may produce heightened levels of internal stimuli experienced as aversive or distressing that in turn may change the stimulus function of co-occurring physical and social events (Carr et al., 1999). Specifically, the presence of these stimulus conditions change previously positive or neutral events into aversive ones or increase the level of noxiousness of events previously viewed as noxious. These changed stimulus elements contribute to the frequency, severity levels, and variability of aggressive responding (Gardner, 2002a). Carr, Smith, Giacin, Whelan, and Pancari (2003) demonstrated these effects in their determination that problem behaviors (aggression, tantrums, and self-injury) among four females with intellectual disabilities were related to the combined effects of menstrual discomfort and task demands. A multicomponent intervention program targeted both sets of antecedents and produced near-zero levels of problem behaviors that were maintained for 15 to 22 months in three of the adults.

In the *Psychiatric Disorders* case formulation paradigm, primary symptoms of various psychiatric syndromes are presumed to exert various influences on aggressive responding in those prone to use aggressive as a means of coping with distress producing conditions (Gardner, 2002a; Reiss & Aman, 1998; Rush & Frances, 2000). As described above, the presence of these symptoms may change the stimulus functions of co-occurring social and physical events. Successful management through medication of such psychiatric symptoms as delusional thought patterns, hallucinations, heightened levels of anger or anxiety, hypomania, and dysphoric affect may serve to reduce or remove these sources of potential influence over aggressive responding. A related model, the *Neurophysiological Dysregulation* paradigm addresses organic irritability arising from neurological or neurochemical abnormalities. Medication to address such organically induced states as irritability, hyperexcitability, and hypersensitivity is used to reduce or remove this potential source of influence on aggressive responding (Barnhill, 1999; Sovner & Fogelman, 1996).

Psychosocial Case Formulation Paradigms

The most frequently used paradigm in analysis and treatment of aggressive acts among persons with intellectual disabilities, especially with those with more severe cognitive and adaptive behavior impairments, is that of *applied behavior analysis*. This case formulation, reflecting a radical behavioral view of human behavior, views aggressive acts as operants that are maintained by contingent environmentally based experiences (Repp & Horner, 1999). As detailed by Gardner (2002a), the application of this case formulation approach to problems of aggression and related disruptive acts, and the types of behavior modification procedures utilized, has evolved over the last few decades from one with a focus on elimination through suppression of aggressive and disruptive acts (Carr & Durand, 1985; Gardner, 1969) into a major focus of providing positive behavioral supports involving functionally equivalent alternative responses and other skills training, altering antecedent conditions, and environmental modifications, (Anderson & Freeman, 2002; Carr, 1997; Koegel, Koegel, & Dunlap, 1996). As noted, this case formulation has offered direction to the majority of the research and clinical studies that specifically address aggressive and related disruptive behaviors in persons with intellectual disabilities.

A number of additional *behavior therapy* systems have paralleled the development of applied behavior analysis. While utilizing reinforcement contingencies as a major construct, these approaches have made use of a range of additional learning and related psychological models. The more notable of these involve social learning concepts and related therapy practices offered by Bandura and colleagues (Bandura, 1969, 1977, 1986; Bandura & Walters, 1963). Bandura's analysis of aggression (1973) offers a range of possible intervention approaches that address potential controlling conditions. Social learning, psychological behaviorism, and related cognitive and cognitive-behavioral views (Bandura, 1986; Craighead, Craighead, Kazdin, & Mahoney, 1994; Staats, 1996) provide direction to assessment and intervention practices that have enjoyed increasing use among clinicians supporting those with intellectual and other developmental disabilities (Gardner, 2002a). These therapy approaches include social skills training, relaxation training, contingency management, token economies, anger management training, aggression replacement training, self-management skills training, systematic desensitization procedures, cognitive-behavioral procedures, coping skills training, and problem-solving/conflict resolution procedures (Alllen 2000; Benson, 2002; Gardner, Graeber, & Cole, 1996; Matson & Duncan, 1997; Nezu & Nezu, 1994; Taylor, 2002; Whitaker, 1993). These social learning and related cognitive-behavioral views of aggressive responding offer a greatly expanded analytic and related treatment armamentarium for the clinician. With these, cognitive and emotional contributions to aggressive responding among persons with intellectual disabilities and mental health issues become direct targets of intervention efforts (Benson, 2002; Gardner, 2002a; Nezu, Nezu, & Gill-Weiss, 1992).

Summary

As is evident, while each of these psychosocial and biomedical paradigms represents a unique case formulation of some of the critical conditions that may influence features of aggressive responding in persons with a dual diagnosis of intellectual disabilities and mental health issues, no single one in isolation provides an adequate integrative account of the possible multiple biomedical, psychological, and environmental conditions that in combination for any specific person may influence occurrence as well as severity, variability over time and conditions, and durability of aggressive responding.

An Alternative Case Formulation

A diagnostic case formulation model is required that reflects the complex of antecedent controlling conditions, the manner in which these are mediated by personal characteristics, and the possible interactions among these. This paradigm should consider (a) the *most salient environmental, psychological, and biomedical stimulus complex* that precedes and serves to initiate the chain of events for specific episodes of aggressive acts, (b) the person's current biomedical and psychological *central processing* risk features that serve to mediate an antecedent activating stimulus complex, as well as (c) those proximate *consequences* that follow occurrences of aggressive and other disruptive activities and combine with a person's motivational states to determine their *functionality and strength*. As noted, the antecedent stimulus complex may include the arousing and activating features of a range of external physical and social environmental as well as internal psychological and biomedical conditions. These antecedent stimulus conditions are processed centrally and transported into the motor tract as acts of aggression and related coping actions. The objective of a comprehensive diagnostic assessment is "to see past" specific psychosocial and biomedical conditions and to ascertain the specific role(s) served by features of each of these conditions in contributing to the *occurrence, severity, fluctuation,* and *chronic recurrence* of aggressive acts. As illustrated earlier, factors that account for frequency of occurrence may differ somewhat from those that influence severity and variability of aggression (Gardner, 2002a). Following a comprehension assessment, informed speculation can be made about the extent of reduction in critical features of a person's aggression that may be expected following effective treatment of each or a combination of the diagnosed psychosocial and/or biomedical controlling conditions (Gardner & Sovner, 1994).

Brief description of one such case formulation model is provided. This case formulation model is described by Gardner and colleagues (Gardner, 1996, 1998a, 2002a; Gardner & Sovner, 1994). This Multimodal (*bio-*, *psycho-*, and *socio-environmental* modalities of influences) Contextual (*instigating*, *central processing*, and *maintaining* conditions that may reflect each of the modalities of influence) Case Formulation approach directs the diagnostician to evaluate both psychosocial and biomedical conditions as possible contributors to occurrence, severity, variability, and habitual recurrence of aggression. The model also provides a means of interfacing various medical and psychiatric diagnostic insights and related diagnostically based interventions with those that involve psychological and social and physical environmental influences.

Context 1: Instigating Influences

As illustrated in previous sections, instigating influences consist of current external (e.g., instructional demands, conflict with peers, blocking of ritualistic or compulsive routines, staff corrective feedback, invasion of personal space) and internal (e.g., high arousal level, anger, pain related distress, deprivation states, dysphoric mood) stimulus conditions that contribute to the occurrence, severity levels, and variability of specific aggressive and related disruptive episodes (Benson & Fuchs, 1999; Carr & Durand, 1985; Lowry & Sovner, 1992; Tsiouris, 2001). These instigating stimulus conditions are highly specific to each person and, when present, represent risk factors for influencing occurrence and related features of aggression for that person (McComas, Hoch, Paone, & El-Roy, 2000; Murphy, Macdonald, Hall, & Oliver, 2000). Similar stimulus conditions may not represent risk factors for aggressive responding in another person. As illustrated previously, it is not unusual for these controlling antecedent conditions to consist of combinations of psychosocial and biomedical influences unique to each person.

Context 2: Central Processing Influences

Central processing influences refer to those personal features of a biomedical and psychological nature that place a person at increased risk for aggressive behaviors

(Gardner 2002a). As noted in an earlier section, the mediating conditions consisting of psychobiological and psychological features determine the specific effects of antecedent instigating conditions on aggressive responding. Knowledge of these influences are central to gaining an understanding of why one person would be at increased risk for aggressive and related disruptive responding when another person of similar cognitive impairments would be at minimal or no risk when both are exposed to similar antecedent conditions.

As further illustration of the personal risk factors described in an earlier section, a significant number of persons with intellectual disabilities who present with chronic problems of impulsive aggression demonstrate an inclination for generalized affective overarousal (also described as hyperexcitability, hyperirritability, hypersensitivity) even to minor conditions of threat or aggravation. This overarousal may involve such emotions as anxiety, irritability, and anger. Also noted are difficulties in modulating the state of overarousal with the result that the person is unable to stabilize or lower the excessive arousal level. A frequent result is that the person is unable to inhibit exaggerated impulsive aggressive reactions directed toward the perceived source of these distressful states. These psychobiological difficulties, and especially a pattern of overreactivity to seemingly minor sources of provocation are present with increased frequency and severity among persons with more severe cognitive and adaptive behavior impairments (Sovner & Fogelman, 1996). Additionally, similar difficulties are present among persons with intellectual disabilities who also present with various psychiatric and personality disorders (Bradley, 2000; Mavromatis, 2000; Reiss, 1994).

Context 3: Maintaining Conditions

As noted earlier, aggressive acts in most instances become functional for a person based on the type of feedback effects of these behaviors that impact on current motivational states of that person. Aggressive acts may result in the removal, reduction, or avoidance of internal or external stimulus conditions experienced by the person as distressful, unpleasant, or aversive (e.g., anxiety level, intrusive medical procedures, taunts from peers, attempt by others to block occurrence of compulsive or ritualistic behavior, denials, parent criticism, unwanted teacher directives or task demands) or may reduce states of deprivation through producing, maintaining, or magnifying internal or external conditions experienced as pleasant or emotionally desirable (e.g., gaining social attention, gaining access to physical, cognitive, or sensory stimulating activities, being included in a valued peer group, creating distress in others) (Carr et al., 1999; Murphy, Macdonald, Hall, & Oliver, 2000; Thompson & Symonds, 1999). A specific contingent consequence serves to strengthen acts of aggression to the extent that the consequence addresses either the specific motivation state giving impetus to the behavior or to an equally or more powerful unmet motivational state. As described by Gardner (2002a), a motivational analysis thus represents a process of identifying the individually unique *motivational states Û consequence dyads*. A number of aberrant motivational features of persons with intellectual disabilities that may require attention in this analysis, especially in persons with significant mental health concerns, has been noted by Gardner (1971, 1977, 2002a) and Reiss and Havercamp (1997, 1998). These become relevant as a specific behavioral consequence frequently has meaning in relation to specific motivational state or states that activates and gives direction to the aggressive act (Gardner, 2002a). A diagnostic hypothesis that acts of aggression serve an "escape" function or a "social attention" function thus is incomplete until the specific motivational states related to the "escape" or "attention" are described (Carr et al., Yarborough, 1999). With this diagnostic information, an individualized intervention program may be designed to reduce the motivational state or states via noncontingent reinforcement procedures (O'Reilly, Lancioni, & Taylor, 1999; Wilder, Fisher, Anders, Cercone, & Neidert, 2001) or in supporting acquisition and/or use of alternative prosocial means of coping with the motivational conditions.

In some instances the diagnosed *motivational states Û consequence dyads* may involve a motivation feature viewed as aberrant in kind, intensity, or duration of each occurrence. In illustration it may be determined through assessment that a number of different events may result in a heightened level of anger that in turn is involved in the instigation of aggressive acts. A program objective in this instance, in addition to teaching alternative means of expressing anger, may include that of reducing or eliminating the excessive level of anger arousal. In other instances, the *motivational states Û consequence dyads* may involve personal features that are viewed at pathological. A person may gain enjoyment out of harming animals, setting fires, or having violent sexual contact with children. In some instances, the presence of a dysphoric mood or delusional thoughts may provide the major impetus for aggressive acts. In these instances, intervention procedures would be selected to reduce or eliminate these pathological features.

From Diagnostics to Interventions

The diagnostic findings about psychosocial and biomedical instigating, central processing, and maintaining conditions presumed to influence occurrence, severity level, variability over time in occurrence and severity, and the habitual recurrence of a person's aggression are translated into a matched set of treatment approaches, that is, all interventions become diagnostically based. In most instances, interventions are required for interrelated sets of antecedent, mediating, and maintaining conditions. Gardner (2002a) provides a detailed description of this case formulation process for the interested reader.

Therapeutic efforts are selected to remove or minimize the influence of biomedical, psychological, and environmental instigating and maintaining influences and to eliminate or minimize related central processing vulnerabilities. These efforts include the reduction or elimination of (a) pathological medical, psychiatric, and psychological conditions that produce or intensify distress levels and (b) impoverished, disruptive, or other aberrant features of the social and physical environments that place a person at continued risk for aggressive acts. Treatment efforts also include program components for addressing psychological deficits, for example, through teaching anger management skills, coping communicative and other socially appropriate alternatives to aggression, the skills to self-manage these prosocial skills, and for increasing the personal motivation to use these newly acquired skills as adaptive functional replacements for the aggressive acts. A skill enhancement program focus to offset psychological central processing vulnerabilities is especially pertinent for those with highly restricted repertoires of coping skills. Acts of aggression may represent the most effective and efficient functional coping reactions to a range of antecedent controlling conditions. As such, these acts must be replaced by equally effective and efficient functionally equivalent prosocial coping skills if aggression is to be minimized or eliminated and treatment effects maintained following termination of interventions (Gardner & Sovner, 1994; Gardner, Graeber-Whalen, & Ford, 2001; Schroeder et al., 1999; Singh et al., 2003).

References

Allen, D. (2000). Recent research on physical aggression in persons with intellectual disability: An overview. *Journal of Intellectual and Developmental Disabilities, 25,* 41-57.

Anderson, C. M., & Freeman, K. A. (2000). Positive behavior support: Expanding the application of applied behavior analysis. *The Behavior Analyst, 23,* 85-94.

Bailey, J., McComas, J. J., Benavides, C., & Lovascz, C. (2002). Functional assessment in a residential setting: Identifying an effective communicative replacement response for aggressive behavior. *Journal of Developmental and Physical Disabilities, 13,* 353-369.

Baker, D. J., Blumbery, E. R., Freeman, R., & Wieseler, N. A. (2002). Can psychiatric disorders be seen as establishing operations? Integrating applied behavior analysis and psychiatry. *Mental Health Aspects of Developmental Disabilities, 5,* 118-124.

Baker, K. L., & Thyer, B. A. (2000). Differential reinforcement of other behavior in the treatment of inappropriate behavior and aggression in an adult with mental retardation at a vocational center. *Scandinavian Journal of Behaviour Therapy, 29,* 37-42.

Baker, W., & Bramston, P. (1997). Attributional and emotional determinants of aggression in people with mild intellectual disabilities. *Journal of Intellectual and Developmental Disabilities, 22,* 169-186.

Bandura, A. (1969). *Principles of behavior modification.* New York: Holt, Rinehart, & Winston.

Bandura, A. (1973). *Aggression: A social learning analysis.* Englewood Cliffs, NJ: Prentice-Hall.

Bandura, A. (1977). *Social learning theory.* Englewood Cliffs, N. J. Prentice-Hall.

Bandura, A. (1986). *Social foundations of thought and action: A social cognitive theory.* Englewood Cliffs, NJ: Prentice-Hall.

Bandura, A., & Walters, R. H. (1963). *Social learning and personality development.* New York: Holt, Rinehart, & Winston.

Barnhill, J. (1999). The relationships between epilepsy and violent behavior in persons with mental retardation. *The NADD Bulletin, 2,* 43-46.

Benson, B. A. (2002). Feeling, thinking, doing: Reducing aggression through skill development. In W. I. Gardner (Ed.), *Aggression and other disruptive behavioral challenges* (pp. 293-323). Kingston, NY: NADD Press.

Benson, B. A., & Fuchs, C. (1999). Anger-arousing situations and coping responses of aggressive adults with intellectual disabilities. *Journal of Intellectual and Developmental Disabilities, 24,* 207-215.

Benson, B. A., Rice, C. J., & Miranti, S. V. (1986). Effects of anger management training with mentally retarded adults in group treatment. *Journal of Consulting and Clinical Psychology, 54,* 728-729.

Berg, W.K., Peck, S., Wacker, D. P., Harding, J, McComas, J., Richman, D., et al. (2000). The effects of presession exposure to attention on the results of assessments of attention as a reinforcer. *Journal of Applied Behavior Analysis, 33,* 463-478.

Bird, F., Dores, P. A., Moniz, D., & Robinson, J. (1989). Reducing severe aggressive and self-injurious behaviors with functional communication training. *American Journal on Mental Retardation, 94,* 37-48.

Borthwick-Duffy, S. A. (1994). Prevalence of destructive behaviors: A study of aggression, self-injury, and property destruction. In T. Thompson & D. B. Gray (Eds.), *Destructive behavior in developmental disabilities* (pp. 3-23). Thousand Oaks, CA: Sage.

Bouras, N., & Drummond, C. (1992). Behavior and psychiatric disorders of people with mental handicaps living in the community. *Journal of Intellectual Disability Research, 36,* 349-357.

Bradley, S. J. (2000). *Affect regulation and the development of psychopathology.* New York: The Guilford Press.

Britton, L. N., Carr, J. E., Kellum, K. K., Dozier, C. L., & Weil, T. M. (2002). A variation of noncontingent reinforcement in the treatment of aberrant behavior. *Research in Developmental Disabilities, 21,* 425-435.

Carr, E. G. (1997). The evolution of applied behvior analysis into positive behvior support. *JASH, 22,* 208-209.

Carr, E. G., & Durand, V. M. (1985). Reducing behavior problems through functional communication training. *Journal of Applied Behavior Analysis, 18,* 111-126.

Carr, E. G., Langdon, N. A., & Yarbrough, S. C. (1999). Linking functional assessment to effective intervention. In A. C. Repp & R. H. Horner (Eds.), *Functional analysis of problem behavior* (pp. 7-31). Belmont, CA: Wadsworth Publishing.

Carr, E. G., Levin, L., McConnachie, G., Carlson, J. I., Kemp, D. C., & Smith, C. E. (1994). *Communication-based intervention for problem behavior.* Baltimore: Paul H. Brookes.

Carr, E. G., Smith, C. E., Giacin, T. A,, Whelan, B. M, & Pancari, J. (2003). Menstrual discomfort as a biological setting event for severe problem behavior: Assessment and intervention. *American Journal on Mental Retardation, 108,* 117-133.

Cole, C. L., Gardner, W. I., & Karan, O. (1985). Self-management training of mentally retarded adults presenting severe conduct difficulties *Applied Research in Mental Retardation, 6,* 337-347.

Craighead, L. W., Craighead. W. E., Kazdin, A. E., & Mahoney, M. J. (1994). *Cognitive and behavioral interventions*. Boston: Allyn and Bacon.

Davanzo, P. A., Berlin, T. R., Widawski, & King, B. H. (1998). Paroxetine treatment of aggression and self-injury in persons with mental retardation. *American Journal on Mental Retardation, 102,* 427-437.

Didden, R., Korzilius, H., van Aperlo, B., van Overloop, C., & de Vries, M. (2002). Sleep problems and daytime problem behaviours in children with intellectual disability. *Journal of Intellectual Disability Research, 46,* 537-547.

Durand, V. M., & Cummins, D. B., (1992). *The Motivational Assessment Scale (MAS) Administration Guide.* Topeka, KS: Monaco & Associates.

Dykens, E. M., Hodapp, R. M., & Finucane, B. M., (2000). *Gentics and mental retardation syndromes: A new look at behavior and intervention.* Baltimore, MD: Paul H. Brookes.

Fredericks, B., & Nishioka-Evans, V. (1999). Functional assessment for a sex offender population. In A. C. Repp & R. H. Horner (Eds.), *Functional analysis of problem behavior* (pp. 279-303). Belmont, CA: Wadsworth Publishing.

Gardner, W. I. (1969). Use of punishment procedures with then severely retarded: A review. *American Journal of Mental Deficiency, 74,* 86-103.

Gardner, W. I. (1971). *Behavior modification in mental retardation.* London: University of London Press.

Gardner, W. I. (1977). *Learning and behavior characteristics of exceptional children and youth.* Boston: Allyn & Bacon.

Gardner, W. I. (1996). Nonspecific behavioral symptoms in persons with a dual diagnosis: A psychological model for integrating biomedical and psychosocial diagnosis and interventions. *Psychology in Mental Retardation and Developmental Disabilities, 21,* 6-11.

Gardner, W. I. (1998a). Initiating the case formulation process. In D. M. Griffiths, W. I. Gardner, & J. A. Nugent (Eds.), *Behavioral supports: Individual centered interventions* (pp. 17-65). Kingston, NY: NADD Press.

Gardner, W. I. (1998b). Teaching skills of self-management. In D. M. Griffiths, W. I. Gardner, & J. A. Nugent (Eds.), *Behavioral supports: Individual centered interventions* (pp. 259-273). Kingston, NY: NADD Press.

Gardner, W. I. (2002a). *Aggression and other disruptive behavioral challenges: Biomedical and psychosocial assessment and treatment.* Kingston, NY: NADD Press.

Gardner, W. I. (2002b). Psychological treatment of persons with mental retardation who present emotional and behavioral challenges. In R. F. B. Gues & D. A. Flikweert (Eds.), *Behandeling van psychische en degragsproblems* (pp. 13-20). Utrecht, The Netherlands: NGBZ/NIZW.

Gardner, W. I., Cole, C. L., Davidson, D. P.,, & Karan, O. C. (1986). Reducing aggression in individuals with developmental disabilities: An expanded stimulus control assessment and intervention model. *Education and Training of the Mentally Retarded, 21*, 3-12.

Gardner, W. I., Graeber, J. L., & Cole, C. L. (1996). Behavior therapies: A multimodal diagnostic and intervention model. In J. W. Jacobson & J. A. Mulick (Eds.), *Manual of diagnosis and professional practice in mental retardation* (pp. 255-269). Washington, DC: American Psychological Association.

Gardner, W. I., Graeber-Whalen, J. L., & Ford, D. (2001). Behavior therapies: Individualizing interventions through treatment formulations. In A. Dosen & K. Day (Eds.), *Treating mental illness and behavior disorders in children and adults with mental retardation* (pp. 69-100). Washington, DC: American Psychiatric Press.

Gardner, W. I., & Sovner. R. (1994*). Self-injurious behaviors: Diagnosis and treatment.* Willow Street, PA: Vida Press.

Gardner, W. I., & Whalen. J. P. (1996). A multimodal behvior analytic model for evaluating the effects of medical problems on nonspecific behavioral symptoms in persons with developmental disabilities. *Behavioral Interventions, 11*, 147-161.

Gedye, A. (1997). *Behavioral diagnostic guide for developmental disabilities.* Vancouver, BC: Diagnostic Books.

Griffiths, D. (2002). Sexual aggression. In W. I. Gardner (Ed.), *Aggression and other disruptive behavioral challenges: Biomedical and psychosocial assessment and treatment* (pp. 325-397). Kingston, NY: NADD Press.

Harris, P. (1993). The nature and extent of aggressive behaviour among people with learning difficulties (mental handicap) in a single health district. *Journal of Intellectual Disability Research, 37*, 221-242.

Jacobson, J. W. (1982). Problem behavior and psychiatric impairment in a developmentally disabled population: I. Behavior frequency. *Applied Research in Mental Retardation, 3*, 121-139.

Kalachnik, J. E., Hanzel, T. E., Harder, S. R., Bauernfeind, J. D., & Engstromn, E. A. (1995). Antiepileptic drug behavioral side-effects in individuals with mental retardation and the use of behavioral measurement techniques. *Mental Retardation, 33*, 374-382.

Kastner, T., Walsh, K. K., & Fraser, M. (2001). Undiagnosed medical conditions and medication side effects presenting as behavioral/psychiatric problems in people with mental retardation. *Mental Health Aspects of Developmental Disabilities, 4*, 101-107.

Kiernan, C., & Kiernan, D. (1994). Challenging behaviour in schools for pupils with severe learning difficulties. *Mental Handicap Research, 7*, 117-201.

Kiernan, C., & Quereshi , H. (1993). Challenging behaviour. In D. Kiernan, (Ed.), *Research to practice: Implications of research on the challenging behaviour of people with learning disabilities* (pp. 53-87). Kidderminster: British Institute of Learning Disabilities.

Koegel, R. L., Koegel, L. K., & Dunlap, G. (1996). *Positive behavioral support.* Baltimore: Paul H. Brookes.

Lindsay, W. R., Marshall, I., Neilson, C., Quinn, K., & Smith, A. H. W. (1998). The treatment of a person with a learning disability convicted of exhibitionism. *Research in Developmental Disabilities, 19*, 295-316.

Lowry, M. A. (1994). Functional assessment of problem behaviors associated with mood disorders. *The Habilitative Mental Healthcare Newsletter, 13*, 79-84.

Lowry, M. A., & Sovner, R. (1992). Severe behaviour problems associated with rapid cycling bipolar disorder in two adults with profound mental retardation. *Journal of Intellectual Disability Research, 36*, 269-281.

Luiselli, J. K., Benner, S., Stoddard, T., Kisowski, K., & Weiss, R. (2002). Behavior support intervention in psychiatric partial hospitalization for adults with mental retardation: Two case studies. *Mental Health Aspects of Developmental Disabilities, 3*, 1-7.

MacLean, W. E., Stone, W. L., & Brown, W. H. (1994). Developmental psychopathology of destructive behavior. In T. Thompson & D. V. Gray (Eds.), *Destructive behavior in developmental disabilities: Diagnosis and treatment* (pp. 68-79). Thousands Oaks, CA: Sage.

Matson, J. L., Bamburg, J. W., Mayville, E. A., Pinkston, J., Bielecki, J., Kuhn, D., et al. (2000). Psychopharmacology and mental retardation: A 10 year review (1990-1999). *Research in Developmental Disabilities, 21*, 263-296.

Matson, J. L., & Duncan, D. (1997). Aggression. In N. N. Singh (Ed.), *Prevention and treatment of severe behavior problems* (pp. 217-236.). Pacific Grove, CA: Brooks/Cole Publishing.

Matson, J. L. & Mayville, E. A. (2001). The relationship of functional variables and psychopathology to aggressive behavior in persons with severe and profound mental retardation. *Journal of Psychopathology and Behavioral Assessment, 23*, 3-9.

Matson, J. L., & Vollmer, T. R. (1995). *The Questions About Behavioral Function (QABF) User's Guide.* Baton Rouge, LA: Scientific Publishers Inc.

Mavromatis, M. (2000). The diagnosis and treatment of borderline personality disorder in persons with developmental disabilities: Three case reports. *Mental Health Aspects of Developmental Disabilities, 3,* 89-97.

McComas, J., Hoch, H., Paone, D., & El-Roy, D. (2000). Escape behavior during academic tasks: A preliminary analysis of idiosyncratic establishing operations. *Journal of Applied Behavior Analysis, 33,* 479-493.

Mikkelsen, E. J., & McKenna, I. (1999). Psychopharmacologic algorithms for adults for developmental disabilities and difficult-to-diagnose behavioral disorders. *Psychiatric Annuals, 29,* 302-314.

Murphy, G., Macdonald, S., Hall, S, & Oliver, C. (2000). Aggression and the termination of "rituals": A new variant of the escape function for challenging behavior? *Research in Developmental Disabilities, 21,* 43-59.

Nezu, C. M., & Nezu, A. M. (1994). Outpatient psychotherapy for adults with mental retardation and concomitant psychopathology: Research and clinical imperatives. *Journal of Consulting and Clinical Psychology, 62,* 34-42.

Nezu, C. M., Nezu, A. M., & Gill-Weiss, M. J. (1992). *Psychopathology in persons with mental retardation.* Champaign, IL: Research Press.

O'Brien, G. (1998). The adult outcome of childhood learning disability. MD thesis. University of Aberdeen, UK.

O'Brien, G. (2000). Learning disabilities. In C. Gillberg & G. O'Brien (Eds.), *Developmental disabilities and behavior, Clinics in Developmental Medicine, No. 149* (pp. 12-26). London: MacKeith Press.

O'Reilly, M. F. (1995). Functional analysis and treatment of escape-maintained aggression correlated with sleep deprivation. *Journal of Applied Behavior Analysis, 28,* 225-226.

O'Reilly, M., Lancioni, G., & Taylor, I. (1999). An empirical analysis of two forms of extinction to treat aggression. *Research in Developmental Disabilities, 20,* 315-325.

Peine, H. A., Darvish, R., Adams, K., Blakelock, H. Jenson, W., & Osborne, J. G. (1995). Medical problems, maladaptive behaviors, and the developmentally disabled. *Behavioral Interventions, 10,* 149-159.

Reichle, J., & Wacker, D. P. (Eds.). (1993). *Communication and language intervention series: Vol 3, Communicative alternatives to challenging behavior: Integrating functional assessment and intervention strategies.* Baltimore: Paul H. Brookes Publishing Co.

Reiss, S. (1994). *Handbook of challenging behavior: Mental health aspects of mental retardation.* Worthington, OH: IDS Publications.

Reiss, S. (1990). Prevalence of dual diagnosis in community-based day programs in the Chicago metropolitan area. *American Journal on Mental Retardation, 94,* 578-585.

Reiss, S., & Aman, M. G. (1998). *Psychotropic medications and developmental disabilities: The international consensus handbook.* Columbus, OH: Ohio State University Nisonger Center.

Reiss, S., & Havercamp, S. M. (1997). Sensitivity theory and mental retardation: Why functional analysis is not enough. *American Journal of Mental Retardation, 101,* 553-566.

Reiss, S., & Havercamp, S. M. (1998). Toward a comprehensive assessment of fundamental motivation: Factor structure of the Reiss Profiles. *Psychological Assessment, 10,* 97-106.

Reiss, S., & Rojahn, J. (1993). Joint occurrence of depression and aggression in children and adults with mental retardation. *Journal of Intellectual Disability Research, 37,* 287-294.

Repp, A. G. (1999). Naturalistic functional assessment with regular and special education students in classroom settings. In A. G., Repp & R. H. Horner (Eds.), *Functional analysis of problem behavior* (pp. 238-258). Belmont, CA: Wadsworth Publishing.

Repp, A. G., & Horner, R. H. (Eds.). (1999). *Functional analysis of problem behavior.* Belmont, CA: Wadsworth Publishing.

Ryan, R. (2000). Posttraumatic stress disorder in persons with developmental disabilities. In A. Poindexter (Ed.), *Assessment and treatment of anxiety disorders in per4sons with mental retardation: Revised and updated for 2000* (pp. 37-45). Kingston, NY: NADD Press.

Rush, A. J., & Frances, A. (2000). Treatment of psychiatric and behavioral problems in mental retardation: Expert consensus guideline series. *American Journal on Mental Retardation, 105,* 159-228.

Schroeder, S. R., Reese, R. M., Hellings, J., Loupe, J., & Tessel, R. E. (1999). The causes of self-injurious behavior and their implications. In N. A. Wieseler, & R. Hanson (Eds.), *Challenging behavior in persons with mental health disorders and severe developmental disabilities* (pp. 65-87). Washington, DC: AAMR Monograph Series.

Scotti, J. R., & Meyer, L. H. (1999). *Behavioral interventions: Principles, models, and practices.* Baltimore: Brookes.

Sheard, M. H. (1984). Clinical pharmacology of aggressive behavior. *Clinical Neuropharmacology, 7,* 173-183.

Singh, N. N., Wahler, R. G., Adkins, A. D., & Myers, R. E. (2003). Soles of the Feet: A mindfulness-based self-control intervention for aggression by an individual with mild mental retardation and mental illness. *Research in Developmental Disabilities, 24,* 158-169.

Sovner, R., & Fogelman. S. (1996). Irritability and mental retardation. *Seminars in Clinical Neuropsychatry, 1,* 105-114.

Sovner, R., Foxx, C. J., Lowry, M. J., & Lowry, M. A. (1993). Floretine treatment of depression and associated self-injury in two adults with mental retardation. *Journal of Intellectual Disabilities Research, 37,* 301-311.

Staats, A. W. (1996*). Behavior and personality: Psychological behaviorism.* New York: Springer Publishing.

Taylor, J. L. (2002). A review of the assessment and treatment of anger and aggression in offenders with intellectual disabilities. *Journal of Intellectual Disaiblity Research, 46 (Suppl 1),* 57-73.

Taylor, J. C., Sisson, L. A., McKelvey, J. L, & Trefelner, M.F. (1993). Situation specificity in attention-seeking problem behavior. *Behavior Modification, 17,* 474-497.

Thompson, T., & Symons, F. J. (1999). Neurobehavioral mechanisms of drug action. In N. A. Wieseler & R. H. Hanson (Eds.), *Challenging behavior of persons with mental health disorders and severe developmental disabilities* (pp. 125-150). Washington, DC: American Association on Mental Retardation.

Tsiouris, J. A. (2001). Diagnosis of depression in people with severe/profound mental retardation. *Journal of Intellectual Disability Research, 45,* 115-120.

Tuinier, S., & Verhoeven, W. M. A. (1993). Psychiatry and mental retardation: Towards a behavioural pharmacological concept. *Journal of Intellectual Disabilities Research, 37,* 16-24.

Vitiello, B., Behar, D., Hunt, J., Stoff, D., & Ricciuti, A. (1990). Subtyping aggression n children and adolescents. *Journal of Neuropsychiatry, 2,* 189-192.

Whitaker, S. (1993). The reduction of aggression in people with learning difficulties: A review of psychological methods. *British Journal of Clinical Psycholoyg, 32,* 1-37.

Wilder, D. A., Fisher, W. W., Anders, B. M., Cercone, J. J., & Neidert, P. L. (2001). Operative mechanisms of noncontingent reinforcement at varying magnitudes and schedules. *Research in Developmental Disabilities, 22,* 117-124.

CONTRIBUTORS

Michael G. Aman, Ph.D.
Nisonger Center,
The Ohio State University

Stephen J. Anderson, Ph.D.
Hammond Developmental Center

Jay W. Bamburg, Ph.D.
Hammond Developmental Center

Rowland P. Barrett, Ph.D.
Emma Pendleton Bradley Hospital,
Brown Medical School

Haven Bernstein
Department of Psychology,
 Queens College and The Graduate
Center, City University of New York

William I. Gardner, Ph.D.
Emeritus Professor,
University of Wisconsin-Madison

Dorothy M. Griffiths, Ph.D.
Professor, Brock University,
St. Catharines, Ontario

Theodore A. Hoch
George Mason University

Steve Holburn, Ph.D.
NYS Institute for Basic Research in
Developmental Disabilities, Staten
Island, NY

John W. Jacobson, Ph.D., B.C.B.A.
Sage Colleges Center for Applied
Behavior Analysis, Troy, NY

Luc Lecavalier, Ph.D.
Nisonger Center,
The Ohio State University

Kristin E. Long
George Mason University

James K. Luiselli, Ed.D.
The May Institute Inc.

Erik A. Mayville
Pathways Strategic Teaching Center

Stephen B. Mayville
Louisiana State University

Megan M. McPeak
George Mason University

Lisa M. Noll, Ph.D.
University of Chicago

Dennis H. Reid
Carolina Behavior Analysis and
Support Center,
Morganton, North Carolina

Johannes Rojahn
George Mason University

Brandi B. Smiroldo, Ph.D.
Hammond Developmental Center

Peter Sturmey Ph.D.
Department of Psychology Queens
College and
The Graduate Center, City University
of New York

Editors

Johnny L. Matson, Ph.D., is a Professor and Distinguished Research Master in the Department of Psychology at LSU. He has published 26 books and 300 book chapters and has a journal devoted to applied research in the area of mental retardation.

Rinita B. Laud is currently a doctoral student in Clinical Psychology at LSU. She received her B.A. from the University of Texas at Austin and her M.A. from LSU. She has been a coauthor on a number of journal articles and book chapters. She has served as a guest reviewer for several journals in the area of intellectual disabilities, as well as a consultant for group homes and developmental centers all over the state of Louisiana.

Michael L. Matson is a student at LSU with primary interests in mental health issues of persons with developmental disabilities. He has published research on psychotropic drug side effects and aggression in children with developmental delays.

Address correspondence to:
Johnny L. Matson, Ph.D.
Department of Psychology
Louisiana State University
Audobon Hall
Baton Rouge, Louisiana 70803-5501